MW01687990

BUSINESS REPLY CARD

FIRST CLASS PERMIT NO. 33107 PHILADELPHIA, PA

POSTAGE WILL BE PAID BY ADDRESSEE

HANLEY & BELFUS, INC.
Medical Publishers
P.O. Box 1377
Philadelphia, PA 19105-9990

NO POSTAGE NECESSARY IF MAILED IN THE UNITED STATES

BUSINESS REPLY CARD

FIRST CLASS PERMIT NO. 33107 PHILADELPHIA, PA

POSTAGE WILL BE PAID BY ADDRESSEE

HANLEY & BELFUS, INC.
Medical Publishers
P.O. Box 1377
Philadelphia, PA 19105-9990

STATE OF THE ART REVIEWS (STARs)

SUBJECT	FREQUENCY	PRICE (U.S.)	PRICE (Foreign)	PRICE (Single)
☐ ADOLESCENT MEDICINE	Triannual	$57.00	$67.00	$25.00
☐ CARDIAC SURGERY	Triannual	$88.00	$98.00	$38.00
☐ OCCUPATIONAL MEDICINE	Quarterly	$68.00	$78.00	$32.00
☐ PHYSICAL MED & REHAB (PM&R)	Triannual	$66.00	$76.00	$29.00
☐ SPINE	Triannual	$78.00	$88.00	$35.00

☐ 1990 subscription ☐ 1989 subscription
Check subject title above.

☐ Single issue
Title ________________

Name ________________
Company/Hospital ________________
Street Address ________________
City/State/Zip ________________

I enclose payment: ☐ Check ☐ Visa ☐ MasterCard
Credit Card # ________________
Expiration Date ________________
Signature ________________

Send order to:
HANLEY & BELFUS, INC.
210 South 13th Street / Philadelphia, PA 19107 / 215-546-7293

STATE OF THE ART REVIEWS (STARs)

SUBJECT	FREQUENCY	PRICE (U.S.)	PRICE (Foreign)	PRICE (Single)
☐ ADOLESCENT MEDICINE	Triannual	$57.00	$67.00	$25.00
☐ CARDIAC SURGERY	Triannual	$88.00	$98.00	$38.00
☐ OCCUPATIONAL MEDICINE	Quarterly	$68.00	$78.00	$32.00
☐ PHYSICAL MED & REHAB (PM&R)	Triannual	$66.00	$76.00	$29.00
☐ SPINE	Triannual	$78.00	$88.00	$35.00

☐ 1990 subscription ☐ 1989 subscription
Check subject title above.

☐ Single issue
Title ________________

Name ________________
Company/Hospital ________________
Street Address ________________
City/State/Zip ________________

I enclose payment: ☐ Check ☐ Visa ☐ MasterCard
Credit Card # ________________
Expiration Date ________________
Signature ________________

Send order to:
HANLEY & BELFUS, INC.
210 South 13th Street / Philadelphia, PA 19107 / 215-546-7293

Occupational Medicine

Shiftwork

Guest Editor:
Allene Jane Scott, MD, MPH
Head, Division of Occupational Medicine
Navy Environmental Health Center
Norfolk, Virginia

Volume 5/Number 2 April–June 1990
HANLEY & BELFUS, INC. Philadelphia

STATE OF THE ART REVIEWS

Publisher: HANLEY & BELFUS, INC.
210 South 13th Street
Philadelphia, PA 19107

OCCUPATIONAL MEDICINE: State of the Art Reviews is included in *Index Medicus, MEDLINE, Bio Sciences Information Service, Current Contents* and *ISI/BIOMED.*

OCCUPATIONAL MEDICINE: State of the Art Reviews **(ISSN 0885-114X)**
April–June 1990 **Volume 5, Number 2** **(ISBN 1-56053-035-9)**

OCCUPATIONAL MEDICINE: State of the Art Reviews is published quarterly by Hanley & Belfus, Inc., 210 South 13th Street, Philadelphia, Pennsylvania 19107. Second-class postage paid at Philadelphia, PA and at additional mailing offices.

POSTMASTER: Send address changes to OCCUPATIONAL MEDICINE: State of the Art Reviews, Hanley & Belfus, Inc., 210 South 13th Street, Philadelphia, PA 19107.

The 1990 subscription price is $68.00 per year U.S., $78.00 outside U.S. (add $40.00 for air mail). Single copies $32.00 U.S., $34.00 outside U.S. (add $10.00 for single copy air mail).

CONTENTS

CONTRIBUTORS

Michael H. Bonnet, PhD
Associate Professor of Medicine, University of California, Irvine; Sleep Laboratory, Veterans Administration Hospital, Long Beach, California

Richard R. Bootzin, PhD
Professor of Psychology, University of Arizona, Tucson, Arizona

Antonio B. Carvalhais, MA
Lecturer, Department of Psychology, University of Connecticut, Storrs, Connecticut

Roger J. Cole, PhD
Postgraduate Research Psychobiologist, University of California, San Diego; Staff, Department of Psychiatry, Veterans Administration Hospital, San Diego, California

Michael J. Colligan, PhD
Division of Training and Manpower Development, National Institute for Occupational Safety and Health, Cincinnati, Ohio

Carlos A. Comperatore, PhD
U.S. Army Aeromedical Research Laboratory, Fort Rucker, Alabama

Charmane I. Eastman, PhD
Associate Professor, Psychology Department, Rush-Presbyterian–St. Luke's Medical Center, Chicago, Illinois

Carl Englund, PhD
Research Psychologist, Sustained Operations Department, San Diego, California

Daniel C. Holley, PhD
Professor of Physiology, Department of Biological Sciences, San Jose State University, San Jose, California

Tamsin L. Kelly, MD
Medical Officer, Sleep Optimization Department, Naval Health Research Center, San Diego, California

H. Donald Kennedy, Jr., MPH, JD
Head, Occupational Health and Preventive Medicine, Naval Medical Command, Southeast Region, Jacksonville, Florida

Kogi K., MD
Occupational Safety and Health Branch, International Labour Office, Geneva, Switzerland

Daniel F. Kripke, MD
Professor of Psychiatry, University of California, San Diego; Staff, Department of Psychiatry, Veterans Administration Medical Center, San Diego, California

Gerald P. Krueger, PhD
U.S. Army Aeromedical Research Laboratory, Fort Rucker, Alabama

Joseph LaDou, MD
Clinical Professor and Chief, Division of Occupational and Environmental Medicine, University of California, San Francisco; Staff, Moffitt Hospital, San Francisco, California

Richard T. Loving, RN, MN
Research Nurse, Department of Psychiatry, Veterans Affairs Medical Center, San Diego, California

David S. Minors, BSc (London), PhD (Manchester)
Senior Lecturer in Physiology, Department of Physiological Sciences, University of Manchester, Manchester, United Kingdom

Timothy H. Monk, PhD
Associate Professor of Psychiatry, University of Pittsburgh; Director, Human Chronobiology Program, Western Psychiatric Institute and Clinic, Pittsburgh, Pennsylvania

Paul Naitoh, PhD
Department Head, Supervisory Research Psychologist, Sleep Optimization Department, Naval Health Research Center, San Diego, California

Ong Choon-Nam, MSc, PhD
Associate Professor, Department of Community Medicine, National University of Singapore, Kent Ridge, Singapore

Patricia E. Penn, PhD
Lecturer, Department of Psychiatry, University of Arizona, Tucson, Arizona

Captain William J. Price
Instructor of Biological Sciences, San Jose State University, San Jose, California

Alain Reinberg, MD, PhD
Fondation A. de Rothschild, Paris, France

Roger R. Rosa, PhD
Research Psychologist, Division of Biomedical and Behavioral Science, National Institute for Occupational Safety and Health, Cincinnati, Ohio

Allene Jane Scott, MD, MPH
Head, Division of Occupational Medicine, Navy Environmental Health Center, Norfolk, Virginia

Michael H. Smolensky, PhD
Professor of Environmental Physiology, School of Public Health, Graduate School of Biomedical Sciences, and Medical School, the University of Texas Health Science Center at Houston; Center for Medical and Public Health Chronobiology, Houston, Texas

Donald I. Tepas, PhD
Professor of Psychology and Director, Graduate Program in Industrial and Organizational Psychology, University of Connecticut, Storrs, Connecticut

James K. Walsh, PhD, ACP
Director, Sleep Disorders and Research Center, Deaconess Hospital, St. Louis; Adjunct Associate Professor, Departments of Psychology, Psychiatry, and Neurology, St. Louis University, St. Louis, Missouri

James M. Waterhouse, BA (Oxon), DPhil (Oxon)
Senior Lecturer, Department of Physiological Sciences, University of Manchester, Manchester, United Kingdom

PUBLISHED ISSUES, 1987–1989

(available from the publisher)

Vol 2/No 1 Jan.–Mar. 1987	**Occupational Cancer and Carcinogenesis** Edited by Paul W. Brandt-Rauf, ScD, MD, DrPH Columbia University, New York, New York
Vol 2/No 2 Apr.–June 1987	**Occupational Pulmonary Disease** Edited by Linda Rosenstock, MD, MPH University of Washington, Seattle, Washington
Vol 2/No 3 July–Sept. 1987	**Health Problems of Health Care Workers** Edited by Edward A. Emmett, MB The Johns Hopkins University, Baltimore, Maryland
Vol 2/No 4 Oct.–Dec. 1987	**Workers with Multiple Chemical Sensitivities** Edited by Mark R. Cullen, MD Yale University, New Haven, Connecticut
Vol 3/No 1 Jan.–Mar. 1988	**Back Pain in Workers** Edited by Richard A. Deyo, MD, MPH University of Washington, Seattle, Washington
Vol 3/No 2 Apr.–June 1988	**Worker Fitness and Risk Evaluations** Edited by Jay S. Himmelstein, MD, MPH and Glenn S. Pransky, MD, MPH University of Massachusetts, Worcester, Massachusetts
Vol 3/No 3 July–Sept. 1988	**The Petroleum Industry** Edited by Neill K. Weaver, MD Washington, D.C.
Vol 3/No 4 Oct.–Dec. 1988	**Psychiatric Injury in the Workplace** Edited by Robert C. Larsen, MD and Jean S. Felton, MD University of California, San Francisco and Irvine, California
Vol 4/No 1 Jan.–Mar. 1989	**The Management Perspective** Edited by L. Fleming Fallon, Jr., MD, MPH, MBA, O.B. Dickerson, MD, MPH and Paul W. Brandt-Rauf, ScD, MD, DrPH Columbia University, New York, New York
Vol 4/No 2 Apr.–June 1989	**Alcoholism and Chemical Dependency** Edited by Curtis Wright, MD, MPH The Johns Hopkins University, Baltimore, Maryland
Vol 4/No 3 July–Sept. 1989	**Occupational Hand Injuries** Edited by Morton L. Kasden, MD, FACS Louisville, Kentucky
Vol 4/No 4 Oct.–Dec. 1989	**Problem Buildings** Edited by James E. Cone, MD, MPH University of California, San Francisco, California and Michael Hodgson, MD, MPH University of Pittsburgh, Pittsburgh, Pennsylvania

1990 ISSUES

Hazardous Waste Workers
Edited by Michael Gochfeld, MD, PhD
and Elissa Ann Favata, MD
University of Medicine and Dentistry of New Jersey
Robert Wood Johnson Medical School, Piscataway, New Jersey

Shiftwork
Edited by Allene J. Scott, MD, MPH
Navy Environmental Health Center
Norfolk, Virginia

Medical Surveillance in the Workplace
Edited by David Rempel, MD, MPH
Hazard Evaluation System and Information Service
California Department of Health Services, Berkeley, California

Worksite Health Promotion
Edited by Michael E. Scofield, PhD
AT&T, Basking Ridge, New Jersey

Additional 1989 special issue:

Occupational HIV Infection:
Risks and Risk Reduction
Edited by Charles E. Becker, MD
University of California, San Francisco, California

Special issue prices:
$14.50—subscribers (add to 1989 subscription rate)
$29.00—nonsubscribers

Ordering Information:
Subscriptions ($68 U.S., $78 outside U.S.) and single issues ($32 U.S., $34 outside U.S.) are available from the publisher—
Hanley & Belfus, Inc., 210 South 13th Street, Philadelphia, PA 19107.
Telephone (215) 546-7293.

PREFACE

My interest in health effects related to shiftwork grew out of personally experiencing symptoms of biological rhythm disruption while doing assembly line type work on a "graveyard" shift. Although that experience occurred many years ago, I still vividly remember the associated chronic state of fatigue, difficulty in staying awake when driving home in the morning, and general persistent malaise. The requirement to complete a thesis for the master's program in public health at the University of Pittsburgh provided an opportunity to review the relevant medical literature dealing with health, safety, and scheduling issues related to irregular shift schedules involving nightwork. From a medical standpoint, these were quite foreign topics. Medical school curricula had essentially ignored chronobiology, chronopharmacology, and chronokinetics. General clinical training, which had not emphasized the importance of including occupational questions in the medical history, completely ignored the possibility that a patient's work schedule might have bearing on medical problems. The belief that many health practitioners have had a similar training experience and thus have limited medical knowledge concerning shiftwork led me to the decision to edit and contribute to this monograph.

The need for occupational health practitioners to be well informed concerning the effects of nightwork and irregular shift schedules on the health and performance of workers is increasing. Safety concerns have been a major impetus behind the growing interest of management, labor, and government in nightwork and extended hours. Safety is an especially important issue for operations such as nuclear power plants, chemical plants, heavy industry, and public transportation. Shiftworkers' failure to correct a stuck valve was considered a significant contributing factor to the Three-Mile Island near meltdown. In the area of transportation, commercial jet travel is of particular concern, since pilots involved in transmeridian flights not only have to deal with rapid crossings of multiple time zones, but with biological rhythm disruption from shiftwork as well. Review of pilot reports submitted to the National Aeronautics and Space Administration under the Aviation Safety Reporting System led to the conclusion that fatigue-associated performance decrements occur and can produce hazardous situations. Major newspapers have raised questions about commercial jet pilot fatigue related to long and irregular hours combined with symptoms of jet lag. The Presidential Commission on the Space Shuttle Challenger Accident found sleep loss and shiftwork to be factors leading to that tragic accident.

Increasingly employers are requesting work schedule evaluations by consultants specializing in the use of chronobiological principles to maximize nightshift performance and minimize medical and psychosocial effects of shiftwork. Employees have sought workers' compensation awards for stress-induced illnesses related to mandatory nightwork and extended hours of work. The general public is becoming aware of the importance of biological rhythms and problems associated with their disruption as evidenced by articles in women's journals and television programs dealing with the topic. On May 23, 1990, the Congress of the United States Office of Technology Assessment held a workshop on shiftwork and extended hours with the purpose of discussing the effects of work schedules other than regular daytime shifts on the health, performance, and social lives of workers and the possible effects on society as a whole. Participants included occupational medicine physicians, a specialist in biocompatible shift scheduling, and professors of law, as well as representatives from the National Transportation Safety Board, the Department of Labor, NASA Ames Research Center, the Service Employees International Union, the International Brotherhood of Teamsters, the United Steel Workers, and the National Institute of Occupational Safety and Health.

Occupational health practitioners can expect to be called upon to give advice to individual employees, management, and unions concerning worker tolerance of shiftwork as it relates to both performance and adverse health effects. The need for preemployment screening and medical surveillance for nightwork is clear.

This issue provides information that should help the practitioner answer questions such as:

How does job performance change with the time of day?

What medical problems are associated with or aggravated by shiftwork?

What type of schedule can improve worker performance and limit medical/social problems related to continuous operations?

How useful are interventions such as meal timing, type of diet, medication, and light therapy?

What individual differences exist with respect to tolerance of and adjustment to shiftwork?

What medical conditions may be incompatible with irregular working hours?

What coping strategies can be suggested to help the shiftworker and his or her family?

What chronopharmacological concerns are related to shiftworkers taking medications?

How does nightwork affect sensitivity to and metabolism of workplace toxins?

Should permissible exposure levels to workplace chemical and physical stressors be modified for nightwork?

This issue is designed not only to deal with these and other questions and to assist in establishing medical surveillance programs for nightworkers, but also to increase the awareness of occupational health professionals of the special problems and needs of shiftworkers.

Many thanks are due the contributors of this issue for their efforts. I also wish to thank Dr. E. Carroll Curtis and Dr. Michael Hodgson for their encouragement, helpful criticism, and professional advice, which helped to lead to the publishing of this issue. Most of all my deepest gratitude is given to my husband, Jeff, for his unending patience and loving support, which enabled me to complete this project.

Allene J. Scott, MD, MPH
GUEST EDITOR

The views expressed here are those of the author and do not reflect the official policy or position of the Department of the Navy, Department of Defense, or the U.S. Government.

DAVID S. MINORS, PhD
JAMES M. WATERHOUSE, DPhil

CIRCADIAN RHYTHMS IN GENERAL

From the Department of Physiological Sciences
University of Manchester
Manchester, United Kingdom

Reprint requests to:
David S. Minors, PhD
Department of Physiological Sciences
University of Manchester
Manchester M13 9PT
UK

Life on our planet has evolved in, and is adjusted to, a rhythmic environment. For most plants and animals, the 24-hour rhythm of light and dark imposed by the sun is a major influence upon their physiology, biochemistry, and ecology. By contrast, humans living in industrialized societies can become independent of natural rhythms of light and food availability. In order to meet socially or for business, however, they need to use artificial clocks that have been synchronized. By convention, these clocks are synchronized to the sun, so that the middle of the day (noon) occurs when the sun is at its zenith. By convention, too, most of us regulate our activities so that the night is for sleep, the daytime for work, and the evenings for leisure. That is, we are, both by design and desire, rhythmic creatures in a rhythmic environment. Rhythmic changes in our physiology that show cycle lengths (termed periods) covering wide intervals of time—from a fraction of a second to a year—have been identified. In this book we are concerned mainly with rhythms having cyclic periods of about 24 hours; they are circadian rhythms.

CIRCADIAN RHYTHMS

The recent development of miniaturized portable data loggers and of radioimmunoassay techniques for the detection of hormones and other substances in very small samples of body fluids has enabled us to determine circadian rhythmicity with comparative ease. Figure 1 illustrates the circadian rhythms in a selection of physiological variables obtained from healthy subjects on a normal schedule of sleep, waking,

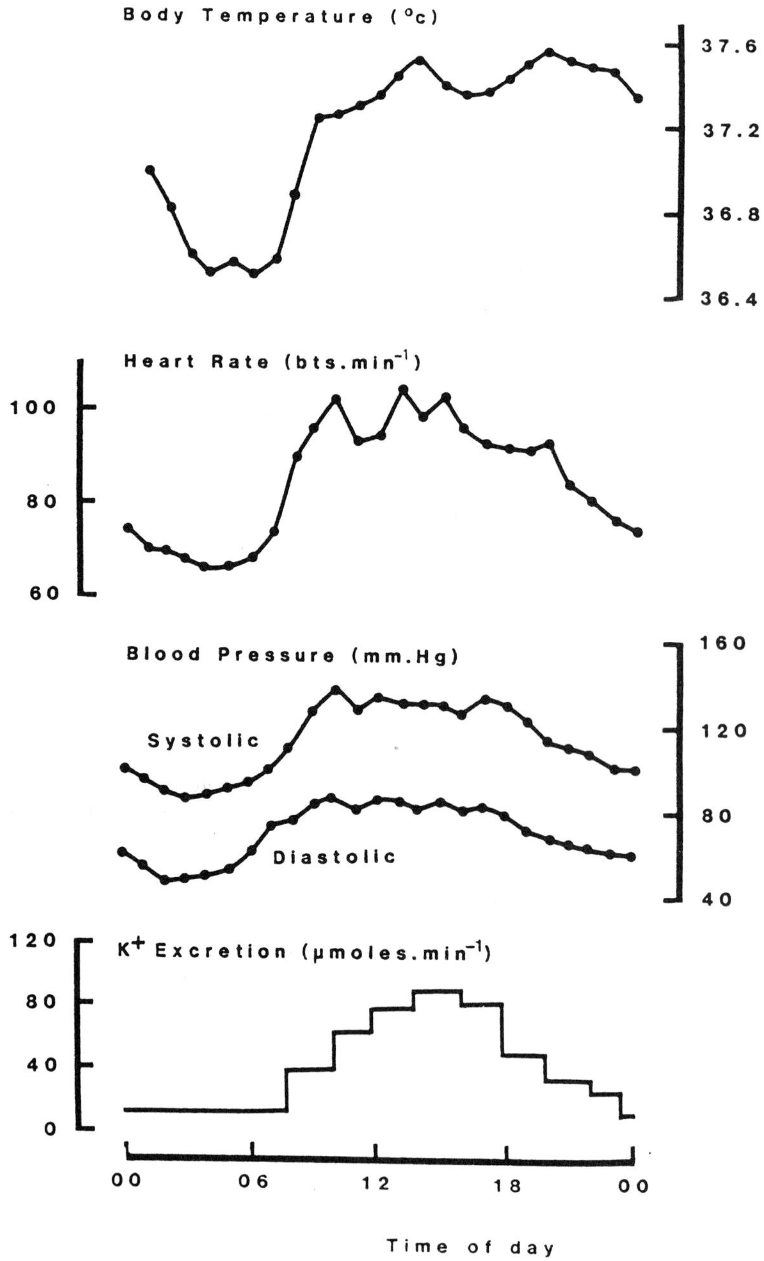

FIGURE 1. Daily changes in deep body temperature, heart rate, blood pressure, and the urinary excretion of potassium. Measurements were made hourly over a single 24-hour period, and the data represent the means from four subjects.

and mealtimes. It can be seen that body temperature, blood pressure, and urinary potassium loss show higher values during the daytime (1200–1800) and lower values during the night, with minimum values in the small hours. Such examples could be added to almost indefinitely; most bodily variables show circadian rhythmicity, usually with a daytime peak. Exceptions are plasma cortisol and other hormones (testosterone and growth hormone, for example) that peak during the hours of nocturnal sleep. Whatever the explanation for the pattern a particular variable follows, we stress that there is little day-to-day variability in its rhythm in healthy individuals.

Describing Rhythms

A quantitative description of a rhythm requires an assessment of: the **mean**—the level about which oscillation takes place; the **range of oscillation**; the **phase** of the rhythm—that is, its placement in time, often described as the time when peak values are found; and the **period** of the rhythm—the time to complete one cycle (in the case of circadian rhythms, the period is always about 24 hours).

Even though the detailed shapes of circadian rhythms can differ considerably among variables (see Fig. 1, for example), they can often be approximated by a cosine curve; fitting a cosine curve to such a data set (cosinor analysis) is a popular method of rhythm analysis.[52] The fitted curve is described in terms of three parameters that are closely related to those given above. They are: the **mesor** or mean value; the **amplitude** or distance between the peak value and the mesor; and the **acrophase** or time of peak (Fig. 2).

EXOGENOUS AND ENDOGENOUS COMPONENTS OF RHYTHMICITY

It might seem at first sight that circadian rhythms could wholly result from the effects of the rhythmic environment upon an individual. Thus, during the daytime people would be awake, active, and taking meals, whereas at night they would be asleep and fasting. One could predict that blood pressure, urinary

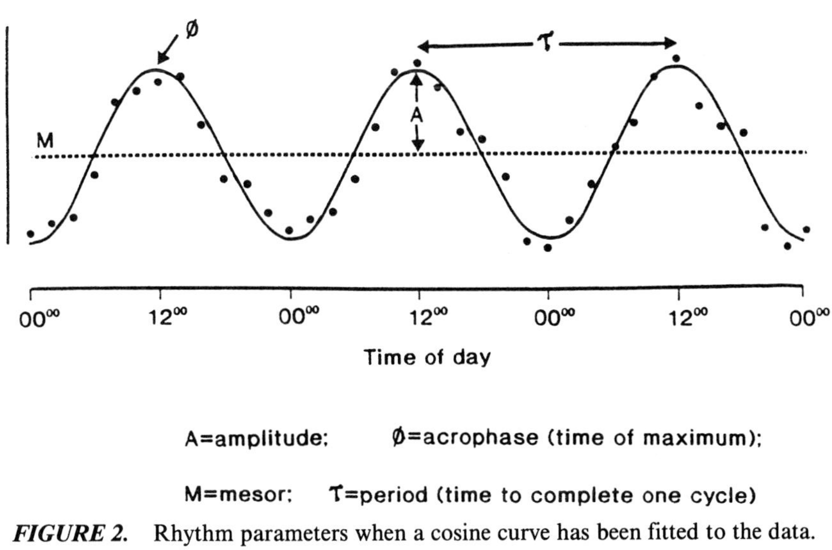

FIGURE 2. Rhythm parameters when a cosine curve has been fitted to the data.

potassium excretion, and temperature would rise during the daytime and fall at night. Such an argument could also explain the nocturnal peak of certain hormones; endocrine function is often associated with growth and repair, which might take place more appropriately when the body is inactive.

Several lines of evidence argue against these explanations, however. Subjective evidence includes our feelings of fatigue if we stay up all night. Even though we have had no sleep, from about 0500 onward we begin to feel less tired, even in an environment that is uniformly noisy and light, that is, uniformly "alerting." Objective evidence[37] is based upon the results of experimental changes in our sleep/wake cycle and environment.

1. As indicated in Figure 1, some changes in the value of a variable cannot easily be explained in terms of a *response* to external changes. Thus, urinary potassium falls in the evening, though we have eaten a large meal, and body temperature and blood pressure fall in the evening before we fall asleep and begin to rise in the morning before we awaken.

2. Changes in lifestyle, as after a time-zone transition or shift to a nightwork schedule, do not result in immediate changes in the rhythms of body temperature or plasma cortisol, for example.

3. Volunteers living in isolation chambers have been studied. (Isolation chambers are rooms constructed in such a way that time cues from the outside—light and noise, for example—are excluded.) The volunteers have lived normally except that the clock, which dictates their lifestyle, has been adjusted to run fast or slow. For example, with a clock that takes 28 (solar) hours to show the passage of a "day," six experimental "days" equal seven real days. Results (Fig. 3) show

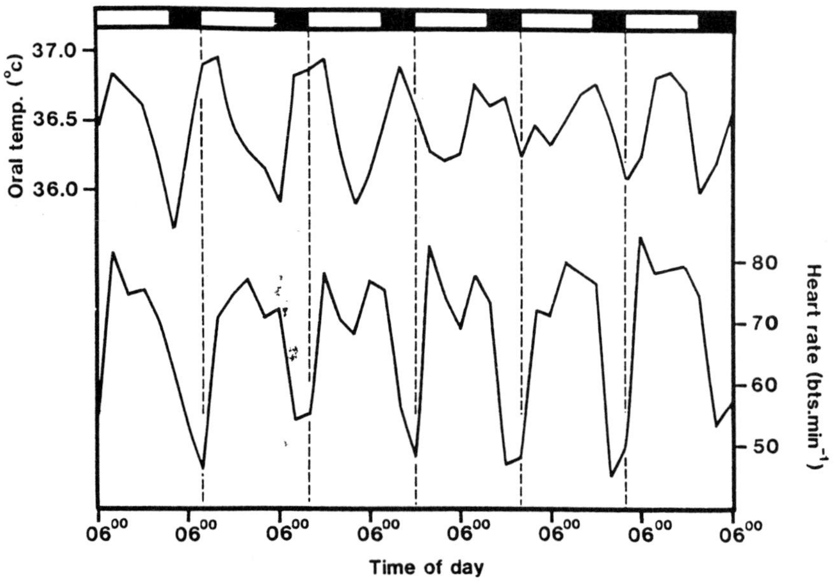

FIGURE 3. Oral temperature and heart rate of a subject living on a 28-hour "day." Real solar days are shown by the times along the bottom, and artificial days are separated by vertical lines. Seven "real" days equal six artificial "days." Black bars indicate sleep times. Note that the heart rate follows the sleep/wake cycle and artificial days, but that oral temperature follows "real" days. Data of Kleitman and Kleitman.[30]

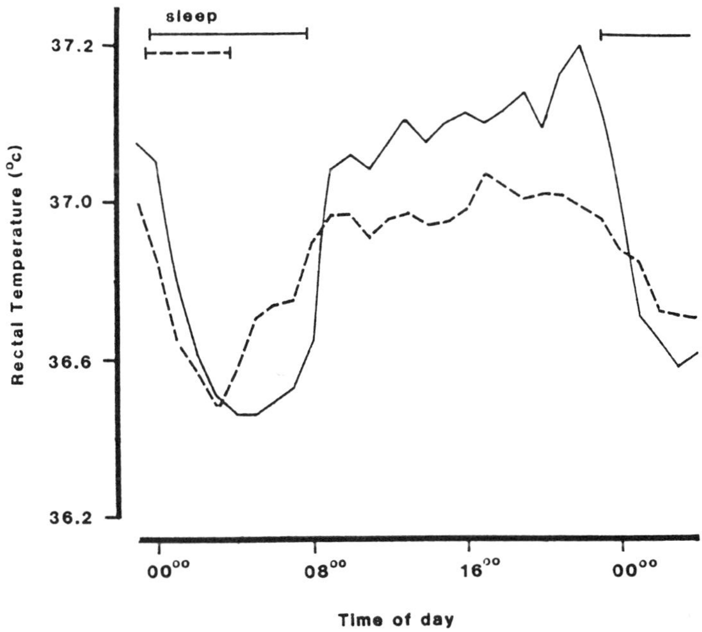

FIGURE 4. Mean circadian changes in rectal temperature measured hourly in eight subjects living a normal sleep/wakefulness cycle (solid line) and in the same subjects woken at 0400 and spending the subsequent 24 hours awake in constant light and taking hourly small identical snacks (broken line). (From Minors DS, Waterhouse JM: Circadian Rhythms and the Human. Bristol, Wright PSG, 1981, with permission.)

that some variables (e.g., heart rate in the figure) follow the new lifestyle, whereas others (e.g., body temperature) continue approximately in synchrony with normal, solar time.

4. A direct test of the hypothesis that circadian rhythms are a reflection of our rhythmic environment and lifestyle is to remove the external rhythms. It is possible to stay awake for 24 hours, take identical snacks at evenly spaced intervals, keep posture constant by remaining in bed or remaining sedentary, and minimize changes in noise, light, and social influences. A protocol that has attempted to control such influences simultaneously has been called the constant routine or Mills's test.[23] Figure 4 shows the average hourly deep body temperature during such a constant routine in a group of eight subjects (broken line). Also shown in this figure is the temperature rhythm when the same subjects slept and ate at conventional times (solid line). A comparison of these two curves yields the following results.

• The temperature rhythm during the constant routine does not disappear; this result is taken to indicate the presence of some **endogenous** component or timing mechanism that is metaphorically called a "body clock."

• There is some effect of the normal alternation of night and day, that is, of a "nychthemeral" existence, because the two sets of data are not identical. This effect, attributed to external factors, is called the **exogenous** component or masking influence.

• In normal circumstances, endogenous and exogenous components are in phase with one another. At night, the low body temperature values dictated by the body's clock are reinforced by inactivity and fasting during sleep; during the daytime, peak activity coincides with the highest temperatures produced by the activity of the body clock.

In addition, the relative size of the two components differs among variables. Results obtained from the protocols described above can be used to compare two variables, A and B, where A is postulated to possess the stronger endogenous component and B the stronger exogenous component. Thus:

• The evening fall and rise *before* awakening would be more marked for A.

• Adjustment to a change in lifestyle would appear to be more rapid for B.

• The rhythm of B would be more likely to follow an abnormal "day" length than would that of A (Fig. 3).

• The difference between the two curves in Figure 4 (normal lifestyle and constant routine) would be more marked for the rhythm of B than for A, and the result obtained during the constant routine would be flatter for rhythm B.

In summary, our circadian rhythms are a mixture of endogenous and exogenous components derived from circadian changes in the load imposed upon our homeostatic mechanisms as well as in the properties of the reflexes that deal with any perturbations.

The advantage of the possession of such rhythms is taken to be that a certain independence of the outside world is achieved. Thus, an internal clock enables the animal to emerge from its hiding place at an appropriate time after the departure of predators and before too much time that can be used for its own activity has been wasted. Another advantage—one that applies equally to man—is that the organism can "pre-adapt" to some forthcoming event. The plant can raise its leaves in preparation for sunrise, and humans can change their hormonal and neuronal status in time for waking and the stresses of the new day. As the evening progresses, they can begin to "tone down" in preparation for sleep. Moore-Ede[45] has described this ability to *prepare* for changes in the environment as "predictive homeostasis," to distinguish it from the more conventional *response* to environmental changes, which he terms "reactive homeostasis."

Having established that normal circadian rhythms in nychthemeral conditions consist of an endogenous component and an exogenous component, it is now necessary to consider each in more detail.

The Exogenous Component

The exogenous component of our rhythmic environment is dominated by the sleep/wake cycle, both directly, through the effects of sleep and exercise, and indirectly, through the association of our waking span with a more dynamic environment, social influences, postural changes, and intake of food and fluid. Since these influences hide from us the activities of the endogenous component, which is of most interest to chronobiologists, they are often called **masking factors**.[4,39] The detailed nature of the masking effect depends upon the variable. Examples are given in Table 1.

The masking influences of the sleep/wake cycle upon the rhythm of body temperature have been investigated in some detail.[39,75] One protocol consists of comparing body temperatures at the same time of day (when that phase of the endogenous component of the circadian rhythm would be the same) under two conditions—when the volunteer is asleep and when the volunteer is awake and

TABLE 1. Examples of Masking Influences in Human Circadian Rhythms

Variable	Masking Influence
Plasma insulin	Plasma glucose (food intake)
Urine flow	Water intake
Plasma antidiuretic hormone	Water intake and posture
Plasma growth hormone	Sleep onset
Plasma prolactin	First episode of REM sleep
Plasma adrenalin	Level of "stress"
Plasma melatonin	Bright light
Blood pressure	Stress and sleep/wake cycle
Body temperature	Sleep/wake cycle and food intake

undertaking different amounts of activity. With a lifestyle that is mainly sedentary, waking values are about 0.2–0.3°C higher than during sleep. This exogenous effect is slightly less if the subject is lying down and greater if the subject is physically active. A large meal increases body temperature by about 0.1–0.2°C for some hours afterwards. Clearly, the combined effects of these factors upon body temperature will mean that the circadian rhythm measured during a normal lifestyle is related to the endogenous component in a complex way (compare the two curves of Fig. 4, for example).

The Endogenous Component—The Body Clock

A study of the endogenous component of a rhythm requires the exogenous component to be minimized for as many consecutive cycles of the endogenous component as possible. One method is to continue the constant-routine protocol beyond 24 hours (see, for example, Froberg et al.,[20] which involved a study of about three days' duration). However, this protocol suffers two disadvantages. First, three cycles are still insufficient to assess the period of the endogenous component, or the effects of external influences, at all accurately. Second, as the experiment progresses, fatigue might begin to predominate over the body clock as an influence.

The method that has yielded most information about the body clock is the free-running experiment.[74] With humans this consists of isolating the subject from any cues regarding the passage of time by conducting the experiment either in a cave or in a specially constructed isolation unit. The subject is allowed to take meals and sleep at will, but these activities are monitored by the experimenter. Samples of urine and plasma can be collected and recordings of deep body temperature and mental performance can be made in order to estimate details of these rhythms. Such experimental protocols routinely last from 10 to 30 days, but experiments lasting several months have been achieved.

With such protocols, even though exogenous influences are generated by the activities of the individual, the lifestyle is *initiated* by the body clock. The results of such experiments and the properties of the body clock that have been deduced from them, are as follows:[13,37,74]

1. Rhythmicity continues—whether it is of sleep, mealtimes, urinary excretion, plasma hormones, or body temperature. Because the individual's temporal structure continues in these circumstances, it is generally inferred that such free-running rhythms must originate from within the individual, from the body clock. It might reasonably be argued, however, that this finding results from a memory of past habits and regular lifestyle, but the findings below refute this alternative.

2. Slight day-by-day variations in sleep times occur, the subject occasionally retiring earlier or later than usual. It is observed that late nights are not accompanied by longer sleeps (as would be the case if sleep length were determined by some stochastic process) but rather by shorter ones. Similarly, early times of retiring result in sleeps that are longer than usual. Such results are most easily explicable in terms of waking up at a set phase of the body clock; going to bed late means that this phase is reached sooner.

3. The rhythms show a period that differs from 24 hours. When groups of individuals are considered there is a normal (Gaussian) distribution of periods with a mean value of 25.0 hours and with tails that extend to the range of at least 24–26 hours. A free-running period as "fast" as 24 hours is unusual, and values less than 24 hours are uncommon. It is because the period of the body clock is only about a day in length that the rhythms it controls are called circadian (Latin: *circa*, about; *diem*, a day).

SITING THE BODY CLOCK

Although the free-running experiment indicates that humans and animals possess a body clock, it does nothing to locate such a structure. Here we will briefly review the evidence indicating where one such structure may reside. Fuller reviews are available.[35,38,44,59,61,62]

If we confine ourselves to mammals, then some of the earliest work in this field indicated that there was a loss of the circadian rhythm in locomotor activity in rodents after ablation of the suprachiasmatic nuclei (SCN) of the hypothalamus, but not after ablation of other areas of the brain (see Rusak and Zucker,[62] for review). At about the same time, the uptake into the SCN of the antimetabolite, 2-deoxyglucose, was found to show circadian rhythmicity.[65] Moreover, infusion into rats of antibody raised against the suprachiasmatic nucleus leads to a loss of drinking and locomotor activity.[51] More recent work has tended to confirm that the SCN shows rhythmicity in an increasing range of variables and species.

One difficulty of interpretation is that such experiments might show no more than that the SCN is part of the pathway through which the clocklike activity must pass. To make a simple analogy: cutting the nerves to a muscle prevents voluntary movement but does not prove that movement *originates* in the motor units of the spinal cord. It was to refute this objection that experiments were carried out upon "hypothalamic islands."[26] In these experiments, groups of hypothalamic cells including the SCN were isolated surgically and left in situ. Such "islands" continued to show circadian rhythmicity, whereas areas outside the islands did not. There still is the possibility, however, that the islands were not the origin of rhythmicity, but rather were receptive to humeral influences reaching them via the cerebrospinal fluid or brain extracellular fluid from adjacent areas of the brain. Such a possibility can be eliminated only by in vitro measurements upon hypothalamic slices. Such preparations show rhythmicity in both the electrophysiological activity of cells[22] and the uptake of 2-deoxyglucose,[53] the phasing of which is predictable from a knowledge of the timing of the light/dark cycle of the animal before removal of the slice. Thus, the neural or metabolic activity of the slices was highest at a time corresponding to the midlight phase in the case of rats. Even though, to date, such preparations have been maintained in a viable state for only a comparatively short period of time (up to 30 hours), they do, nevertheless, indicate strongly that the SCN contains an autonomous circadian oscillator.

Recent work has shown that circadian rhythmicity can be restored to arrhythmic hamsters (rendered as such by ablation of the SCN) by transplantation of sections of fetal brain containing the SCN.[31] Particularly impressive are reports of work in which the fetal donors possessed mutant clocks that were known to produce circadian rhythms with abnormal periods when expressed in adults. The transplant recipients regained rhythmicity but with a period indistinguishable from that of the donor.[36,48]

Such a position—that the SCN are the site of the body clock—has become complicated by a series of results indicating the need for more than one body clock. These results can be summarized briefly as follows:

1. Humans in time-free experiments can show spontaneous internal desynchronization, in which a rhythm shows two periods simultaneously.[74] This phenomenon has not been described in other animals, but "splitting"—the development of two bursts of activity, one corresponding to the light/dark transition and the other to the dark/light transition—is not uncommon.

2. SCN ablation does not always result in the loss of all rhythmicity. The animal may continue to show an ultradian rhythm (one with a period of 3–12 hours) in its activity pattern.[60] In the rat, some experimenters,[64] but not all,[18] have shown that SCN lesions did not eliminate circadian rhythmicity in body temperature. Also in the rat, rhythmic food-anticipatory behavior persists following SCN lesions.[12] Similar results, indicating that the circadian rhythms of body temperature and plasma cortisol levels are more resistant than those of activity and drinking after SCN ablation, have been found in squirrel monkeys.[43,44,68] It has been suggested that the source of this remaining circadian rhythmicity is part of the ventrolateral area of the hypothalamus.

3. In some passerine birds, ablation studies indicate that the pineal gland also acts as an autonomous clock. In mammals it is not yet clear exactly what role is played by the pineal gland in the generation of circadian rhythms.[3,6,24,56,68]

Whether two (or even more) clocks exist in the brain is an issue that still needs resolution. However, the further indirect evidence, namely that the SCN send outputs to many areas including the ventrolateral hypothalamus and (via the sympathetic nervous system) the pineal body,[35] and that there are receptors for melatonin and other neuropeptides in the SCN,[35,47,57] all suggests that the concept of a single circumscribed area of the brain acting alone as the body clock needs modification.

One solution[9,47,59] is to suggest that the time-keeping role can be shared by two or more areas of the brain, one of which includes the SCN. These areas are normally synchronized and together produce the endogenous component of circadian rhythms. It seems to us that, under certain experimental circumstances, these different areas can become separated functionally, as during internal desynchronization, or one of them can take on a more dominant role, if, for instance, the SCN are ablated. Considered this way, "endogenous component" and "body clock" are concepts devised to account for experimental findings. The important point is that, even though such concepts must, at any time, have a neuronal basis, the assumption that the anatomical counterpart(s) are always identical might be unwarranted. Even so, interest in the body clock in mammals has centered on the SCN, as indicated in the discussion above.

When the detailed mode of action of the cells in the SCN is considered, the question arises whether the individual cells behave as a series of identical clocks or whether their integrated output is different from that of the individual cells.[19,35,68] By way of an analogy, consider the case of the mechanical clock. It works because the escapement regulates the release of energy from a wound spring, which is used to turn a series of intermeshing cogwheels. A reductionist experimental approach would direct attention to the individual cogs. The structure and properties of the cog and its inputs and outputs could be determined, as could the effect upon the clock of removing a cog, of stopping it from turning, or of interfering with it in some other way. What such an approach would show is that the hands of the clock—and the indicators on other dials if we were investigating a clock that showed the phases of the moon as well as solar hours, minutes, and seconds—are *not* simply related to the periods of rotation of either most of the cogwheels or the original escapement mechanism. We could not easily deduce the period of the individual components of the clock from a knowledge of the movement of its hands or vice versa. In the same way, we need to know not only details of the neuroanatomy, neurochemistry, neurophysiology, and neuropharmacology of the cells that constitute the body's timing system, but also *how these constituents interact* to form the system as a whole. These are all areas where much work remains to be done, and the recent development of techniques to culture SCN cells[33] would be expected to make an important contribution.

ADJUSTING THE BODY CLOCK

Even though the inherent period of the body clock differs from 24 hours, the period is exactly 24 hours under normal conditions. This adjustment of the clock is termed **entrainment** and is necessary to prevent a continuing mismatch between internal and external time.

Entrainment of the body clock to 24 hours is achieved by rhythmic changes in the external environment called **zeitgebers** (German: *zeit*, time; *geber*, giver). In most animals the light/dark cycle associated with the solar day is the major zeitgeber, although food availability might play a role in some predatory species.

Zeitgebers in Humans

What are the zeitgebers in humans and how do they exert their effects? There is still some controversy in this field, the debate centering on whether the main zeitgeber is the light/dark cycle or social rhythms.

Wever and his colleagues[74] originally advanced the view that alternations of light and dark were a weaker zeitgeber than were rhythmic cues provided by social influences. Briefly, they found that subjects in free-running experiments were not entrained to a 24-hour day by a light/dark schedule alone but by a light/dark schedule supplemented by gong strokes to summon the subjects to perform tasks. The researchers interpreted the result to indicate that the subjects perceived the gong strokes as social contacts from the experimenters. One problem in interpreting these experiments is that subjects were free to use auxiliary lighting during the imposed "night." Thus there was no real need to make use of the rhythmic information provided by the light/dark cycle alone. When the gong strokes were added, however, and because they were more frequent in the "day" than during the "night," it would have been inconvenient to ignore the information they gave.

Czeisler and colleagues[16] have argued that the light/dark cycle, rather than social influences, acted as a synchronizer. They showed that humans entrained to an imposed light/dark cycle when no auxiliary lighting was allowed during the dark phase. In considering a detailed interpretation of these results, it should be remembered that the protocol was such that it would have been inconvenient for the subjects not to adjust their sleep/wake cycle to accord with that of the imposed dark/light regimen and that, as a result, other potential zeitgebers—activity/inactivity and feeding/fasting—would automatically arise from the response of the subjects. By contrast, the role of social factors as a zeitgeber cannot be deduced, since social interaction with the experimenters appears to have been possible *at any time*, rather than imposed as a present or absent regimen. This protocol would not appear to impose the *rhythmicity* that is necessary for a zeitgeber.

More recently, there has been interest in the role of *bright* light as a zeitgeber, and Czeisler's group[14,15] have published a set of data showing very clearly that humans can respond to bright light as they would to a zeitgeber. (This work on a phase-response curve to light in humans will be discussed more fully below.) Even though the physical activity of subjects can be controlled in such studies, mental activity and the effects it might be supposed to exert upon the release of adrenaline and other hormones cannot. As a result, one can never be sure that the effects of light are wholly due to light per se rather than, or in addition to, increased mental activity.

It is our view that, in a normal environment, a group of zeitgebers acts simultaneously, some derived directly from the environment and others arising as a consequence of behavioral responses (see also Griffiths[21]). For example, the scenario could be: people go to bed because they know they need a certain amount of sleep to prepare for the rigors of the next day. Because domestic (e.g., shopping) and business commitments require one to be awake during the daytime, it is convenient to arrange waking time to coincide with daytime. Once the sleep/wake cycle has been established, all other potential zeitgebers (light/dark, feeding/fasting, social mixing/social isolation, noise/quiet, etc.) are adjusted to coincide.

Recent work upon hamsters, in which several factors that adjust the body clock (drugs, light, activity, for example) have been studied, has been independently interpreted as indicating that many of these zeitgebers might act through the common mechanism of adjusting an animal's pattern of activity.[49,50,69,70] This is an interesting convergence of ideas about means by which the body clock is adjusted.

Even though we have stressed how several zeitgebers might act together, we still find valuable attempts to study single zeitgebers in isolation. Information from this latter approach will enable us to strengthen our "zeitgeber package" and so promote entrainment of the body clock after time-zone transitions or during nightwork, for instance.

Zeitgeber Mechanisms

Recent work has concentrated upon the means by which a single zeitgeber might adjust the body clock in humans. Several groups[40] have shown that pulses of bright light (approaching the strength of natural rather than domestic lighting) can adjust the circadian rhythms of sleep, body temperature, and plasma melatonin. The amount and direction of adjustment depends upon when the pulse is given in relation to the phase of the body clock. Pulses in the hours around waking advance the clock, those in the hours about retiring delay it, and those in the middle of the day have no effect. This relationship between the phase at which the light pulse is given and the effect upon the body clock is called a phase-response curve (PRC). By far the most complete set of data for humans so far is that of Czeisler's group, though only Honma et al.[25] and Minors et al.[41] have studied phase changes induced during a "classical" free-running protocol. Since the free-running period of the body clock in humans shows a period in excess of 24 hours, it is assumed that the important part of the PRC is that at the end of sleep when a pulse of light advances the clock by the one hour each day that is required. The demonstration that a PRC to light exists in humans brings us into line with other species, in which, however, PRCs from several other zeitgebers and drugs also have been measured.

A pathway by which light might exert a direct effect upon the body clock is the retinohypothalamic tract, which runs directly between the eyes and the SCN.[7,63,68] Bright light suppresses the secretion of melatonin by the pineal gland in humans[32] and might produce a number of behavioral changes—in drinking, eating, and activity, for example—that might themselves act as zeitgebers.[76] The detailed pathways and mechanisms by which the zeitgeber information is transmitted to and within the central nervous system remain to be established. Recently, there has been an increasing interest in the effects of neurotransmitters, their agonists and antagonists, upon the body clock.[54,69,71] At the moment, we can say little more than that pathways are known to exist among areas believed to be more or less closely associated with the body clock and between the periphery and these areas.

Adjusting the Rest of the Body Clock

How is information about body time transmitted from the body clock throughout the body? This might be achieved by several general mechanisms, including the effects of body temperature, blood-borne hormones, and the ubiquitous ramifications of the sympathetic nervous system. All evidence is indirect at the moment. Nevertheless, by way of some examples, striking parallels among the following groups of rhythms indicate some sort of link.

Rhythms of Body Temperature, Metabolic Rate, Alertness, and the Ability to Sleep. Higher temperatures are associated with a higher metabolic rate, decreased fatigue, increased alertness, better performance at many types of mental activity, decreased ability to fall asleep, and increased tendency to wake up.

Rhythms of Heart Rate, Blood Pressure, Plasma Adrenaline, and Airway Patency. Increased sympathetic nervous system activity raises all these variables, and the time of peak of these rhythms (about 1800–2000) is associated with best athletic performance.[5]

Rhythms of Plasma Cortisol, Arthritic Pain, Response to Allergens, Asthmatic Attacks, and Urinary Potassium Excretion. The natural immunosuppressive and anti-inflammatory properties of cortisol seem to account for most of these circadian effects, but its action upon the kidney is somewhat different.[46] It appears to influence the flux of potassium ions between the intra- and extracellular compartments, a function which, when applied to renal tubular cells, alters the amount excreted in the urine.

These examples show possible ways in which the SCN and any associated areas comprising the body clock could control all circadian rhythms. They also show means by which any tendency for individual cells to show autonomous rhythms—and it is known that many cells, tissues, and organs will do this if they are studied in isolation from the body—can be subordinated to a "master oscillator."[44]

The exact means by which the circadian rhythms in sympathetic nervous system activity, plasma cortisol, other hormones, and body temperature could synchronize all rhythmic processes in the body is unknown. One possibility is through changes in reflex pathways. There are circadian rhythms in the activities of neuromodulators and in the number and affinity of receptors for transmitters and hormones.[54,55] These phenomena alter the threshold and sensitivity of reflex pathways, and this, in turn, alters the "set-point" at which variables are controlled homeostatically by feedback loops. Examples of these principles include renal responses to vascular expansion,[28] to thermoregulatory reflexes and preferred ambient temperature,[8,34,66,67] and to the hypothalamico-hypophyseal-adrenocortical axis and the control of plasma cortisol.[1,2,17,27]

DIFFERENCES AMONG INDIVIDUALS

We are no more equal with regard to circadian rhythms than we are with regard to any other variable. We make different uses of potential zeitgebers, and our circadian rhythms have different phases with reference to solar time and amplitudes. Because some people choose to ignore many social factors, their zeitgebers can be weak enough for circadian rhythms to free-run with a period different from 24 hours. At times, these people are asleep during the daytime and awake throughout the night. Less extremely, an individual might go to bed progressively later until bedtime is at about 0600 but then miss a night's sleep and next go to bed *early* at about 2100; then the sequence starts all over again. For those whose work requires them to be available at conventional times, such a lifestyle is impossible or highly inconvenient, of course.[11] Treatment consists of rendering the person's zeitgebers more effective, whether by requiring him to take more notice of conventional ones or by strengthening conventional zeitgebers with regular routines and exposure to bright light.

Less extreme abnormalities, but ones that are not less inconvenient, are two unusual forms of insomnia.[73] The more common of these is called delayed sleep phase syndrome (DSPS) and the rarer, advanced sleep phase syndrome (ASPS). In DSPS the sufferer shows an entrained sleep/wake cycle with a 24-hour period, except that it is phased very late. During the weekends and holidays, the sleep times (0300–1100) cause only a minor inconvenience and sleep loss does not occur, but weekdays entail a loss of sleep because the sufferers have to rise at what to them is a very early hour. In ASPS, the problem is that sleep onset occurs unusually early, say between 1800 and 2100, so that a normal social life is not possible.[42] Insofar as entrainment to a 24-hour period has occurred, these syndromes indicate a lesser degree of abnormality than the free-running behaviors described above.

Even closer to "normal" are the examples of "morning types" (or larks) and "evening types" (or owls), which make up 10–20% of the total population.[29] Morning types show rhythms that are phased earlier than average; they rise early, work best early in the day, and "fade away" in the evening. By contrast, the evening types are late to rise, slow to get going, and often at their peak in the evening.

It seems reasonable to speculate that all these types can be placed on a scale that considers the interactions between the free-running period of the body clock and the efficacy of zeitgebers, an efficacy that can be reduced by weaker zeitgebers, poorer transmission pathways, or a body clock that is less sensitive to zeitgebers. Some of these relationships are indicated in Figure 5.

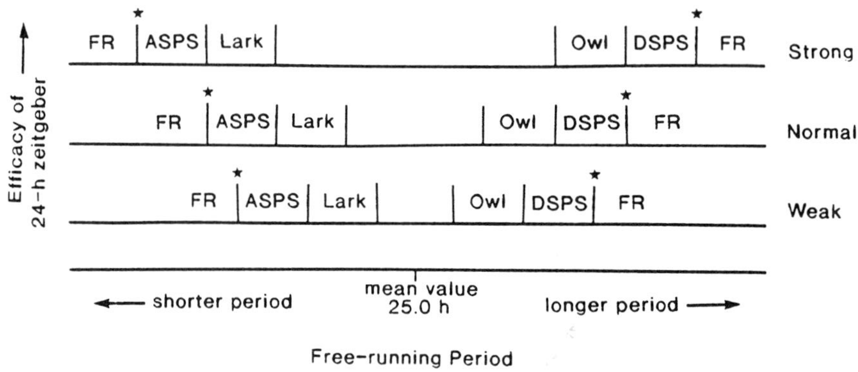

FIGURE 5. The relationship between the free-running period of the body clock, the effectiveness of 24-hour zeitgebers, and some circadian abnormalities. ASPS, advanced sleep phase syndrome; DSPS, delayed sleep phase syndrome; FR, free-running rhythm. *, individuals with a free-running period outside these limits will not be entrained to the 24-hour day.

These factors suggest that individuals differ in the ease with which they adjust to changes in the timing of their lifestyle. For example, larks and those with ASPS would find less difficulty with changes requiring their circadian rhythms to be advanced (as after an eastward time-zone transition or working an early shift, for example), whereas they would find westward time-zone transitions and nightwork particularly troublesome. For evening types, the opposite position would be predicted. We stress that these "abnormalities" are produced by either clock or zeitgeber disorders. Once again, it is the *interaction* between the environment and the body clock that is important.

In the above examples, the different rhythms adjusted together. That is, in DSPS, the "evening fall" in body temperature is delayed by the same amount as is sleep onset. Any abnormality is not between different rhythms within the body but rather between the body as a whole and its environment. This is in contrast to some forms of depression in which there is evidence for a mismatching in the timing of different rhythms within the body.[10,72]

Various factors also affect the amplitude of our circadian rhythms. A low amplitude can result from one of three causes. First, the endogenous component (the clock) may be weak. Second, there may be little polarity in our lifestyle or environment, for example, because our sleep is fractionated and we take several daytime naps or we are rather inactive when awake. Thirdly, there may be a clash between the timing of endogenous and exogenous components of a rhythm so that the normal additive effect of the amplitudes of the two components is missing. This would occur during nightwork and transiently after a time-zone transition (see below).

IMPLICATIONS

It can be seen that, under normal circumstances, a multitude of circadian rhythms resulting from the simultaneous presence of external and internal influences interact with each other. Under normal conditions the rhythms are phase-locked (that is, their relative timings are constant) both when different physiological and psychological variables are considered and when internal and external rhythms are compared. There is a stability in the whole temporal structure of an organism.

An outline of some of the effects of this timing system upon healthy individuals has been given. It is reasonable to suppose that this outline might be relevant also to a study of the symptoms and treatment of disease processes. For example, the observations that the natural tendency for blood to coagulate is greatest in the hours immediately after waking, that airway resistance is highest in the late evening and during the night, and that the concentration of the anti-inflammatory agent, cortisol, is lowest in the evening would lead one to inquire if there were circadian rhythms in disease processes associated with these factors. (In fact, the possible links between plasma cortisol, arthritic pain, and asthma have already been described.) Moreover, since the pharmacokinetics of a drug depend upon its uptake from the gut, metabolism by the liver, and elimination by the kidneys—and all these processes have rhythmic components—it is reasonable to investigate the importance of circadian changes in drug treatment.

In addition, abnormal sleep/wake schedules upset the normal temporal structure of an individual, including associated factors such as mealtimes and social influences. The problem arises because the body clock is stable and unable to adjust its timing rapidly. Such stability is normally advantageous, in that it prevents the clock from adjusting unnecessarily in response to, say, a brief spell of darkness or a short sleep. It means, however, that shiftwork and time-zone transitions produce temporary "mismatching" between the new environment—and the exogenous components of rhythms the new environment is responsible for—and the endogenous component, the body clock. Such abnormalities coincide with, and are believed to be in some way responsible for, fatigue, poor performance, feelings of general malaise, and gastrointestinal disorders. After time-zone transitions, such a group of symptoms is known as "jet lag syndrome," but it is found also in shiftworkers who are required to sleep at abnormal times. Indeed, the persistence of such symptoms is one of the reasons why workers leave shiftwork. There might even be some link between this imposed abnormality of circadian rhythms and the observation that shiftworkers as a group are more liable than nonshift-working controls to suffer from duodenal ulcers. Moreover, the mismatching between the sleep/wake cycle and other circadian rhythms that is found in some forms of depression might indicate that the two are linked in some way.

A knowledge of the properties of the circadian system should help ameliorate some of these problems. First, it should enable advice to be given to time-zone travelers, shiftworkers, and those who devise shift schedules to enable individuals to work with their body clock instead of against it. Second, this knowledge should enable us to make attempts to strengthen zeitgebers or render them more effective. It might lead to the development of drugs or treatments that speed up the adjustment of the circadian timing system.

Subsequent chapters will deal in detail with investigations of some of these predictions together with the ways in which our knowledge of circadian rhythms has aided an understanding and treatment of many of the problems associated with abnormal sleep/wake schedules and chronopathology.

SUMMARY

Circadian rhythms in humans are a mixture of endogenous and exogenous components that are derived from the body clock and the interaction between our environment and lifestyle. Inherently, the body clock tends to run slow (by solar time) with a period of about 25 hours. Under normal circumstances, however, zeitgebers adjust it to run with a period of exactly 24 hours. The important zeitgebers in humans appear to be a mixture of bright light and social factors. Recent evidence favors the hypothalamic suprachiasmatic nuclei as a site of the body clock in mammals, though other sites, including the pineal gland, might also play some role.

Circadian rhythms not only enable us to adjust better to our rhythmic environment but also influence our responses to disease processes and drugs. Moreover, when our lifestyles are altered abruptly, our body clock is slow to adjust. The result is the symptoms associated with "jet lag" and the general malaise suffered by many nightworkers.

REFERENCES

1. Akana SF, Cascio CS, Levin J-ZDN, Dallman MF: Reset of feedback in the adrenocortical system: An apparent shift in sensitivity of adrenocorticotropin to inhibition by corticosterone between morning and evening. Endocrinology 119:2325–2332, 1986.
2. Angeli A: Glucocorticoid secretion: A circadian synchronizer of the human temporal structure. J Steroid Biochem 19:545–554, 1983.
3. Arendt J: Mammalian pineal rhythms. Pineal Res Rev 3:161–213, 1985.
4. Aschoff J: Exogenous and endogenous components in circadian rhythms. Cold Spring Harb Symp Quant Biol 25:11–28, 1960.
5. Baxter C, Reilly T: Influence of the time of day on all-out swimming. Br J Sports Med 17:122–127, 1983.
6. Binkley S: Yearly review. Circadian organisation in mammals and birds. Photochem Photobiol 35:887–890, 1982.
7. Brandenberg J, Bobbert AC, Eggelmeyer F: Evidence for the existence of a retino-hypothalamo-retinal loop in rabbits. Int J Chronobiol 8:13–29, 1981.
8. Cabanac M, Hildebrandt G, Massonnet B, Strempel H: A study of the nycthemeral cycle of behavioural temperature regulation in man. J Physiol (London) 257:275–291, 1976.
9. Cassone VM, Menaker M: Is the avian circadian system a neuroendocrine loop? J Exp Zool 232:539–549, 1984.
10. Checkley S: The relationship between biologial rhythms and the affective disorders. In Arendt J, Minors DS, Waterhouse JM (eds): Biological Rhythms in Clinical Practice. London, Wright, 1989, pp 160–183.
11. Chiba Y: A school-refuser: His rest activity rhythm involved multiple circadian components. Chronobiologia 11:21–27, 1984.
12. Clarke JD, Coleman GJ: Persistent meal-associated rhythms in SCN-lesioned rats. Physiol Behav 36:105–113, 1986.
13. Czeisler CA: Human circadian physiology: Internal organisation of temperature, sleep-wake and neuro-endocrine rhythms monitored in an environment free of time cues. PhD Thesis, Stanford University, CA, 1978.
14. Czeisler CA, Allan JS, Strogatz SH, et al: Bright light resets the human circadian pacemaker independent of the timing of the sleep-wake cycle. Science 233:667–671, 1986.
15. Czeisler CA, Kronauer RE, Duffy JF, et al: Bright light induction of strong (Type O) resetting of the human circadian pacemaker. Science 244:1328–1333, 1989.
16. Czeisler CA, Richardson CR, Zimmerman JC, et al: Entrainment of human circadian rhythms by light-dark cycles: A reassessment. Photochem Photobiol 34:239–247, 1981.
17. De Cherney GS, DeBold CR, Jackson RV, et al: Diurnal variation in the response of plasma adrenocorticotropin and cortisol to intravenous ovine corticotropin-releasing hormone. J Clin Endocrinol Metab 61:271–279, 1985.
18. Eastman CI, Mistlberger RE, Rechtschaffen AE: Suprachiasmatic nuclei lesions eliminate circadian temperature and sleep rhythms in the rat. Physiol Behav 32:357–368, 1984.
19. Enright JT: Temporal precision in circadian systems: A reliable neuronal clock from unreliable components? Science 209:1542–1545, 1980.
20. Froberg J, Karlsson C-G, Levi L, Lidberg L: Circadian variations in performance, psychological ratings, catecholamine excretions, and diuresis during prolonged sleep deprivation. Int J Psychobiol 2:23–36, 1972.

21. Griffiths RA: Natural environmental cues and circadian rhythms of behaviour—a perspective. Chronobiol Int 3:247–253, 1986.
22. Groos GA, Hedricks I: Circadian rhythms in electrical discharge of rat suprachiasmatic neurons recorded in vitro. Neurosci Lett 34:283–288, 1982.
23. Halberg F: Obituary. Professor John Mills, Chronobiologia 5:91–93, 1987.
24. Hastings MH, Vance G, Maywood E: Some reflections on the phylogeny and function of the pineal. Experientia 45:903–908, 1989.
25. Honma K, Honma S, Wada T: Phase-dependent shift of free-running human circadian rhythms in response to a single bright light pulse. Experientia 43:1205 1207, 1987.
26. Inouye ST, Kawamura H: Persistence of circadian rhythmicity in a mammalian hypothalamic "island" containing the suprachiasmatic nucleus. Proc Natl Acad Sci USA 76:5962–5966, 1979.
27. Kaneko M, Hiroshige T, Shinsako J, Dallman MF: Diurnal changes in amplification of hormone rhythms in the adrenocortical system. Am J Physiol 239:R309–R316, 1980.
28. Kass DA, Sulzman FM, Fuller CA, Moore-Ede MC: Renal responses to central vascular expansion are suppressed at night in conscious primates. Am J Physiol 239:F343–F351, 1980.
29. Kerkhof G: Individual differences in circadian rhythms. In Folkard S, Monk TH (eds): Hours of Work. Temporal Factors in Work-Scheduling. Chichester, John Wiley, 1986, pp 29–35.
30. Kleitman N, Kleitman E: Effect of non-24-hour routines of living on oral temperature and heart rate. J Appl Physiol 6:283–291, 1953.
31. Lehman MN, Silver R, Gladstone WR, et al: Circadian rhythmicity restored by neural transplant. Immunocytochemical characterization of the grafts and its integration with the host brain. J Neurosci 7:1626–1638, 1987.
32. Lewy AJ, Wehr TA, Goodwin FK, et al: Light suppresses melatonin secretion in humans. Science 210:1267–1269, 1980.
33. Marani E, Rietveld WJ, Windhorst W, Corino M: Properties of cultured suprachiasmatic nucleus cells. In Pauly JE, Scheving LE (eds): Advances in Chronobiology A. New York, Alan R Liss, 1987, pp 215–221.
34. Marotte H, Timbal J: Circadian rhythms of thermoregulating responses in man exposed to thermal stimuli. Chronobiologia 9:375–387, 1982.
35. Meijer JH, Rietveld WJ: Neurophysiology of the suprachiasmatic circadian pacemaker in rodents. Physiol Rev 69:671–707, 1989.
36. Miller JA: Clockwork in the brain. Bioscience 39:75–78, 1989.
37. Minors DS, Waterhouse JM: Circadian Rhythms and the Human. Bristol, Wright PSG, 1981.
38. Minors DS, Waterhouse JM: Circadian rhythms and their mechanisms. Experientia 42:1–13, 1986.
39. Minors DS, Waterhouse JM: Masking in humans: The problem and some attempts to solve it. Chronobiol Int 6:29–53, 1989.
40. Minors DS, Waterhouse JM: The influence of light in the entrainment of the circadian system: An introduction. In Proceedings of the Ninth International Symposium of Night and Shiftwork. In press.
41. Minors DS, Waterhouse JM, Wirz-Justice A: Establishing a human phase-response curve: Some problems. Abstracts of the Ninth International Symposium on Night and Shiftwork. Verona, September 1989, p 78.
42. Moldofsky H, Musisi S, Phillipson EA: Treatment of a case of advanced sleep phase syndrome by phase advanced chronotherapy. Sleep 9:61–65, 1986.
43. Moore RY: Organisation and function of a central nervous system oscillator: The suprachiasmatic hypothalamic nucleus. Fed Proc 42:2783–2789, 1983.
44. Moore-Ede MC: The circadian timing system in mammals: Two pacemakers preside over many secondary oscillators. Fed proc 42:2802–2808.
45. Moore-Ede MC: Physiology of the circadian timing system: Predictive versus reactive homeostasis. Am J Physiol 250:R737–R752, 1986.
46. Moore-Ede MC, Brennan MF, Ball MR: Circadian variations of intercompartmental potassium fluxes in man. J Appl Physiol 38:163–170, 1975.
47. Morgan PJ, Williams LM: Central melatonin receptors: Implications for a mode of action. Experientia 45:955–965, 1989.
48. Mrosovsky N: Mutant hamsters in a hurry. Nature 337:213–214, 1989.
49. Mrosovsky N: Nonphotic enhancement of adjustment to new light-dark cycles: Masking interpretation discounted. J Biol Rhythms 4:365–370, 1989.
50. Mrosovsky N, Reebs SG, Honrada GI, Salmon PA: Behavioural entrainment of circadian rhythms. Experientia 45:696–702, 1989.

51. Nagai K, Mori T, Nakagawa H: Application of an immunological technique to behavioural studies: Anti-suprachiasmatic nucleus Y-globulin-induced loss of the circadian rhythm. Biomed Res 3:294–302, 1982.
52. Nelson W, Tong YL, Lee J-K, Halberg F: Methods for cosinor-rhythmometry. Chronobiologia 6:305–323, 1979.
53. Newman GC, Hospod FE: Rhythm of suprachiasmatic nucleus 2-deoxyglucose uptake in vitro. Brain Res 381:345–350, 1986.
54. Redfern PH, Campbell IC, Davies JA, Martin KF (eds): Circadian Rhythms in the Central Nervous System. London, Macmillan, 1985.
55. Redfern PH, Waterhouse JM, Minors DS: Introduction: Definition and measurement of rhythms. Pharmacol Ther, in press.
56. Reiter RJ: Intrinsic rhythms of the pineal gland and associated hormone cycles in body fluids. Annu Rev Chronopharmacol 44:77–105, 1988.
57. Reppert SM, Weaver DR, Rivkees SA, Stopa EG: Putative melatonin receptors in a human biological clock. Science 242:78–81, 1988.
58. Roelfsema F: The influence of light on circadian rhythms. Experientia 43:7–13, 1987.
59. Rosenwasser AM, Adler NT: Structure and function in circadian timing systems: Evidence for multiple coupled circadian oscillators. Neurosci Biobehav Rev 10:431–448, 1986.
60. Rusak B: The role of the suprachiasmatic nuclei in the generation of circadian rhythms in the golden hamster. J Comp Physiol [A] 118:145–164, 1977.
61. Rusak B: The mammalian circadian system: Models in physiology. J Biol Rhythms 4:121–134, 1989.
62. Rusak B, Zucker I: Neural regulation of circadian rhythms. Physiol Rev 59:449–526, 1979.
63. Sadun AA, Schaechter JD, Smith LEH: A retinohypothalamic pathway in man: Light mediation of circadian rhythms. Brain Res 302:371–377, 1984.
64. Satinoff E, Prosser R: Suprachiasmatic nuclear lesions eliminate circadian rhythms of drinking and activity, but not of body temperature, in male rats. J Biol Rhythms 3:1–22, 1988.
65. Schwartz WT, Gainer H: Localisation of the "biological clock" in the brain. JAMA 246:681, 1981.
66. Stephenson LA, Wenger CB, O'Donovan BH, Nadel ER: Circadian rhythm in sweating and cutaneous blood flow. Am J Physiol 246:R321–R324, 1984.
67. Terai Y, Asayama M, Ogawa T, et al: Circadian variation of preferred environmental temperature and body temperature. J Therm Biol 10:151–156, 1985.
68. Turek FW: Circadian neural rhythms in mammals. Annu Rev Physiol 47:49–64, 1985.
69. Turek FW, Losee-Olsen S: Entrainment of the circadian activity rhythm to the light-dark cycle can be altered by a short-acting benzodiazepine, triazolam. J Biol Rhythms 2:249–260, 1987.
70. Van Reeth O, Turek FW: Simulated activity mediates phase shifts in the hamster circadian clock induced by dark pulses or benzodiazepines. Nature 339:49–51, 1989.
71. Van Reeth O, Vanderhaeghen JJ, Turek FW: A benzodiazepine antagonist, Ro 15-1788, can block the phase-shifting effects of triazolam on the mammalian circadian clock. Brain Res 444:333–339, 1988.
72. Wehr TA, Rosenthal NE: Seasonality and affective illness. Am J Psychiatr 146:829–839, 1989.
73. Weiztman ED: Sleep and its disorders. Annu Rev Neurosci 4:381–417, 1981.
74. Wever R: The Circadian System of Man. Results of Experiments under Temporal Isolation. Berlin, Springer-Verlag, 1979.
75. Wever RA: Internal interaction within the human circadian system: The masking effect. Experientia 41:332–342, 1985.
76. Wurtman RJ, Lieberman HR: Melatonin secretion as a mediator of circadian variations in sleep and sleepiness. J Pineal Res 2:301–303, 1985.

TIMOTHY H. MONK, PhD

SHIFTWORKER PERFORMANCE

From the Sleep Evaluation Center
Western Psychiatric Institute
University of Pittsburgh School of Medicine
Pittsburgh, Pennsylvania

Reprint requests to:
Timothy H. Monk, PhD
Sleep Evaluation Center
Western Psychiatric Institute
3811 O'Hara Street
Pittsburgh, PA 15213-2593

HUMAN CIRCADIAN PRINCIPLES

From the discussion of circadian rhythms given by Drs. Minors and Waterhouse in Chapter 1, it is clear that the human being differs in physiological makeup from one time of day to another. Whether one remains awake or sleeps at night, body temperature falls, melatonin is in the bloodstream, and cortisol is suppressed until the early morning, to name but a few changes. It is therefore not surprising that the individual's *psychological* milieu like the *physiological* milieu may be "as different as night and day" at different times.

These differences have vital importance for any consideration of the safety and performance of the shiftworker. We energetically prevent employees from operating dangerous machinery with more than the legal limit of alcohol in their bloodstream. Shouldn't we be equally concerned when large decrements in performance might arise from *circadian* principles? Perhaps the melatonin circulating in the blood of an unadjusted nightworker is potentially as lethal as the alcohol circulating in the blood of an inebriated dayworker. Importantly, moreover, nightshift performance decrements do not spring only from the *direct* influence of the biological clock. One must also consider *indirect* influences from changes in sleep attainment, mood, and subjective alertness. Both direct and indirect routes can be vitally important in determining the safety and productivity of the shiftworker and thus the profitability or social worth of the enterprise he or she is employed in.

SHIFTWORKER SAFETY

While greater environmental risks are occasionally associated with shiftwork than with daywork—for example, because of the absence of daylight or of increased chemical exposure on 12-hour shifts[7]—they are usually outweighed by the reduction in human traffic during shiftwork hours. Indeed, when the accident rate is not expressed as a percentage of "traffic load," it is lower on the nightshift than on the others.[45] However, when accidents are expressed in terms of number per worker on the job, the nightshift often comes out worst.[10] This illustrates the point that it is primarily the unadjusted shiftworker who is the agent of risk, rather than the work environment.

Maladjusted shiftworkers can become agents of risk to themselves and others in a number of different ways. The first way is through sleepiness at work,[1] the etiology of which is discussed below. Sleepiness at work can lead to the problem of missed signals (e.g., a red light, a dial going critical) or of inappropriate responses to correctly perceived signals (e.g., landing an airplane on the wrong runway) as well as that of actually dozing on the job.[32] These effects are also important causes of accidents in the commute to and from work.

Although it is tempting to regard all dangerous shiftworkers as being overly sleepy, in fact, certain groups of maladjusted shiftworkers are not sleepy at all but may be just as dangerous. These workers are too upset and angry to be sleepy. Their anger may be either biological (circadian dysfunction, sleep loss) or social (an imminent divorce). Such mood changes can lead to a cavalier (or directly aggressive) attitude toward the handling of dangerous machinery and to an absence of concern for the safety of others.

The third means by which shiftworkers can become agents of risk is through simple performance decrements. Although not subjectively sleepy, workers may be suffering circadian-related performance decrements that might lead to personal injury because of the critical nature of the work (e.g., in the meat-packing industry).

In considering the total "social cost" of shiftwork, one must realize that not only the worker, but also his or her family and indeed the surrounding community face hazards to their safety and well-being as a result of shiftwork. In evaluating these hazards one must recognize the multifaceted nature of the shiftwork issue. At one extreme are rare but highly significant events, such as a near meltdown at a power plant, a chemical plant explosion, or a train derailment. These highly visible events can affect thousands of lives and have a massive impact on the safety and well-being of surrounding communities. At the other end of the spectrum are comparatively frequent events with limited consequences, such as vehicular accidents on the drive home from work and minor injuries at work. Because of their lower profile in the news media, these events tend to be relatively ignored. In dollars and cents terms (and, indeed, overall human misery) it is quite possible, however, that the sum total of the frequent small events is as important to society as that of the occasional dramatic ones. Both are often the result of shiftworker errors, and both should be factored in when society evaluates the cost-effectiveness of shiftwork.

It is false, however, to think that shiftwork is necessarily accompanied by high risk. Discussions of safety, and probably also of health, are concerned primarily with shiftworkers who are not coping for one reason or another, rather than with the entire population of shiftworkers. Measures that reduce either the stress on the shiftworker (e.g., by the adoption of more benign schedules) or the resulting strain (e.g., by the provision of support systems and education) will undoubtedly improve safety both at the workplace and on the drive home from it.

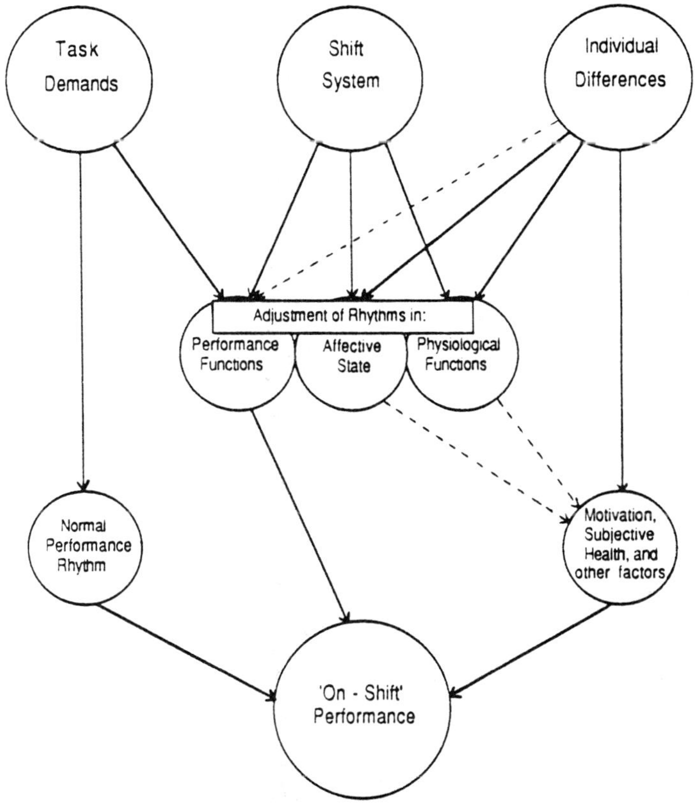

FIGURE 1. A conceptual model of the factors affecting "on-shift" performance. Solid lines represent known influences, and dashed lines probable ones.[15]

PERFORMANCE CONSEQUENCES OF SHIFTWORK

While safety and performance are inextricably linked, it is quite possible for performance efficiency (and thus productivity and competitiveness) to be impaired without an accompanying change in *safety* risk. This complexity stems not only from the influence of task demands on both time-of-day effects in performance efficiency and the oscillatory control underlying them, but also from the influence of sleep deprivation effects, subjective and objective health effects, motivation effects (which are influenced by social and family problems), and the effects of individual differences on both normal rhythm parameters and the rate at which these parameters adjust to a change in routine.

Although it represents something of an oversimplification, the conceptual model of Folkard and Monk,[15] which is illustrated in Figure 1, represents a useful framework in which to consider these effects. Essentially, this model (like the later one of DeVries-Griever and Meijman[10]) reinforces the point that the "on-shift" performance of the shiftworker is the product of many different factors, some interacting directly, others operating through changes in the adjustment process.

The three major inputs to the system are task demands (i.e., the levels of vigilance and of physical and cognitive work required), the particular shift system used (very different effects spring from fixed or permanent shifts than from rotating schedules, for example), and individual differences (including the worker's personality, age, health, sleep needs, and behavior patterns[41]). These factors serve to affect the adjustment process in performance function (circadian performance rhythms), affective state (circadian rhythms in subjective vigilance, mood, and well-being), and physiological functions (sleep being the most crucial, but also the circadian rhythms in temperature and neuroendocrine function). The interaction of those adjustment effects then influences the worker's on-shift performance, both directly and through indirect effects on his or her subjective health and well-being. Thus, one cannot simply assert that a nightshift performance will be poor because the worker is then "at a low ebb." That assertion may be quite wrong for some tasks[37] and is remiss in leaving out the sleep deprivation, health, and motivational effects that can often outweigh the strictly circadian ones.[44,10]

This chapter discusses human circadian performance rhythms, how they arise, and how they differ according to the task being performed. It will then discuss circadian rhythms in subjective alertness/sleepiness and their relationship to the circadian system and the sleep/wake cycle. Following this consideration of *laboratory-based* studies of circadian performance rhythms, it will conclude with a discussion of actual "on-the-job" shiftworker performance.

CIRCADIAN PERFORMANCE RHYTHMS

Circadian performance rhythms are not merely the step function resulting from poor performance at night by comparison with better performance during the day; nor are they of trivial magnitude or always peculiar to the individual. They are robust fluctuations of significant magnitude that are (for about 80% of the population) predictable in form, given knowledge of the task being tested.[17] Even over the normal waking day, fluctuations in performance efficiency can equal those induced by ingesting the "legal limit" of alcohol or restricting the previous night's sleep to three hours.[18]

Performance has to be measured carefully if valid circadian performance rhythms are to be obtained. One major contaminant is the "practice effect" whereby people perform better and better as they become more and more practiced at the task. Performance improvements may last weeks or even months.[26] Also, differences in such chance factors as the subject's motivation, perception of the task, and distraction by some nontask event, can render performance measurement notoriously inaccurate. This means that a single performance reading cannot meaningfully measure performance. To accurately measure circadian performance rhythms sufficient replications must be made to even out such inaccuracies. Thus, each trial should contain a large number of measured events (e.g., reactions) and each time of day should be associated with a large number of trials, coming from different subjects, from different days, or, preferably, from different subjects and different days.

An example of the care needed to cope with all these problems is provided by an early study of scholastic performance carried out by Laird.[31] Laird used 112 subjects divided into seven squads that were matched for intelligence. Six weeks' experimentation was necessary, with each squad attending at six times of the day, in a design that enabled both time of day and day of week to be studied independently of each other and without contamination by either practice effects or the actual material given. At each session a battery of nine different tasks was given, and some tasks were often represented by several different instances (e.g., about 50 computations for the "simple addition" task). To avoid contamination due to personal prejudices, the subjects were misled to believe that the experiment was a study of temperature changes. The study was successful in demonstrating reliable day-of-week and time-of-day trends in various cognitive tasks, including a time-of-day effect in immediate memory, which was replicated by Folkard and Monk[16] half a century later (see Fig. 4).

It is, perhaps, chastening to realize that, even in this age of electronic data analysis and on-line experimental control, the care and elegance of Laird's study have seldom been approached, let alone surpassed. All too often performance measures, sometimes of the most trivial sort, have simply been inserted into shiftwork studies as part of a battery of otherwise physiological tests, without their special needs and controls being taken into account.

The Work of Kleitman and Colquhoun

As Lavie[33] points out in his comprehensive historical review, the study of circadian performance rhythms has an illustrious history, predating (by about half a century) even the invention of the term "circadian." These early studies presaged the importance of intertask differences in diurnal rhythm, with Gates[21] concluding that "in general, the forenoon is the best time for strictly mental work . . . while the afternoon may best be taken up with school subjects in which motor factors are predominant." Most influential in the present age, however, have been Nathaniel Kleitman from the United States and W. Peter Colquhoun from England.

In contrast to the earlier work, studies carried out in Chicago in the 1930s by Kleitman and reported in his book *Sleep and Wakefulness*[29] were concerned mainly with simple repetitive tasks, such as card dealing, which had a comparatively small cognitive load. Perhaps because of the task chosen, there was strong evidence for a parallelism between the circadian rhythms of body temperature and performance speed. Kleitman believed there was a causal relationship between the two, even asserting that one could infer the performance rhythm from the oral temperatures, thus avoiding the use of "time-consuming performance tests which, in themselves, interfere with, or disrupt, the scheduled activities of the persons studied."[30]

When, in the 1960s, Colquhoun and co-workers at Cambridge addressed the problem of circadian performance rhythms, the emphasis was still very much on simple repetitive tasks and on a parallelism between temperature and performance rhythms. However, the notion of a causal relationship between the two was carefully avoided; instead, a mechanism involving a rhythm in basal arousal (or the inverse of sleepiness) was invoked as a mediating factor.[9,24]

This arousal rhythm was never specified in fine detail, but it was held to parallel the temperature rhythm and to mediate changes in performance level through an "inverted U" relationship, whereby rises in arousal level are associated with improvements in performance up to a certain arousal level, after which performance starts to decline. (A good example of superoptimal arousal is the difficulty in unlocking one's car door when a downpour of rain has made speed imperative.) From outside the circadian rhythms area, the Yerkes-Dodson law has postulated an inverted U relationship in which the optimal arousal level of a task is dependent on its complexity, the more complex tasks having lower optimal arousal levels.

The mechanism of the inverted U was needed because of a finding the Cambridge group frankly regarded as anomalous—namely, the decline in performance over much of the waking day that they had observed in the memory task of digit span.[5] By invoking the arousal model, this apparent anomaly could be explained by the postulation that digit span has a low optimal arousal and the time-of-day variation thus occurs on the falling arm of the inverted U. A further advantage was that time of day could then be regarded as just another arousing agent, such as white noise or knowledge of results. A series of experiments involving combinations of these agents could then be carried out, and the various interactions explored in detail.[6] These experiments produced results that were in agreement with the model, but because one of the problems of the inverted U concept is tautology, the positive results are perhaps not entirely surprising. More recently we have quantified the predictions of the arousal model,[35] testing its fit to circadian performance rhythms in a variable memory-load task. Although some fits were impressively good, the fact that a phase shift was also required casts doubt on a *unitary* arousal model of time-of-day effects.

Thus, through the 1960s and early 1970s, the notion was of a single performance rhythm usually parallel to the temperature rhythm, except in memory tasks such as digit span, whose rhythms were explained in terms of superoptimal arousal. As can be seen in Figure 2, for some tasks, at least, the parallelism with temperature is quite striking. This notion persisted until the mid-70s when Folkard[13] (who, like me, was at the time a member of Colquhoun's group) studied the time-of-day effect in two complex cognitive tasks—namely, logical syllogisms and the Baddeley[2] logical reasoning test. These tasks represented a departure from previous efforts in that they involved the subject in fairly complex thought processes and could not simply be worked through in a mindless, routine

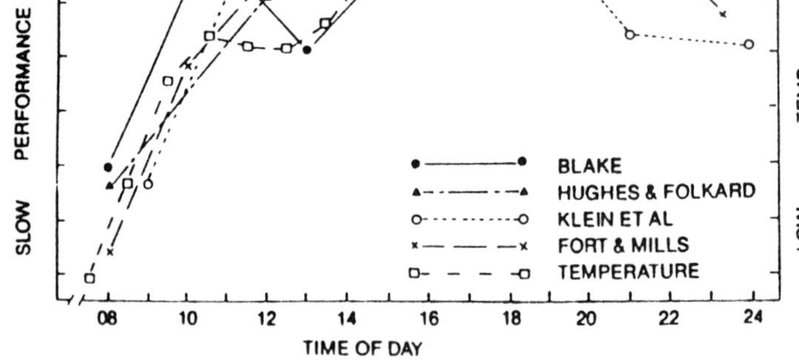

FIGURE 2. The time-of-day function for a series of studies involving serial search tasks, plotted together with the time-of-day function in temperature.[17]

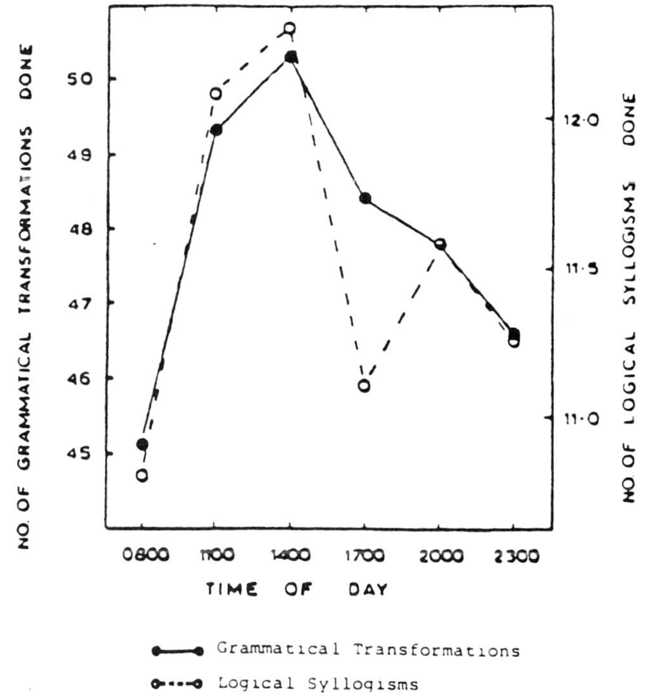

FIGURE 3. The time-of-day function for performance in a logical syllogisms (0---0) and grammatical transformation (●—●) task.[13]

fashion. The results are shown in Figure 3, which reveals time-of-day curves with a midday peak, unlike either the digit span or simple repetitive-task time-of-day function. This result heralded a new approach to the study of circadian performance rhythms, with more emphasis on the *differences* between circadian performance rhythms than on their similarities and greater theoretical richness in considering the mechanisms by which circadian performance rhythms might occur.

Later circadian performance rhythm research focused on both "pure memory" and "working memory" tasks. With regard to the former, it was clear even from the early studies that the time-of-day function for memory was very different from that for other tasks. Research by Baddeley et al.[3] and Hockey et al.[25] confirmed that for relatively "pure" tasks of immediate memory (i.e., memory tested within a few minutes of presentation), performance was better in the morning than in the afternoon or evening. This result was explained in terms of the arousal model by postulating that immediate memory was interfered with by evening high arousal. This agreed with evidence from outside the time-of-day area that arousing manipulations such as anxiety could produce decrements in immediate memory performance. In contrast, a more robust finding from these arousal manipulation studies was that high arousal was actually beneficial to long-term memory of the material.[28] Thus, if one waited a few days rather than a few minutes before testing the memory, the high-arousal presentation condition might result in superior performance.

These experiments suggested that the time-of-day function for long-term memory might be very different, in terms of time-of-day presentation effects, from that of immediate memory. Thus the time of day giving an arousal level that was optimal for immediate memory might be associated with a suboptimal arousal level for long-term memory. That prediction was tested by Folkard,[18] who presented a story to groups of schoolchildren at either morning (0900) or afternoon (1500) sessions. Memory for the material was tested either immediately after presentation or after one week's delay. The predictions of the model were perfectly validated. The morning presentation group performed better than the afternoon group on the immediate test but worse on the delayed test, regardless of what time of day either test was given. Interestingly, the magnitudes of the time-of-day effects for immediate and delayed tests were 64% and 44%, respectively, of the difference in performance due to the week's delay. Clearly, even when one is considering differences between 0900 and 1300, time-of-day effects are important and striking. In practical terms, of course, this study has ramifications for the scheduling of school timetables, which had been the focus of the early studies. Thus, for good long-term retention, afternoon teaching might be more efficient.

The schoolchildren study was later validated at more extreme times of day. Night nurses were compared for memory of material in a training film presented at either 0400 or 2030. Again, the conclusions of the arousal model were validated by a crossover between immediate and delayed memory. Short-term memory was better for the 0400 presentation, long-term memory for the 2030 presentation,[38] and time of recall again proved to be irrelevant. This has ramifications supporting students who "burn the midnight oil." In the early hours of the morning, when arousal is low, good immediate memory might hoodwink the student into thinking the material has been successfully memorized, whereas long-term retention might actually be rather poor.

A time-of-day function for immediate memory was determined by Folkard and Monk.[16] As can be seen in Figure 4 (taken from their article), the observed decline over the waking day coincided very well with that found by Laird more than half a century earlier and was markedly different from the rise over the day observed in body temperature.

Not only does the circadian performance rhythm differ between memory and nonmemory tasks, but it also changes when the memory load within the same task varies. Thus, by increasing the working memory load (the number of target letters to be remembered) in a performance test given as part of a rapidly rotating shift-schedule (laboratory) study, Folkard et al.[14] were able to totally transform the circadian performance rhythm (Fig. 5). The good parallelism between temperature and performance rhythms (top panel) was seen to break down (middle panel) and eventually become inverted (bottom panel) as the memory load of the task was increased. Thus, even with the same basic task—in this case, a serial search task—increasing the memory load can totally alter the associated time-of-day function.

CIRCADIAN ALERTNESS RHYTHMS

Just as there are circadian rhythms in *objective* performance, so too are there rhythms in the *subjective* ratings of how wide awake or sleepy a person feels. The existence of circadian alertness rhythms fits in nicely with the notion that psychological circadian rhythms act as an interface between the physiological

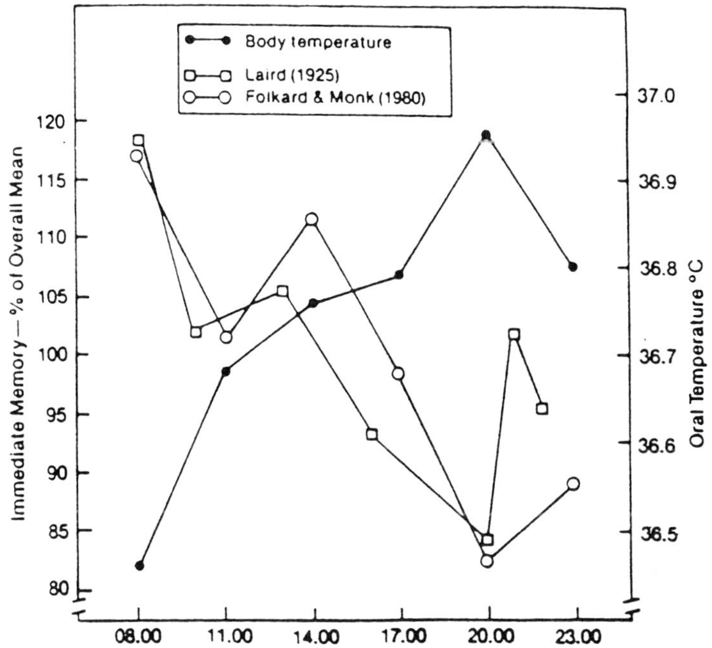

FIGURE 4. The time-of-day effect in immediate memory for information presented in prose.[16]

circadian processes and the particular (sleeping and waking) behaviors that those processes are intended to elicit.[40] It would, indeed, be strange in a normal diurnal routine if drops in alertness did not precede the decision to go to bed at night. However, the relation between subjective alertness and the sleep/wake cycle is not a simple one.

On the basis of common sense, it can be predicted that for people working during normal daytime hours, subjective alertness is likely to be reduced as they emerge from sleep at the beginning of the waking day and as they approach sleep at the end of it. What is less obvious is the time-of-day function in between these extremes. Figure 6 presents a collection of time-of-day functions from several different studies using different subject pools; all the studies were subjective ratings of alertness from people who were asleep at night and awake during the day. The most striking finding is that all studies showed a well-defined peak in subjective alertness occurring in the late morning or early afternoon. Only one of the studies showed the classic "post-lunch dip" that is present in some performance rhythms[5] and in objective sleepiness as measured by the Multiple Sleep Latency Test (MSLT),[43] and none showed the early evening peak that typically appears in body temperature.[9] Figure 7 presents the time-of-day functions in subjective alertness and body temperature in a study of 38 subjects in whom the two measures were taken concurrently.[39]

The problem of subjective alertness as related to body temperature is an interesting one. When the sleep/wake cycle is suspended and subjects are kept

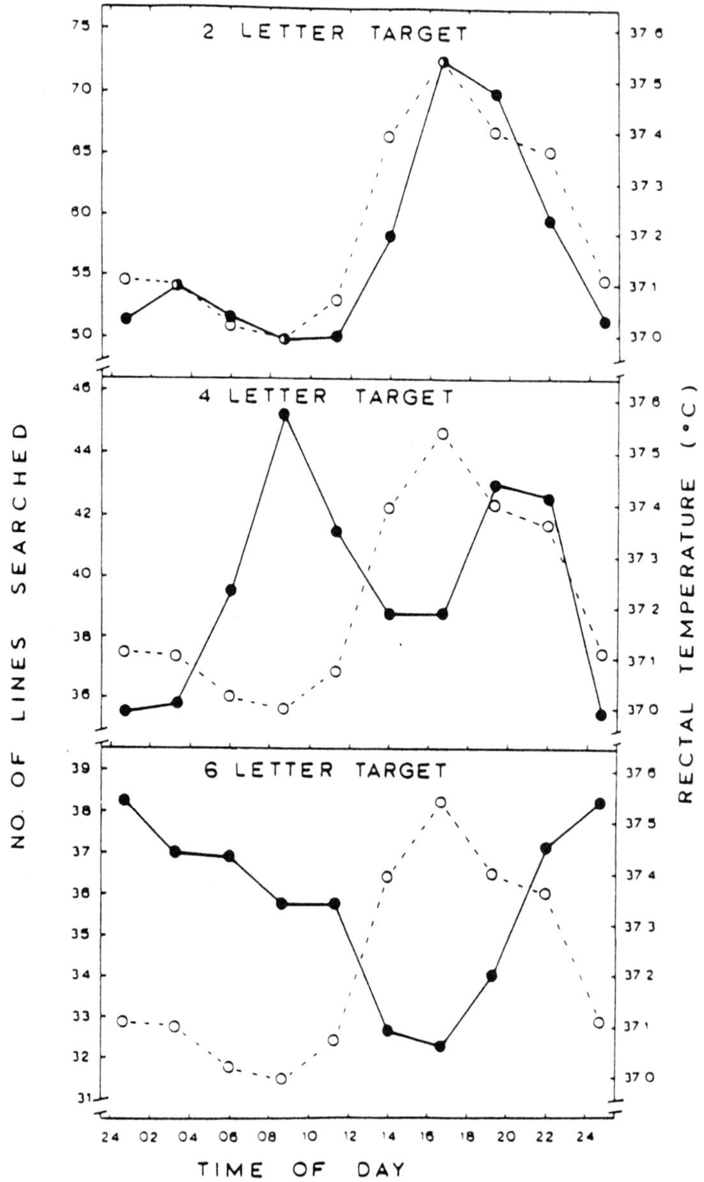

FIGURE 5. The time-of-day function for low- (two-letter), medium- (four-letter), and high- (six-letter) memory load versions of a serial search task (●—●) plotted together with rectal temperature (0---0).[15]

in wakeful temporal isolation, the circadian rhythms in subjective alertness and body temperature that clearly emerge are superimposed upon the gradual decline observed in both measures as the vigil progresses. The data of Froberg[20]

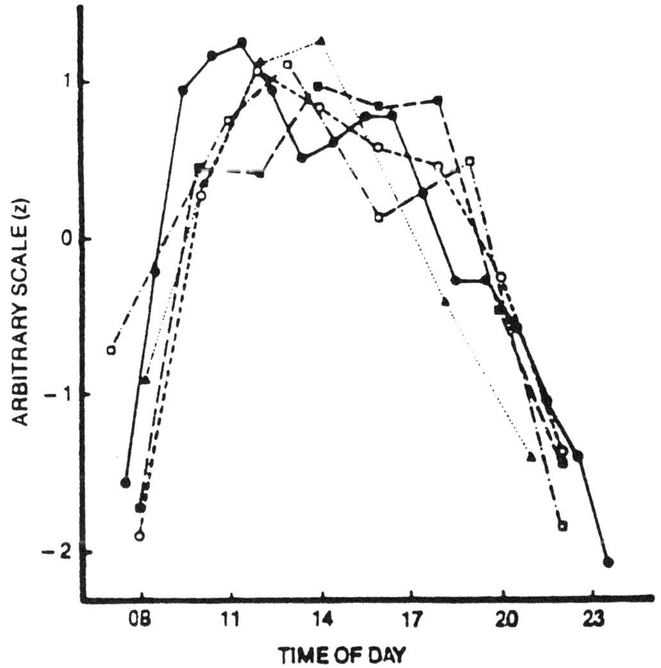

FIGURE 6. The time-of-day function in self-rated alertness/activation level from a number of different studies.[18]

(collected from 15 female subjects), illustrating this nicely, show a clear parallelism between the two measures ($r = 0.7, p < 0.01$), with coincidence in both times of peak and times of trough (Fig. 8). Therefore, when the sleep/wake cycle is suspended, there is a parallelism between the two measures that agrees with the coincidence in body temperature and subjective alertness troughs observed in nightworkers.[37]

To explore the influence of the temperature rhythm on subjective alertness, I and my colleagues undertook a series of "forced desynchronization" studies.[36,40] In these studies, abnormally long or short day lengths were imposed in temporal isolation studies lasting several months at a time. Thus, the subject was unaware of time of day but was told when to go to bed, get up, and take meals, according to a strict routine that corresponded to some non-24-hour day length (e.g., 23 hours, 26 hours).

Under such conditions, a desynchronization in period can emerge. When the sleep/wake cycle is driven at a period that is beyond the range of entrainment of the circadian oscillator controlling the temperature rhythm (the deep "biological clock"), the oscillator then assumes a period length close to that observed in "free-running" studies in which temporally isolated subjects choose their own bedtimes and waketimes (typically around 25 hours in young male subjects). Thus, the data have two periodicities. Examination of the subjective alertness rhythms at those two periodicities revealed that both the temperature rhythm oscillator and the sleep/wake cycle influenced subjective alertness. Moreover, at the temperature rhythm oscillator period, there was a parallelism between body

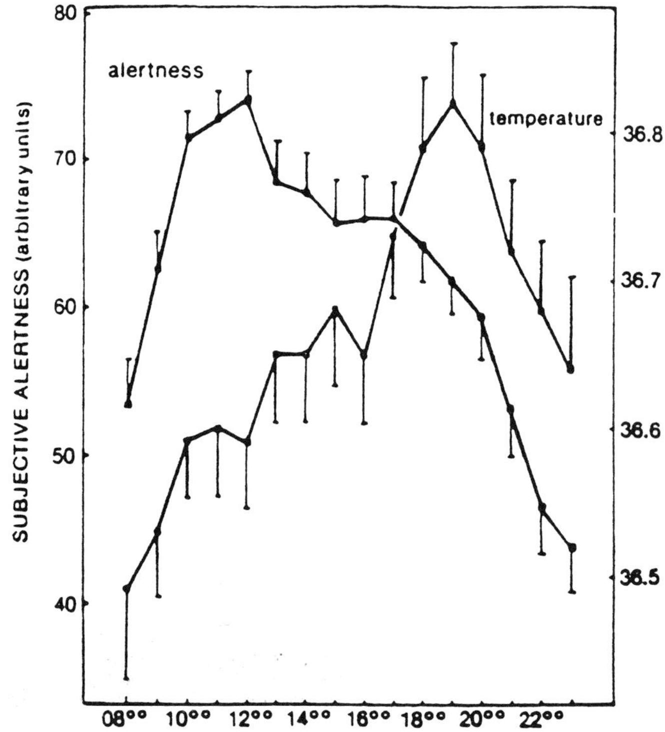

FIGURE 7. The time-of-day functions of subjective alertness and oral temperature for 38 subjects studied over eight days (± 1 standard error).[39]

temperature and subjective alertness, and at the sleep/wake cycle period, the maximal subjective alertness was found to occur about 8 to 10 hours after waking, thus coinciding quite nicely with the early afternoon peak in alertness usually found (see Figs. 6 and 7). Therefore, we can explain the relationship between subjective alertness and body temperature by postulating control by both the temperature rhythm oscillator and the sleep/wake cycle mechanism, with the latter tending to predominate under normal sleep/wake patterns.

Having *two* rhythmic processes underlying the generation of subjective alertness rhythms complicates the picture when it comes to understanding the subjective alertness (or, more usually, sleepiness) of shiftworkers on the job. We cannot simply use the status of the temperature oscillator as a predictor of sleepiness but must also take into account the status of the sleep/wake cycle processes—processes that are considerably more labile in phase adjustment than the temperature oscillator. Further research is needed in order to understand how the two underlying processes might interact in a phase adjustment situation.

ON-THE-JOB SHIFTWORKER PERFORMANCE

There are major problems in trying to determine intershift differences in "real task" performance. The most important of these is the difference in working environments. Not only lighting levels, but also supervision levels, group morale,

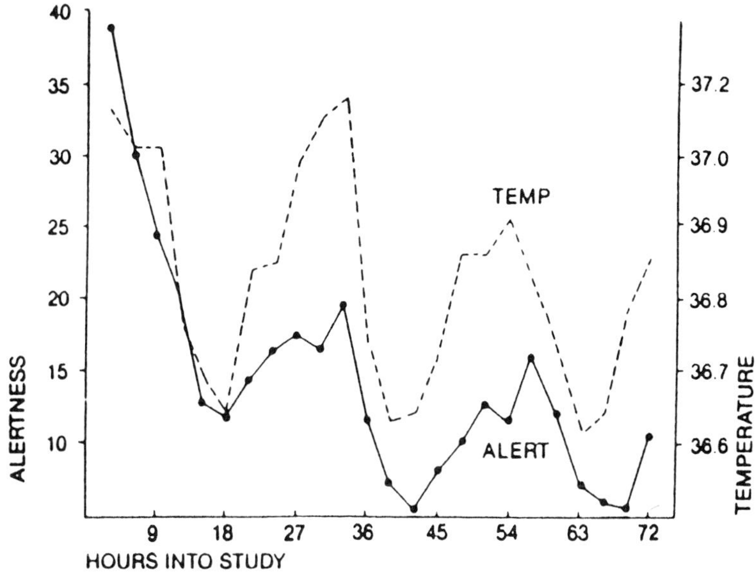

FIGURE 8. Average subjective alertness and body temperature of 15 subjects experiencing 72 hours of sleep deprivation under temporal isolation.[20]

and distractions can all be very different indeed between nightshifts and dayshifts. Also, poorer performance can occur on the nightshift simply because nobody is there to repair broken machines.[34] Not only the work environment, but the work itself may be quite different between night and day. Very often particular parts of the job are actually saved for the nightshift, either in response to the demands of the process (preparing things for shipment in the morning), or to make life easier for the nightworkers (e.g., long-running computer jobs may be held back to be run at night). Even in continuous-process operations, complicated development work may be permitted to intrude during the day but not at night.[10]

Despite such problems and complications, a few studies have been able to obtain relatively continuous 24-hour "real task" data, and indeed these studies show a remarkable similarity in time-of-day function (Fig. 9). The six studies can be divided into three that actually measure the speed[8,46] or accuracy[4] with which the primary task is done and three that measure the consequences of lapses in attention or vigilance.[4,23,15] All six agree in showing performance to be worse during the night hours, although in three of them there is also evidence of a pronounced postlunch dip that almost equals the nighttime dip. In a recent study of truck drivers[22] the risk of accidents at the 2400–0200 time interval was found to be more than double the normal risk.

Thus, it would seem reasonable to assert that, in general, nightshift job performance is inferior to dayshift job performance. However, as we have been careful to point out, nightshift performances can be degraded in a number of different ways, not all of them directly circadian. It is possible that differences in motivation level can affect time-of-day functions, as Khaleque and Verhaegen[27] showed in a comparison of cigar-making speeds between morning and afternoon

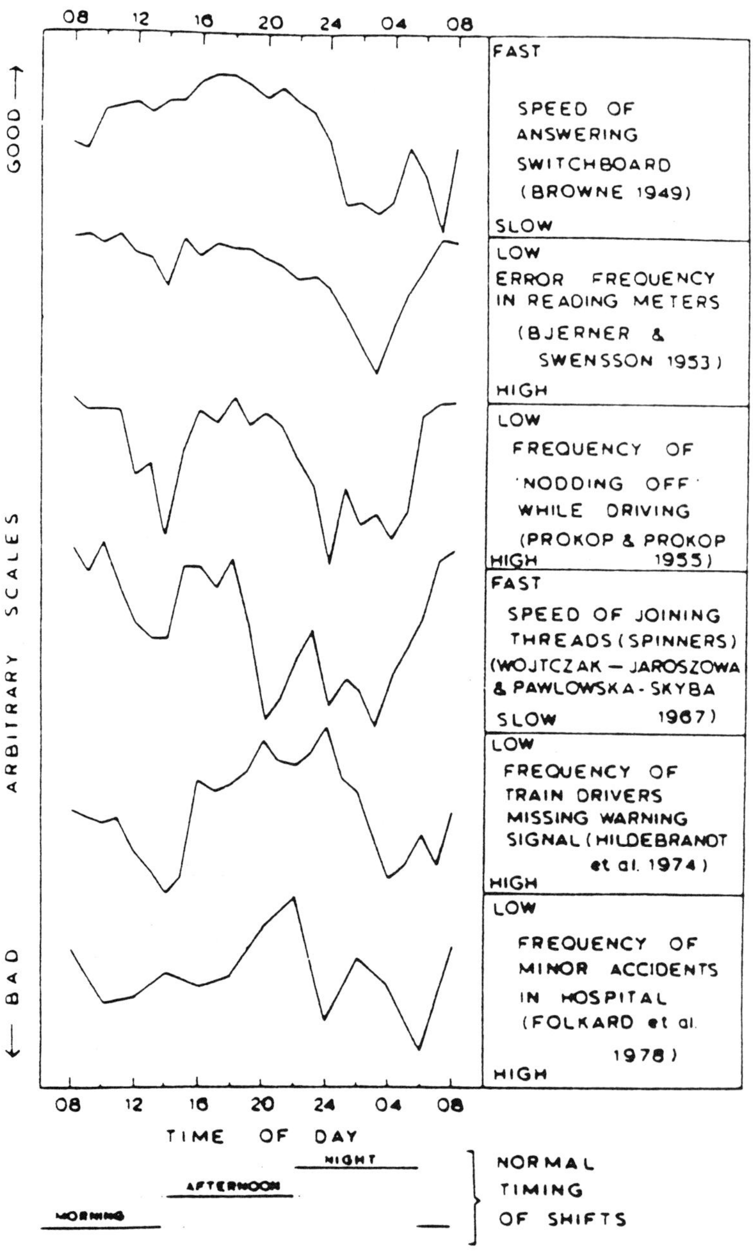

FIGURE 9. Variations in "real job" measures over the 24-hour period.[15]

shifts. Significantly, time-of-day differences appeared only in highly stressed workers who were making considerable effort to gain piecework bonuses. Thus, it is possible that circadian effects can only "show through" when workers are under pressure. In the absence of pressure, workers may be able to equate dayshift and nightshift performance because both are considerably suboptimal. In that case, overall intershift differences in productivity are more likely to be due to absenteeism and tardiness than to individual performance.[12,11]

CONCLUSIONS

The performance rhythms of shiftworkers are the result of complex, multifaceted processes. As well as tapping into the "low ebb" of certain circadian performance rhythms, nightwork involves sleep disruption, social and domestic disruption, and the chronic equivalent of jet lag, all of which can radically affect performance and safety. Thus, the amelioration of the problem must be equally multifaceted, lessening not only the stress on the shiftworker (e.g., by the selection of more benign shift schedules) but also the resultant strain (e.g., through health, education, and counseling programs).

REFERENCES

1. Akerstedt T: Sleepiness as a consequence of shift work. Sleep 11:17–34, 1988.
2. Baddeley AD: A three-minute reasoning test based on grammatical transformation. Psychonom Sci 10:341 341, 1968.
3. Baddeley AD, Hatter JE, Scott D, Snashall A: Memory and time of day. Q J Exp Psychol 22:605–609, 1970.
4. Bjerner B, Swensson A: Shiftwork and rhythm. Acta Med Scand 278:102–107, 1953.
5. Blake MJF: Time of day effects on performance in a range of tasks. Psychonom Sci 9:349–350, 1967.
6. Blake MJF: Temperament and time of day. In Colquhoun WP (ed): In Biological Rhythms and Human Performance. London, Academic Prress, 1971, pp 109–148.
7. Brief RS, Scala RA: Occupational health aspects of unusual work schedules: A review of Exxon's experience. Am Ind Hyg Assoc J 47:199–202, 1986.
8. Browne RC: The day and night performance of teleprinter switchboard operators. Occup Psychol 23:121–126, 1949.
9. Colquhoun WP: Circadian variations in mental efficiency. In Colquhoun WP (ed): Biological Rhythms and Human Peformance. London, Academic Press, 1971, pp 39–107.
10. DeVries-Griever AHG, Meijman TF: The impact of abnormal hours of work on various models of information processing: A process model on human costs of performance. Ergonomics 30:1287–1299, 1987.
11. Farrell D, Stamm CL: Meta-analysis of the correlates of employee absence. Hum Relations 41:211–227, 1988.
12. Fischer FM: Retrospective study regarding absenteeism among shiftworkers. Int Arch Occup Environ Health 58:301–320, 1986.
13. Folkard S: Diurnal variation in logical reasoning. Br J Psychol 66:1–8, 1975.
14. Folkard S, Knauth P, Monk TH, Rutenfranz J: The effect of memory load on the circadian variation in performance efficiency under a rapidly rotating shift system. Erognomics 19:479–488, 1976.
15. Folkard S, Monk TH: Shiftwork and performance. Hum Factors 21:483–4492, 1979.
16. Folkard S, Monk TH: Circadian rhythms in human memory. Br J Psychol 71:295–307, 1980.
17. Folkard S, Monk TH: Circadian performance rhythms. In Folkard S, Monk TH (eds): Hours of Work: Temporal Factors in Work Scheduling. New York, John Wiley, 1985, 37–52.
18. Folkard S, Monk TH, Bradbury R, Rosenthall J: Time of day effects in school children's immediate and delayed recall of meaningful material. Br J Psychol 68:45–50, 1977.
19. Folkard S, Monk TH, Lobban MC: Short- and long-term adjustment of circadian rhythms in "permanent" night nurses. Ergonomics 21:785–799, 1978.
20. Froberg JE: Twenty-four-hour patterns in human performance, subjective and physiological variables, and differences between morning and evening active subjects. Biol Psychol 5:119–134, 1977.
21. Gates AI: Diurnal variations in memory and association. University of California Publications in Psychology 1:323–344, 1916.
22. Hamelin P: Lorry driver's time habits in work and their involvement in traffic accidents. Ergonomics 30:1323–1333, 1987.
23. Hildebrandt G, Rohmert W, Rutenfranz J: Twelve- and 24-hour rhythms in error frequency of locomotive drivers and the influence of tiredness. Int J Chronobiol 2:175–180, 1974.

24. Hockey GRJ, Colquhoun WP: Diurnal variation in human performance: A review. In Colquhoun WP (ed): Aspects of Human Efficiency: Diurnal Rhythm and Loss of Sleep. London, English Universities Press, 1972, pp 39–107.
25. Hockey GRJ, Davies S, Gray MM: Forgetting as a function of sleep at different times of day. Q J Exp Psychol 24:389–393, 1972.
26. Holding DH: Principles of Training. Oxford, Pergamon Press, 1965.
27. Kahleque A, Verhaegen P: Circadian effects in short-cycle repetitive work in a two-shift system. In Reinberg A, Vieux N, Andlauer P (eds): Night and Shift Work: Biological and Social Aspects. Oxford, Pergamon Press, 1981, pp 409–416.
28. Kleinsmith LJ, Kaplan S: Paired-associate learning as a function of arousal and interpolated interval. J Exp Psychol 65:190–193, 1963.
29. Kleitman N: Sleep and Wakefulness. Chicago, University of Chicago Press, 1963.
30. Kleitman N, Jackson DP: Body temperature and performance under different routines. J Appl Physiol 3:309–328, 1950.
31. Laird DA: Relative performance of college students as conditioned by time of day and day of week. J Exp Psychol 8:50–63, 1925.
32. Lauber JK, Kayten PJ: Sleepiness, circadian dysrhythmia, and fatigue in transportation system accidents. Sleep 11:503–512, 1988.
33. Lavie P: The search for cycles in mental performance from Lombard to Kleitman. Chronobiologia 7:247–256, 1980.
34. Meers A: Performance on different turns of duty within a three-shift system and its relation to body temperature: Two field studies. In Colquhoun P, Folkard S, Knauth P, Rutenfranz J (eds): Experimental Studies of Shiftwork. Opladen, Westdeutscher Verlag, 1975, pp 188–205.
35. Monk TH: The arousal model of time of day effects in human performance efficiency. Chronobiologia 9:49–54, 1982.
36. Monk TH: Subjective ratings of sleepiness: The underlying circadian mechanisms. Sleep 10:343–353, 1987.
37. Monk TH, Embrey DE: A field study of circadian rhythms in actual and interpolated task performance. In Reinberg A, Vieux N, Andlauer P (eds): Night and Shift Work: Biological and Social Aspects. Oxford, Pergamon Press, 1981, pp 473–480.
38. Monk TH, Knauth P, Folkard S, Rutenfranz J: Memory-based performance measures in studies of shiftwork. Ergonomics 21:819–826, 1978.
39. Monk TH, Leng VC, Folkard S, Weitzman ED: Circadian rhythms in subjective alertness and core body temperature. Chronobiologia 10:49–55, 1983.
40. Monk TH, Moline ML, Fookson JE, Peetz SM: Circadian determinants of subjective alertness. J Biol Rhythms 4:393–404, 1989.
41. Moog R: Optimization of shift work: Physiological contributions. Ergonomics 30:1249–1259, 1987.
42. Prokop O, Prokop L: Ermunudung und Einschlafen am Steuer. Zentralbl Verkehrs-Med Verkehrs-Psychol angrenzende Gebiete 1:19–30, 1955.
43. Richardson GS, Carskadon MA, Orav EJ, Dement WC: Circadian variation of sleep tendency in elderly and young adult subjects. Sleep 5:S82–S94, 1982.
44. Tilley AJ, Wilkinson RT, Warren PSG, et al: The sleep and performance of shift workers. Hum Factors 24:629–641, 1982.
45. Wojtczak-Jaroszowa J, Jarosz D: Chronohygienic and chronosocial aspects of industrial accidents. Prog Clin Biol Res 227B:415–426, 1987.
46. Wojtczak-Jaroszowa J, Pawlowksa-Skyba K: Night and shift work. I: Circadian variations in work. Med Pr 18:1, 1967.

DONALD I. TEPAS, PhD
ANTONIO B. CARVALHAIS, MA

SLEEP PATTERNS OF SHIFTWORKERS

Division of Industrial and Organizational Psychology
Department of Psychology
University of Connecticut
Storrs, Connecticut

Reprint requests to:
Donald I. Tepas
Department of Psychology
Box U-20
University of Connecticut
406 Babbidge Road
Storrs, CT 06269-1020

Like many animals, humans are *circadian* in that their behavior and biology vary in a fairly regular periodicity of approximately 24 hours. Workdays are usually partitioned into three separate periods: time spent in the workplace, sleep time, and off-time with activities at the individual's discretion. One way of considering the sleep patterns of shiftworkers is to examine the sequence, duration, and time of day of these work, sleep, and off-time periods. We refer to these patterns as sleep strategies.

Sleep strategies can be studied from at least three perspectives. First, we can study when the major sleep time period occurs within a day—that is, within a 24-hour period. This is a **circadian sleep strategy.** Second, we can study sleep microstructure (polysomnographic sleep-stage architecture) within sleep periods—that is, changes with a higher frequency than one per 24 hours. These changes yield **ultradian sleep-stage sequencing.** Third, we can study sleep period changes that occur over a number of days—that is, changes with a lower frequency than one per 24 hours. These are **infradian sleep strategies.** Circadian sleep strategies, ultradian sleep-stage sequencing, and infradian sleep strategies are all manifest in the sleep of employed people working the nightshift.

This chapter briefly reviews early efforts to understand the sleep patterns of shiftworkers. It then describes the current model of circadian, infradian, and ultradian shiftworker sleep changes. Studies and data supporting the model are presented, and the implications and limitations of the model are discussed. Finally, techniques and instruments for evaluating shiftworker sleep habits and strategies reliably and validly are presented, and pitfalls of their use are considered.

BACKGROUND

Historic View

In 1897 Marie de Manaceine wrote, "We owe everything to light; without it life is impossible; it is light that we are searching for all our lives everywhere and in everything, and it is natural that we should so act as to awaken every day in the midst of light and not darkness. It is unnecessary to add that the habit of people in society of going to bed when day is dawning and rising at midday, or even later, is extremely hurtful. As a general rule it is well to go to sleep at no later hour than eleven, though the contemporary life of great cities is so organised that it is often very difficult to carry out this hygienic rule."[3] Clearly, de Manaceine was not the first to suggest that humans are diurnal animals, but she is a good historical example of how sleep scientists have linked daytime sleep with bad hygiene.

This perception among scientists that daytime sleep is bad hygiene has sustained itself over the years, and it has often harbored the idea that daytime sleep is (literally) unhealthy. Workers developed a similar bias. The industrial revolution produced fuel for that bias. Although it eventually led to shorter work hours, the industrial revolution's early innovations were the time clock, rigid work hours, and more required nightwork. These innovations decreased worker flexibility and were often associated with an ugly and dirty workplace. It is not surprising that the nightshift became known as the "graveyard shift," an overt association with death and illness.

Modern History

After World War II, advances in electronic technology made the electrophysiological assessment of human sleep (polysomnography) practical. The scientific study of human sleep expanded, and sleep quantity and quality were objectively measured under a wide range of conditions. At about the same time, chronobiology developed as a discipline. With time, sleep scientists began to incorporate expanded chronobiological notions into their conceptions and to examine practical applications of chronobiological theory.

One human problem area submitted to chronobiological analysis was shiftwork. Early polysomnographic studies of shiftwork issues centered on the effects of *acute* changes in ultradian sleep stage sequencing. That is, subjects were brought into the laboratory and subjected to abrupt changes in work/sleep time schedules, or they were placed on unusual laboratory work schedules for brief periods of time. In general, the reports from these studies of acute shifts to daytime sleep emphasized effects in keeping with the historic conceptions mentioned earlier. For these studies, changes within ultradian sleep stage sequencing periods that resulted from acute shifts to daytime sleep were interpreted to show and extrapolated to suggest that the sleep of most night shiftworkers should be viewed as a "disturbance." These studies did not consider infradian sleep strategies. Shiftworker sleep seemed to be a clinical problem, just as insomnia, in the classic view, was.[10]

Shiftworker Studies

In the context of history, it is not surprising that early studies of ultradian sleep-stage sequencing of shiftworkers emphasized its disruption and did not consider the nature of sleep sequencing with chronic exposure. Subsequent studies of *chronic* ultradian sleep-stage sequencing, as manifested in the polysomnographic sleep-stage sequencing of *experienced* shiftworkers,[8,19,21] suggest a different primary conception or model of the effects of daytime sleep. The most consistent finding of these studies is that sleeping during the day results in a *decrease* in sleep length. In general, the ultradian sleep-stage sequencing of experienced shiftworkers is in keeping with what has been observed in normal human subjects who have intentionally reduced their usual sleep length over a period of time.[9,22] Thus, chronic changes in sleep strategy that include daytime sleep appear to have only modest effects on ultradian sleep-stage sequencing.

The view that a major effect of night shiftwork is a chronic reduction in sleep length (but not a change in ultradian sleep-stage sequencing) is supported by behavioral data collected from experienced shiftworkers. Using standard performance tasks shown to be sensitive to the effects of sleep deprivation, studies have demonstrated that under controlled testing night shiftwork is associated with significant decrements in performance.[16,19] In addition, it is important to note that little if any evidence supports the notion that workers with experience adjust to night shiftwork with unique changes in circadian strategies or ultradian sleep-stage sequencing that allow them to get normal sleep. Even workers who most prefer nightwork and appear to have reasonable coping skills report reductions in their usual sleep length.[13]

CIRCADIAN AND INFRADIAN SLEEP STRATEGIES

Although the ultradian sleep-stage sequencing of shiftworkers has been extensively studied, less is known about the circadian and infradian sleep strategies elected by experienced shiftworkers. Workday sleep strategies have been investigated in both rotating and permanent shiftworkers.[1,12,14] As noted earlier, most working days can be partitioned into three periods: time spent in the workplace, sleep time, and off-time. Day shiftworkers use a sequence of sleep, work, and then off-time. Afternoon/evening shiftworkers use the sequence of sleep, off-time, and work. Night shiftworkers use the same sequence as afternoon/ evening workers. Night shiftworkers differ from other workers in that their sleep periods are shorter and occur during the day.

It can be argued, however, that by looking only at workday data we ignore significant nonworkday differences that result in fairly regular infradian variations. There is evidence that some rotating shiftworkers change their sleep behavior as they alternate between workdays and nonworkdays.[6,20] It is argued that without the constraint of fixed work hours, shiftworkers alter their sleep strategies on nonworkdays. For many workers these alterations may reflect significant changes in sleep behavior. In order to examine this question further, we have studied the workday and nonworkday sleep times of *permanent* shiftworkers. This area has not been extensively studied.

Method

The data for this study were collected from a confidential work/sleep survey in four plants of a Fortune 500 company in the rubber and plastics industry category. The overall response rate was 90.4%. The survey methods and characteristics of this data base have been described previously.[4,18] The self-report measures of sleep length used in this analysis correlate 0.83 with polysomnographic total sleep time.[17] The sample for this analysis included all permanent, discontinuous hourly shiftworkers working on 8-hour shifts with complete survey data on workday as well as nonworkday sleep behavior.

Subjects. One thousand two hundred sixty-two workers met the criteria outlined above. Their mean age was 33.5 years, with a range of 18–65 years and a standard deviation of 10.23 years. This sample was 70% male. The mean time on the job was 4.36 years, and 79% reported that they had been on a particular shift more than 6 months. Mean educational level was 12.1 years, with a standard deviation of 1.6 years.

Procedure. These workers were classified into three shift groups on the basis of reported working hours. Those working at least 7 consecutive hours between 0600 and 1600 were assigned to the permanent day (PD) group. Those working at least 7 consecutive hours between 1500 and 0100 were assigned to the permanent afternoon/evening (PA) group. And those working at least 7 consecutive hours between 2200 and 0700 hours were assigned to the permanent night (PN) group. All of the workers studied were on *permanent* and *discontinuous* shifts in that: (1) they worked the same shift time every week; and (2) their nonworkdays were on the weekend, as opposed to continuous shiftworkers, whose nonworkday could be a weekday.

In this survey, respondents were asked to fill in the appropriate times for the statement, "I usually go to sleep at ______ and get up at ______," for both workdays and nonworkdays. The following values were computed from the survey reports of usual bedtimes and arising times: workday sleep length (WSL), nonworkday sleep length (NWSL), workday sleep onset (WSON) time of day, workday sleep offset (WSOFF) time of day, nonworkday sleep onset (NWSON) time of day, and nonworkday sleep offset (NWSOFF) time of day. Owing to the circular scaling of time-of-day reports, simply calculating ordinary arithmetic means results in significant estimation errors. To avoid these errors, a logarithmic geometric algorithm was used to calculate sleep onset and offset times.

Results

Sleep Length. Table 1 shows the reported mean sleep length and standard deviation in minutes on workdays and nonworkdays for each shift group. The results of a 3 × 2 repeated measures, mixed factorial analysis of variance with shift as a between-subjects independent variable containing two levels (workday and nonworkday) and *sleep length* as the dependent variable indicate that for this sample of permanent, discontinuous shiftworkers, there are: (1) statistically significant differences for sleep length between shifts ($F = 9.47$, $df = 2$, $p < 0.001$); (2) statistically significant differences between workday and nonworkday sleep lengths ($F = 901.56$, $df = 2$, $p < 0.001$); and, (3) a significant interaction effect ($F = 44.99$, $df = 2$, $p < 0.001$), indicating that the magnitude of workday and nonworkday sleep length differences is dependent on shift.

Tukey tests for WSL confirmed significant differences among all the various combinations of shifts ($p < 0.05$). However, NWSL comparisons did not result in significant differences between any of the shift combinations. For all shift groups, NWSL was significantly increased from WSL. A comparison of the data in Table 1 indicates that the PN group had the largest increase, 1.95 hours; PD and PA groups increased 1.31 and 0.83 hours, respectively. Pearson correlations

TABLE 1. Means and Standard Deviations of Sleep Length in Minutes for All Workshift Groups on Workdays (WSL) and Nonworkdays (NWSL)

	Shift	N	Mean	SD
Workday sleep (WSL)	PD	566	434.10	50.43
	PA	355	462.63	73.10
	PN	341	409.35	85.35
	ALL	1262	435.44	70.69
Nonworkday sleep (NWSL)	PD	566	512.66	80.37
	PA	355	512.19	81.37
	PN	341	526.45	100.35
	ALL	1262	516.25	86.64

PD, permanent dayshift; PA, permanent afternoon/evening shift; PN, permanent nightshift.
Additional tables of workday sleep length by age, gender, and shift are available upon request from the authors.

between WSL and NWSL for PD, PA, and PN are 0.37, 0.43, and 0.09, respectively. All are positive and significant at the 0.05 level or better.

Sleep Onset Time of Day. Table 2 shows the mean sleep onset time of day and standard deviations in 24-hour military times for workdays and nonworkdays across shifts. The results of a 3 × 2 analysis of variance for sleep onset indicate a significant difference in sleep onset time of day between shifts ($F = 520$, $df = 2$, $p < 0.001$), significant differences between WSON and NWSON ($F = 107.08$, $df = 2$, $p < 0.001$), and a significant interaction between shift and time ($F = 259.23$, $df = 2$, $p < 0.001$). Tukey tests for WSON were all significant ($p < 0.05$), indicating a significant difference among the various cells. Tukey tests for NWSON resulted in significant differences only between PD and PA groups and PA and PN groups ($p < 0.05$).

Sleep Offset Time of Day. Table 3 shows the mean sleep offset time of day and standard deviations in 24-hour military time for workdays and nonworkdays across shifts. The results of a 3 × 2 analysis of variance for sleep offset time of day are all statistically significant, indicating a significant difference in sleep offset time of day among shifts ($F = 220.17$, $df = 2$, $p < 0.001$), significant differences between WSOFF and NWSOFF ($F = 41.44$, $df = 2$, $p < 0.001$), and a significant interaction between shift and time ($F = 238.01$, $df = 2$, $p < 0.001$). Tukey tests for WSOFF were statistically significant ($p < 0.05$), indicating a significant difference among the various cells. Tukey tests for NWOFF resulted only in significant differences between PD and PA groups and PD and PN groups ($p < 0.05$).

TABLE 2. Means and Standard Deviations for Sleep Onset Time of Day for All Workshift Groups on Workdays (WSON) and Nonworkdays (NWSON)

	Shift	N	Mean	SD
Workday sleep (WSON)	PD	567	2206	3.60
	PA	355	0130	4.02
	PN	341	0931	1.78
	ALL	1263	1259	9.00
Nonworkday sleep (NWSON)	PD	567	2301	9.59
	PA	355	0008	10.46
	PN	341	2330	9.57
	ALL	1263	2343	10.23

PD, permanent dayshift; PA, permanent afternoon/evening shift; PN, permanent nightshift.

TABLE 3. Means and Standard Deviations of Sleep Offset Time of Day for All Workshift Groups on Workdays (WSOFF) and Nonworkdays (NWSOFF)

	Shift	N	Mean	SD
Workday sleep (WSOFF)	PD	566	0530	.63
	PA	355	0901	1.44
	PN	341	1616	2.33
	ALL	1262	0922	4.72
Nonworkday sleep (NWSOFF)	PD	566	0747	1.94
	PA	355	0859	1.65
	PN	341	0852	3.25
	ALL	1262	0807	2.40

PD, permanent dayshift; PA, permanent afternoon/evening shift; PN, permanent nightshift.

Discussion

As expected, most permanent shiftworkers on discontinuous shifts alter their sleep behavior on nonworkdays. Not being constrained by work hours, people are free on nonworkdays to select whatever sleep/wake strategy they prefer. The data presented support the theory that we are diurnal animals. Workers in this sample who work diurnal hours do not make major alterations in the time of day they sleep. Those who do not work diurnal hours shift to a diurnal orientation when provided with the opportunity on nonworkdays. Thus, infradian sleep strategies vary with workshift schedule.

When feasible, people do elect circadian sleep strategies. The return to a diurnal orientation on nonworkdays fits with chronobiological explanations. These explanations stress two concepts: appropriate or inappropriate chronobiological timing, and chronobiological desynchronization.[7] Appropriate chronobiological timing is the time of day at which the position of the biological clocks or circadian systems results in maximal potential for a particular activity. Inappropriate chronobiological timing is the time of day at which the position of the biological clocks or circadian systems results in minimal potential for a particular activity. For example, the appropriate chronobiological sleep time is at night, and the inappropriate chronobiological sleep time is in the morning. When sleep behavior is altered to a new time, say from day to night, the various circadian components change at different rates, resulting in circadian desynchronization.

These chronobiological explanations are an attractive approach to understanding shiftworker sleep behavior. However, another useful approach emphasizes *societal* factors (such as parental roles, community activities, and environmental distractions) in assessing variable sleep behavior.[11] This explanation stresses social factors that exert pressure on the individual to alter sleep behavior in order to fulfill societal roles. It can be argued that the nonworkday change in shiftworker sleep behavior indicates that some social needs are not being met by the worker's workday sleep strategy. These two explanations, chronobiological and social, are not mutually exclusive, and neither can fully explain all the behavior of shiftworkers.

A widely held notion about the reduced WSL of PN shiftworkers is that people on this shift are self-selected.[12] That is, people may select the PN shift because they are naturally short sleepers. This position is difficult to defend if NWSL is considered. PN workers would not be expected to increase their NWSL. However, a comparison of the data in Table 1 indicates that the PN group has the largest increase in reported sleep duration from workdays to nonworkdays. The PN group increases an average of 1.95 hours, the PD group 1.31 hours, and the PA group 0.83 hour.

Perhaps the increase in NWSL fully compensates for reduced WSL. If this is the case, there should be a significant *negative* correlation between WSL and NWSL. However, as noted earlier, the actual correlations are all positive and account for no more than 20% of the variance. Most important is the finding that all of these correlations are in the opposite direction from what compensatory notions would predict.

If the total weekly sleep duration of workers is calculated by combining WSL and NWSL, PN shiftworkers, on the average, sleep 237 minutes less per week than PA and 96 minutes less than PD shiftworkers. Therefore, even with an increase in NWSL, PN shiftworkers sleep less. This increase in NWSL for PN does not appear to compensate fully for reduced WSL and thus supports the suggestion that PN workers suffer from chronic sleep deprivation.[10,13]

The results clearly demonstrate that most permanent shiftworkers frequently change their sleep behavior as they alternate between workdays and nonworkdays. Thus, they show infradian variations in the timing of their sleep. From this sleep perspective, it could be argued that few workers are in fact on permanent shifts. It could also be argued from this perspective that the PN schedule may result in more adverse effects than many rotating shift schedules, since most PN workers use infradian sleep strategies that, *in effect, place them on rotating shifts.* If the direction of shift rotation is a significant factor,[8] it might also be proposed that an additional impact is associated with PN schedules. Again from the sleep perspective, most PN workers appear to rotate forward from night wakefulness to day wakefulness when going to nonworkdays, and backwards from day wakefulness to night wakefulness when going to workdays. Given the sleep strategies currently selected by most workers, it might be argued that *discontinuous* PN shiftwork is perhaps the worst possible rotation schedule.

IMPROVING SHIFTWORKER SLEEP

It is important to note that many of the shiftworker sleep characteristics reported here are *self-selected.* Except during work hours, workers are free to go to bed when they choose. Data also indicate that by far the majority of workers use an alarm or other device to terminate sleep.[10,18] That is, workers have *elected* these strategies for a variety of reasons, and in many cases the strategy they elect may promote poor sleep habits. Improved assessment methods, education with regard to good sleep hygiene, and increased sensitivity to chronobiological mechanisms may be ways the occupational health practitioner can reduce potential health and safety hazards traditionally associated with shiftwork.

Sleep Disorders and Napping

We have argued that the major problem facing most night shiftworkers is obtaining enough sleep, rather than having undisturbed sleep. The occupational health practitioner, however, is often faced with worker complaints about sleep. Obviously, some night shiftworkers suffer from sleep disorders, just as some day shiftworkers do. When clear signs of a sleep disturbance are evident, referral to an accredited sleep disorders center is appropriate. Drug treatments for insomnia, depression, or stress reduction should *not* be prescribed without formal assessment by a specialist in sleep disorders.

A related question we must also consider, however, is whether the incidence of sleep disorders is higher in night shiftworkers. Indeed, survey data indicate that night shiftworkers report difficulty falling or staying asleep more frequently than do day shiftworkers.[18] Whether these complaints about sleep represent a higher incidence of sleep disorders remains to be determined. Sleep disorders may be a secondary effect promoted by unusual work hours and the fact that sleep-deprivation–induced sleepiness makes napping easier.

Night shiftworkers report a high incidence of frequent napping.[18] Napping is often viewed as a strategy some workers use to get additional sleep. Certainly, naps are one way of overcoming *acute* sleep deprivation effects. However, napping, as a way of overcoming *chronic* sleep deprivation effects, may very well be a bad strategy. Permanent nightshift workers who do not report frequent workday and nonworkday napping do not report elevated difficulty falling or staying asleep.[15]

Just as napping is often not recommended for people suffering from insomnia, frequent napping by night shiftworkers is probably a bad strategy. The occupational health practitioner might very well be advised not to recommend napping as a solution for chronic nightshift-related sleep deprivation. Obviously, a recommendation to avoid frequent napping should be made with care. Naps are often a good way to overcome sleep reductions associated with unusual or infrequent extended work schedules. For some workers, naps may be the only way to get the minimal sleep needed to function. When this is true on a regular basis, the primary recommendation should be a change in work schedule, not a reduction in napping.

Assessing Sleep

When confronted with sleep complaints from individual shiftworkers, it is appropriate for the occupational health practitioner to assess the worker's sleep behavior. As noted earlier, subjective reports of sleep length can be highly correlated with polysomnographic recordings of sleep. Such a correlation exists for the method we use, which asks workers when they usually go to sleep and get up on workdays and nonworkdays. However, not all subjective sleep length estimates have significant predictive value. Simply asking workers how long they sleep, perhaps the more common approach used in the field, yields sleep length estimates with minimal or no polysomnographic predictive value.[17]

Obtaining accurate subjective estimates of sleep onset latency is very difficult, if not impossible, for some workers. General estimates of sleep latency frequently do *not* correlate with polysomnographic sleep latency measures, and specific subjective sleep latency measures may show only a minimal correlation with immediate sleep period polysomnographic measures.[2] For nonclinical populations, people most frequently rate the quality of their sleep on the basis of how they feel when they wake up, rather than on the basis of any criterion directly related to ultradian sleep sequencing.[5] Thus, considerable care must be taken in interpreting responses of workers to questions about their sleep.

Infradian Sleep Strategies

The data presented clearly indicate that for many shiftworkers sleep timing and duration on workdays may be quite different from nonworkdays. When attempting to assess the impact of work schedules on an individual, it is important to determine the infradian sleep and nap strategies the worker uses. There are several reasons to look at these strategies: (1) As noted earlier, frequent napping on both workdays and nonworkdays may be a sign of a sleep problem other than insufficient sleep. (2) Infradian sleep strategies that deviate significantly from the model suggested by the times presented here may point to unusual societal factors that make it difficult for the worker to adapt to a work schedule. For example, a worker may have a second job that limits the usual increase in "nonworkday" sleep length. (3) As we have pointed out, the infradian sleep strategies employed by our subjects are not ideal from a chronobiological viewpoint. Because many dimensions of this sleep behavior are elected by the individual, it may be possible to get some workers to adopt sleep habits that are closer to the chronobiological ideal.

SUMMARY

Work hours affect sleep because the sleep behavior of people on nonworkdays differs from that on workdays. For most workers, workday sleep is shorter than nonworkday sleep. On nonworkdays most workers sleep at night. Work schedule interacts with the effects of work hours on workday sleep. On workdays, people on the nightshift sleep the least, people on the afternoon/evening shift sleep the most, and people on the dayshift sleep less than those on the afternoon/evening shift but more than those on the nightshift. Thus, the infradian sleep strategy elected by a shiftworker is ordinarily related to the schedule worked.

Despite historical preconceptions that nightshift work disturbs sleep, the primary problem appears to be a workday reduction in sleep length, which most workers do *not* usually compensate for by getting more sleep on their nonworkdays. Polysomnographic studies of workers on the nightshift show ultradian sleep-stage sequencing similar to that of people who have chronically reduced their usual sleep duration. This chronic reduction in sleep length is evident in data from experienced night shiftworkers, including those who most prefer to work nights. Experienced night shiftworkers also manifest decrements in performance of the sort expected of people suffering from chronic sleep deprivation. It seems reasonable to suggest that chronic sleep deprivation of night shiftworkers may often be a productivity, safety, or health hazard.

Sleep disorders may be a secondary problem also facing night shiftworkers. In general, shiftworkers who do night shiftwork report difficulty falling asleep or staying asleep at rates higher than workers who do not work nights. Data suggest that this may be due to the regular practice of inappropriate infradian sleep strategies or to chronic napping habits. At this point in our study of shiftworker sleep behavior, there is as yet no clear evidence that night shiftworkers suffer from clinical sleep disorders at a higher rate than other workers.

It is reasonable to suggest that occupational health professionals can make initial assessments of the sleep complaints made by night shiftworkers. Subjective measurements can be used for these assessments if care is taken to use appropriate methods. It is recommended that this data be collected by asking workers quite literal and concrete questions about the time of day they usually elect to go to sleep and get up. A sleep survey of this sort should gather main sleep period and napping times for both workdays and nonworkdays, so that the infradian sleep strategy of the worker can be identified. Regular reductions in sleep length or frequent napping are good signs that some changes are needed.

The average sleep times reported here provide a model of typical shiftwork sleep behavior. This is not to suggest that the usual behaviors practiced by most shiftworkers are adequate or provide good rules for chronobiological hygiene. They do provide a data base that the occupational health professional can use as a reference to suggest changes in a worker's sleep strategy or make referrals for diagnosis. Since the tables presented include data from permanent shiftworkers who are on the dayshift or afternoon/evening shifts, they may also be of help when considering the complaints of workers who do not work the nightshift.

The sleep strategies of rotating shiftworkers require further study, but the data currently available suggest that their sleep strategies parallel those of permanent shiftworkers.[14] When individual worker assessment suggests the possibility of a sleep disorder, the worker should be referred to an accredited sleep disorders center for diagnosis and treatment when appropriate. Prescription of drugs to treat worker sleep complaint symptoms without diagnosis by a sleep disorders professional is *not* appropriate because some drugs may exacerbate workplace performance and safety problems. When many people in the workplace manifest persistent sleep problems, a change in the work schedule system used is probably warranted and consultation with a human factors work schedule specialist is appropriate.

REFERENCES

1. Armstrong D, Tepas DI, Moss PD: Sleep reports from two samples of rotating shift workers. Sleep Res 9:267, 1980.
2. Armstrong D, Tepas DI, Byrnes EA, et al: Sleep latencies: Watch what you ask and when! Sleep Res 10:133, 1981.
3. de Manaceine M: Sleep: Its Physiology, Pathology, Hygiene, and Psychology. London, Walter Scott, 1897, p 185.
4. Gordon GC, Tepas DI, Stock CG, Walsh JK: Gaining access to shift workers through labor unions. Behav Res Methods Instrum 11:14–17, 1979.
5. Kamens L, Carlson ML, Falkin S, et al: Relative importance of subjective criteria for judging sleep quality. Sleep Res 11:201, 1982.
6. Knauth P, Rutenfranz J: Duration of sleep related to the type of shift work. In Reinberg A, Vieux N, Andlauer P (eds): Night and Shiftwork: Biological and Social Aspects. New York, Pergamon, 1980, pp 161–168.
7. Monk TH: Advantages and disadvantages of rapidly rotating shift schedules—A circadian viewpoint. Hum Factors 28:688–689, 1986.
8. Monk TH, Tepas DI: Shift work. In Cooper CL, Smith MJ (eds): Job Stress and Blue Collar Work. Chichester, John Wiley, 1985, pp 65–84.
9. Mullaney DJ, Johnson LC, Naitoh P, et al: Sleep during and after gradual sleep reduction. Psychophysiology 14:237–244, 1977.
10. Tepas DI: Work/sleep time schedules and performance. In Webb WB (ed): Biological Rhythms, Sleep and Performance. Chichester, John Wiley, 1982, pp 175–204.
11. Tepas DI: Adaptation to shiftwork: Fact or fallacy? J Hum Ergol 11(suppl):1–12, 1982.
12. Tepas DI: Shiftworker sleep strategies. J Hum Ergol 11(suppl):325–336, 1982.
13. Tepas DI, Mahan RP: The many meanings of sleep. Work & Stress 3:93–102, 1989.
14. Tepas DI, Walsh JK, Armstrong D: Comprehensive study of the sleep of shift workers. In Johnson LC, Tepas DI, Colquhoun WP, Colligan MJ (eds): Biological Rhythms, Sleep and Shift Work. New York, Spectrum, 1981, pp 347–356.
15. Tepas DI, Carvalhais AB, Popkin SM: Shiftworker nap strategies. Sleep Res, in press.
16. Tepas DI, Walsh JK, Moss PD, Armstrong D: Polysomnographic correlates of shift worker performance in the laboratory. In Reinberg A, Vieux N, Andlauer P (eds): Night and Shift Work: Biological and Social Aspects. New York, Pergamon, 1981, pp 179–186.
17. Tepas DI, Canning PH, Moss PD, et al: How should one measure human sleep length in surveys? Sleep Res 9:266, 1980.
18. Tepas DI, Armstrong DR, Carlson ML, et al: Changing industry to continuous operations: Different strokes for different plants. Behav Res Methods Instrum Comput 17:670–676, 1985.
19. Tilley AJ, Wilkinson RT, Warren PSG, et al: The sleep and performance of shift workers. Hum Factors 24:629–641, 1982.
20. Van Loon JH: Diurnal body temperature curves in shift workers. Ergonomics 6:267–273, 1963.
21. Walsh JK, Tepas DI, Moss PD: The EEG sleep of night and rotating shift workers. In Johnson LC, Tepas DI, Colquhoun WP, Colligan MJ (eds): Biological Rhythms, Sleep and Shift Work. New York, Spectrum, 1981, pp 371–381.
22. Webb WB, Agnew HW Jr: The effects of chronic limitation of sleep length. Psychophysiology 11:265–274, 1974.

PAUL NAITOH, PhD
TAMSIN L. KELLY, MD
CARL ENGLUND, PhD

HEALTH EFFECTS OF SLEEP DEPRIVATION

From the Naval Health Research Center
San Diego, California

Reprint requests to:
Paul Naitoh, PhD
Naval Health Research Center
P.O. Box 85122
San Diego, CA 92138-9174

Report No. 89-46, supported by the Naval Medical Research and Development Command under Work Unit M0096.002-5301. The views presented in this paper are those of the authors and do not reflect the official policy or position of the Department of the Navy, the Department of Defense, or the U.S. Government.

Early to bed and early to rise, makes a man healthy, wealthy and wise.

Poor Richard's Almanac

Effects of sleep loss on job performance are well documented in many review papers and a recently published monograph.[118] In contrast, health consequences of acute and chronic sleep loss have been poorly documented except in a few social and epidemiological surveys on shift- and nightwork. The purpose of this chapter is to survey and critically review the results of laboratory and field studies on health consequences of sleep loss. Three kinds of sleep loss are identified: total, selective, and partial sleep loss. The most critical information for practitioners of occupational medicine is the health consequences of loss of several hours of sleep repeatedly every day over many days or months—that is, chronic partial sleep deprivation. Unfortunately, this survey found that very few chronic partial sleep loss studies were conducted owing to the prohibitive cost of running them and, more importantly, to the apparently minimal health effects of sleep loss. This paper describes and evaluates the currently available data base to determine the effects of different kinds of sleep loss on the functional integrity of the human organism. The factors discussed include: adrenomedullary activity, adrenocortical activity, metabolism, hematological and immunological changes, autonomic nervous system activity, epilepsy, physical working capacity, antidepressant effects, and mental health.

BACKGROUND

It is commonly believed that we need approximately 7–8 hours of sleep every night and that sleep serves a restorative function. Some people think that missing this period of restoration of mind and body may present an immediate threat to health, or that chronic sleep deprivation may shorten life span or increase morbidity. When we stay awake all night, our body misses the surge of putatively restorative human growth hormone (hGH) that occurs during nocturnal sleep and, at the same time, gets an overabundance of "stressor substance," such as norepinephrine and corticosteroids.

However, everybody has experienced going without sleep at one time or another, either totally for one or two nights, or for a few hours nightly over several days. Many ordinary life events, such as working to meet deadlines, earning a living as a night- or shiftworker, or managing family and business emergencies, can lead to temporary total or partial sleep deprivation. Can such a common life experience be dangerous or fatal?

A series of reports on sleep deprivation studies in rats by Rechtschaffen and his group[25,26,33–35,91,152,153,239,240] suggests that it might. Rats subjected to total sleep deprivation or to selective rapid eye movement (REM) sleep deprivation died in approximately three or five weeks, respectively. Rechtschaffen and others[240] speculated on the basis of energy requirements that humans would "survive sleep loss about 3.7 times longer than rats, or about 77 days of total sleep deprivation versus 21 days of rats, and 135 days of partial sleep deprivation versus 37 days of rats" (p. 80). Horne[118] raises serious doubts about generalizing the findings in rats to humans. The rat's small body requires much more constant effort, or larger energy expenditures, to maintain core body temperature than the much larger human body with its more adequate thermoregulatory mechanisms. Death in severely sleep-deprived rats might be due more to thermoregulatory failure, which would not be expected to occur in humans, than to sleep loss itself.

During World War II, greater London over a six-year period experienced frequent air raids with nightly disruptions of sleep, but Pai[218] reported no ill effects of sleep loss among a large number of people. Progressively increasing sleepiness serves as a built-in safety valve that works to prevent accumulation of an inordinate sleep loss (as hunger and thirst prevent us from going too long without food and water). Because of this, it takes great personal effort or vigorous social support to remain awake for more than 48 hours.

Our impression is that direct detrimental health consequences of sleep loss are probably minimal.[107,128,141–143] The reports of healthy insomniacs who need little or no sleep[128,180,181] seem to support this view. Nonetheless, it is possible that sleep loss interacts with stressful environments or biological weaknesses to the detriment of health. This might explain the cases of "sleep loss psychosis" reported in early literature.[43,319] In what follows we will summarize research findings on the health consequences of sleep loss and attempt to separate fact from myth in this somewhat controversial area.

The purpose of this report is to provide medical professionals who are responsible for maintaining the health of men and women in shift and irregular work environments with background information on the medical consequences of sleep loss. There is an increasing need for such knowledge because more and more military and civilian personnel are involved in shiftwork and round-the-clock sustained/continuous operation (SUSOP/CONOP). The increase in SUSOP/CONOP in the military is documented in a technical report by U.S.

Army Combined Arms Combat Development Activity on "Continuous Operations Study (CONOPS) Final Report," published in 1987 and available to U.S. Government Agencies (AD-B111424L). We will not here discuss the effects of partial and total sleep deprivation on psychomotor and cognitive tasks, because many readily available reviews[118,170,188,192,198,200,204,325,327] have been produced since the publication of the *Handbook of Human Engineering Data* in 1952 by Tufts College.

Before we discuss biomedical effects of sleep loss, we need to define what we mean by sleep deprivation. Researchers have, so far, recognized three kinds of sleep deprivation:

(1) Total sleep deprivation
(2) Partial sleep deprivation
(3) Selective sleep deprivation.

Total sleep deprivation means getting no sleep during at least one 24–hour cycle. For example, if a person who usually sleeps from 2300 to 0700 awakens one morning at 0700 and stays awake until 2300 of the following day, that person has gone 40 hours without sleep. During this 40-hour period, one 8-hour sleep period has been missed. Strictly speaking, 8 hours of total sleep deprivation have occurred. However, in general practice, we use the hours of continuous wakefulness—40 hours in this example—as the amount of total sleep deprivation.[197,200]

We frequently experience **partial sleep deprivation**. Partial sleep deprivation means sleeping less than usual.[198,274,316,325,326] In research, partial sleep deprivation has been created in two ways: (1) a gradual reduction in sleep duration; for example, a reduction by 30 minutes every two weeks, providing sleepers with an ample opportunity to adjust to longer waking hours each day,[100,125] or (2) a sudden reduction in sleep duration, for example, from a customary 8 hours to 5. The short sleep regimen is tried out for a few days[57,108,111,120,209,273] or continued for a long period of time so that sleepers can adapt to the new life-style.[100,315,325]

Unlike total and partial sleep deprivation, clear-cut **selective sleep deprivation** does not occur in real world situations. It is created only as a result of manipulation of sleep in a laboratory, where changes in sleep stages can be observed as they take place. When sleep is observed electrophysiologically, it is classified into seven states: wake; sleep stages 1, 2, 3, 4; REM sleep; and movement time. Often, sleep stages 3 and 4 are combined and designated as slow wave sleep (SWS), which is contrasted to the amount of REM sleep. Sleep stage 1 is thought to be a transition stage, when we are neither asleep nor awake.[131] Sleep stage 2 has a unique brain wave signature, "sleep spindles," indicating that at this stage we are fully asleep. Although the functions of sleep and the various sleep stages are not fully understood,[40,116–118] it has been suggested that SWS is needed for "body repair," whereas REM sleep is needed for "mind repair."[77–80,88,217,302] In nocturnal sleep of adults with no sleep disorders, these sleep stages follow each other in a fairly fixed pattern, creating a fairly predictable sleep profile. (For a more complete discussion of the sleep stages, see Rechtschaffen and Kales.[241])

Selective sleep deprivation consists of preventing the occurrence of a particular sleep stage. In REM sleep (or SWS) stage deprivation, sleepers are prevented from getting REM sleep (or SWS) by being awakened whenever they begin to enter that sleep stage.[5,13,77,305]

The sleep deprivation we experience in daily life is likely to be a mixture of these three types. For example, we may simultaneously experience both partial and REM sleep deprivation when we curtail our sleep by waking up a couple of hours earlier in the morning, thus missing the early morning sleep that is rich in REM sleep. Taking antidepresssants or hypnotics has also been shown to reduce REM or SWS.[12,132,217] In this report, we are mostly concerned with health effects of total sleep deprivation, because that is what the majority of the research has dealt with.

SLEEP LOSS AND ADRENOMEDULLARY ACTIVITY

The adrenomedullary system produces two separate catecholamines, epinephrine (EP) and, in small quantities, norepinephrine (NE). These hormonal secretions are rapidly increased by stressors such as cold, pain, anoxia, shock, hypoglycemia, hypotension, physical exercise, psychological stimuli, and drugs in common use, such as caffeine, nicotine, and alcohol. Both EP and NE act on all organs of the body, causing "sympathetic activation," a collection of effects generally serving to improve physical effectiveness for "fight or flight" emergency situations.[116,118] These effects include increased heart rate, strengthened cardiac contraction, constriction of arterioles in the skin, and both vasodilation and constriction of voluntary muscle arterioles. NE is generally more powerful in raising blood pressure, while EP is generally more powerful in the mobilization of glucose and fat and the relaxation of smooth muscles. Urinary EP shows a strong circadian rhythm, but urinary NE shows no significant circadian rhythm.[9,102,103,110,116] Thus any changes in EP during sleep deprivation must be analyzed to partition out the circadian component.

Fiorica et al. observed no significant changes in total urinary catecholamines during 85 hours of total sleep deprivation.[95] Levi[158,159] also found no consistent changes in EP or NE up to 75 hours of total sleep deprivation, when he did not take experimental subjects' age into account. No significant increase in 24-hour urinary EP was seen in his older subjects (49–64 years, average age 56). However, 24-hour urinary EP increased in the young group (20–44 years, average age of 29). Levi attributed the results to differences observed in self-pacing between the young and old. Early in the experiment, the young subjects mobilized more physical and mental resources to achieve superior performance, but subsequently they slackened their work pace owing to exhaustion. The old subjects seemed more in control of and less reactive to the study environment and kept a more even pace throughout the experiment. Froberg found that "morning-type" people did not differ from "evening-type" people in circadian rhythms of urinary EP secretion during 72 hours of total sleep deprivation. Sleep loss neither disrupted circadian rhythm nor increased urinary EP excretion. Excretion of vanillylmandelic acid, a major metabolite of NE, did not change during a total of 205 hours of sleep deprivation.[102]

From these studies we could conclude, as previous review papers have,[110,116,199] that no consistent significant increase in the adrenomedullary activity occurs during total sleep deprivation. In other words, total sleep deprivation in itself does not cause "stress" in the usual sense.

Some studies, however, have suggested an adrenomedullary activation during total sleep deprivation. Steinberg and others[279] studied the effects of total sleep deprivation, sleep, and immobility on the levels of EP, NE, metanephrine, normetanephrine, and vanillylmandelic acid under a strictly controlled diet. They found higher urinary catechalomine excretion during nights of sleep deprivation when subjects lay on a bed (but remained awake) than during nights of normal sleep. Other urinary substances showed no change. They concluded that wakefulness caused significant elevation in EP and NE. Kuhn and his group performed a series of studies[148] examining the effects of 5 days of total sleep deprivation on 24-hour urine levels of metanephrine, normetanephrine, and vanillylmandelic acid. They observed a significant increase of normetanephrine during sleep deprivation days (except day 2), a significant increase in metanephrine on day 3, and a significant increase in vanillylmandelic acid on the last day of the study. These responses were interpreted as reflecting stress caused by enforced sleep loss of 5 days. However, Kuhn et al. imposed greater psychological and physical demands and other situational factors on their subjects than the previously discussed studies. These stressors, rather than the sleep loss itself, may have caused the adrenomedullary activation.

Hasselman et al.[112] reported higher urinary EP and NE during bicycle ergonometric work after one night of sleep loss than after a normal night's sleep. It appears that sleep-deprived subjects may be able to perform the same amount of physical work as usual, but in doing so, they must increase adrenomedullary activity for greater mobilization of energy resources. They also found that ambient temperature is an important situational factor affecting adrenomedullary output. They observed a dramatic increase of urinary catecholamines when the sleep-deprived subjects worked with a bicycle ergonometer under high ambient temperature. Thus, sleep deprivation appears to interact with other stressors rather than directly affecting adrenomedullary activation.

In summary, total sleep loss of 3 days or less causes neither significant increases in adrenomedullary activity nor circadian disruption of EP rhythm if sleep deprivation is conducted under physically and mentally nondemanding, experimental environments. When total sleep deprivation takes place in high physical and mental workloads under uncomfortable ambient temperature, or the subjects are particularly energetic in their efforts to maintain top performance by adopting a high work pace, a significant activation of the adrenomedullary system may be reflected in increased urinary catecholamines.

SLEEP LOSS AND ADRENOCORTICAL ACTIVITY

The pituitary-adrenocortical system produces glucocorticoids, mineralocorticoids, and androgenic steroids. The main glucocorticoid is cortisol. Production of cortisol increases in response to many stressors—for example, surgery or illness. Cortisol increases hepatic glycogenesis, suppresses protein synthesis, and has anti-insulin action in peripheral tissues, thus providing energy needed for coping with prolonged, stressful circumstances. The cortisol level sensitively reflects psychological states, increasing with arousal and anticipation of stress.

Because of difficulties in assaying serum cortisol, early studies used the quantity of eosinophils, lymphocytes, and urinary 17-ketosteroids and electrolytes (factors affected by adrenal steroids) to indirectly monitor activation of the pituitary-adrenocortical system. Attempts to determine whether total sleep deprivation would activate the pituitary-adrenocortical system were further complicated by the presence of a strong circadian rhythm in these hormones.

Urinary 17–ketosteroids have been found to show no change after 72 hours of total sleep deprivation[43] and were even reported to decrease on the second, third, and fourth days of total sleep deprivation.[190,293,324] Urinary 17–hydroxycorticosteroids were also observed to show no change after 72 or 120 hours of total sleep deprivation,[43,143] and one night of total sleep deprivation did not change the time of the circadian peak of plasma 17-hydroxycorticoid.[98] Rubin et al.[252] found that plasma and urinary 17-hydroxycorticosteroid decreased from the baseline value to a low point after 170 hours of total sleep deprivation. These differences in results probably reflect more the varied psychological and physical demands imposed on the subjects than the effects of sleep loss itself.[191,198] Opstad and Aakvaag[209] observed levels of serum cortisol during 5-day-long training field exercises. These training courses required heavy and continuous physical activities with less than a total of 2 hours of sleep per 24 hours. Serum cortisol decreased from a relatively high level on day 1 to a low level on day 5. Similarly, a reduced cortisol level was observed at the end of 48 hours of sleep deprivation among subjects who did not experience heavy physical work. Kant et al. observed slight decreases in urinary cortisol levels during sleep loss of 72 hours.[132]

In contrast, Kuhn et al.[148] reported an increase of urinary 17–hydroxycorticosteroid for the first two days of total sleep deprivation.

Briefly, total sleep deprivation of up to 72 hours has little effect on glucocorticoids, especially compared with the large increases in 17-hydroxycorticoid sometimes observed during baseline periods when subjects are experiencing pre-experiment excitement and anxiety. Total sleep loss does not cause the classical nonspecific emergency reaction.

SLEEP LOSS AND METABOLISM

People expend more metabolic energy during a sleepless day than during a normal 24-hour cycle. The metabolism slows down during sleep, and this energy conservation does not occur during sleep deprivation.

Biological energy is based on the adenosine triphosphate (ATP) system. Thus, total sleep loss might be anticipated to affect ATP. Luby et al. reported that after 4 days of sleep deprivation energy production (as measured by specific activity of ATP after whole blood was incubated with radioactive phosphorus) increased, while the ATP level dropped.[166] After 7 days of total sleep deprivation (TSD), energy production had dropped almost to baseline, whereas the level of ATP had risen but was still below baseline. Unfortunately, this study involved only one subject and has never been replicated.

When the ATP reserve is depleted, phosphocreatine is used as a high energy source. Under these conditions the level of urinary creatinine may indirectly signal the degree of energy expenditure. However, a number of studies have found that total sleep deprivation of up to 120 hours does not change the urinary creatinine level.[95,143,270] Resting metabolism as assessed by oxygen consumption also remain unchanged during total sleep deprivation of up to 120 hours.[95]

If total sleep deprivation is a catabolic state, it might cause an acceleration of protein turnover, which should be reflected by an increase in the urinary total nitrogen. However, total sleep deprivation of up to 126 hours did not affect the 24-hour urinary total nitrogen level.[148] Scrimshaw et al.[270] observed a decrease of urinary nitrogen on the first day of total sleep deprivation and an estimated 12% increase in protein requirement over the basal need during the second day. Kant et al.[132] found an increased urea excretion within 24–48 hours of sleep deprivation, and it stayed high during the remainder of a 72–hour sleep deprivation. This finding was interpreted to reflect the increased protein catabolism to supply energy needs. Adam and Oswald, studying rats' brains, found less protein synthesis during 13 hours of total sleep loss but increased protein synthesis during the subsequent recovery sleep.

Under some circumstances, where sustained physical activities are required, the body may convert from carbohydrates to lipids as the primary fuel for biological energy. It appears that total sleep deprivation in environments requiring constant mental alertness and physical activity falls in this category.[249,250] The research findings of Kuhn et al.[110,148] indicate that lipids are a preferred energy source during total sleep deprivation. They found that plasma-free fatty acids increased by 130% and 182% after 48 hours and 72 hours of total sleep deprivation respectively. They detected a much slower fall in the blood glucose level after glucose ingestion after sleep loss than before; after 3–4 days of total sleep loss, a "glucose tolerance curve" resembled the curve for borderline diabetics. Vondra et al. found that hyperglycemia in response to an oral glucose tolerance test was prolonged after 120 hours of sleep deprivation.[311] This result was accompanied by a decreased input of pyruvate into the Krebs cycle. Van Helder et al.[297] believe that this change in glucose metabolism is a prediabetic type of metabolic state. They found that subjects who were deprived of sleep for 60 hours and physically exercised developed insulin resistance. Their proposal that sleep loss results in decreased insulin sensitivity at peripheral insulin receptor sites, eventually leading to "insulin exhaustion at pancreatic sites," needs confirmation because the receptive role played by physical exercise was not clearly separated from the role of sleep loss in itself. Unlike Kuhn et al.[148] and Vondra et al.,[311] they observed no protracted glycemia, possibly because of the relatively short (60 hours) sleep deprivation against that of 120 hours. Fiorica et al.[95] showed that the respiratory quotient also reflected a shift from carbohydrate- to lipid-dominated metabolism on the second and third days of total sleep deprivation.

Total cholesterol in plasma and in the vastus lateralis muscle and plasma triglycerides decreased during a 120-hour sleep deprivation.[311] The changes resembled alterations in cholesterol metabolism observed in cardiovascular diseases or the conditions preceding them.

Sleep deprivation was reported to increase plasma levels of thyroid (T_3, T_4, and rT_3) hormone,[214,220] increasing metabolic rate. Opstad and Aakvaag[211] found that the combined effect of sleep deprivation, prolonged heavy physical work, and caloric deficiency caused thyroxine to increase on day 1 but to decrease from day 2 to day 5, the end of the training course. Triiodothyronine showed a similar trend to T_4. Palmblad et al.[220] found very small increases of about 10% for T_3 and T_4 plasma levels after 48 hours of sleep deprivation.

Sleep loss reduces androgens.[68] Serum testosterone decreased during a 5-day training course involving sleep loss, hard physical work, and caloric deficiency.[1,210,211] Testosterone decreased to below 25% of precourse levels after 48 hours of sleep loss. This decrease reflected reduced production of testosterone, not increased metabolism.

Briefly, these findings suggest that, as total sleep loss continues, skeletal muscles and other tissues begin to derive more energy from the use of free fatty acids. Total sleep loss of two nights or more may result in switching the main energy substrate from carbohydrates to lipids to meet energy demands, resulting in increased plasma-free fatty acids, increased plasma glucose, and sluggish plasma glucose use.

SLEEP LOSS AND HEMATOLOGICAL AND IMMUNOLOGICAL CHANGES

Total sleep deprivation changed neither the erythrocyte count[98,138] nor the hematocrit level.[95,143] However, a drop in plasma iron was reported in humans[147,161,300] and in rats.[83,84] Kuhn et al.[148] reported that plasma iron dropped to one-half its normal level during 120 hours of total sleep loss. Their report showed that the plasma iron decline was sharp during the first 48 hours of sleep loss and subsequently much more gradual. Return to the normal value was slow, taking roughly one week. Intestinal absorption and excretion rates of iron, as measured by radioactive iron uptake, showed no changes during total sleep loss. There was no evidence of impaired erythropoiesis. Thus the reduction in plasma iron was attributed to a failure of the reclamation process of removal of iron from plasma into the splenic-hepatic reticuloendothelial system and the erythropoietic tissue in the bone marrow.[110] Lindemann et al. used a 4- to 5-day training course involving continuous physical activities, limited caloric intake, and partial sleep deprivation (1 to 3 hours of sleep loss per night) and observed changes in hemoglobin, hematocrit, serum iron, bilirubin, and other values. Both hemoglobin and hematocrit decreased during the course. The serum iron increased until day 4 but decreased sharply to 50–60% below initial values on day 5. The bilirubin levels increased markedly, but they came down to the precourse value immediately after the training course. The elevated iron and bilirubin levels were attributed to damage to erythrocytes from the mechanical stress of heavy, continuous physical activities, and not to sleep loss itself. Similar results are reported during Japanese ranger training lasting 93 hours.[333]

The level of serum ferritin, which returns iron to the erythropoietic tissues in the bone marrow, was elevated during a 4- to 5-day training course.[300] The increase of ferritin was correlated with decreased hemoglobin values and increased total bilirubin. Iron released from disintegrated erythrocytes increased ferritin synthesis in the reticuloendothelial system and subsequently increased release of ferritin in blood. The effects of sleep deprivation itself on erythrocytes remain unclear. Levi[159] reported that total sleep deprivation of 24 hours resulted in serum iron decreases of 26% in older subjects (average age, 56), while iron decreased by 52% in younger subjects (average age, 29). Erythrocyte sedimentation rate (a measure that can be affected by many things, including anemia and inflammation) of the older subjects increased by 38% and that of the younger subjects by 168%.

Drucker-Colin[83] and Drucker-Colin et al.[84] found that normocytic anemia can be induced in rats by administration of phenylindanedione (PID, an indirect anticoagulant) during total sleep loss. Administration of parachlorphenylalanine (PCPA, a serotonin synthesis inhibitor) along with PID during sleep loss aggravated the anemic process; anemia without evidence of PID-induced internal bleeding was detectable after 3 days of treatment. These drugs do not produce anemia when administered without accompanying sleep loss, and, as Drucker-Colin emphasized, even an 8-day-long period of sleep deprivation without the drugs does not produce anemia, indicating that sleep loss interacts with the drugs rather than acting directly to produce anemia. Earlier animal studies reported decreases in erythrocyte count, down to as low as 60% of normal.[138] The studies of Drucker-Colin et al.[84] suggest vulnerability of the hemopoietic system to combined sleep loss and drug administration.

It is common belief that the "stress" of losing sleep causes us to catch cold. Immunodeficiency may follow stressful life changes.[118,219]

Palmblad[221] observed an increased production of interferon and decreased phagocytosis during 77 hours of total sleep deprivation. These changes were too small to be of clinical significance. In a subsequent study,[222] the immunological measure of the rate of proliferation of white blood cells in response to an antigen was used. The proliferation of polymorphonuclear leukocytes and monocytes after antigen exposure was reduced after total sleep deprivation of 48 hours, but it remained within normal range; the drop appears to be of no clinical significance.

Briefly, no serious immunological changes follow sleep deprivation. Reduced lymphocyte stimulability and neutrophil phagocytosis and gradually increasing interferon production are expected after 48–72 hours of sleep deprivation,[219] but these changes in cell-mediated immunity would be too small to be of clinical significance. The body's iron equilibrium may be altered during sleep deprivation, and the addition of certain drugs or other stressors may lead to anemia.

SLEEP LOSS AND AUTONOMIC ACTIVITY

Mean core body temperature gets lower during total sleep deprivation. The circadian variation remains but its amplitude is reduced. Homeostatic ability to maintain core body temperature when exposed to cold is not impaired by 84–86 hours of total sleep deprivation,[95] but Sawka et al. suggest some degraded thermoregulation during exercise after total sleep deprivation.[260]

Resting systolic and diastolic blood pressures do not change during total sleep deprivation.[54,199] Resting heart rate has generally been found to show little systematic change during sleep loss,[67,116,198,203,324] except Bjerner reported general systematic slowdown of resting heart rate.[42] Fenz and Craig[94] reported that heart rate increased on day 2 of total sleep deprivation, but the increase was found only in one of the two daily measures. On the third day, heart rate dropped. Total sleep deprivation caused a progressive increase in heart rate variability, much of it related to an increase in the normal tendency of the heart rate to vary with respiration—"respiratory sinus arrhythmia."[116]

Endogenously depressive patients have a lower amplitude circadian heart rate curve than normal subjects. Twenty-four hours of total sleep deprivation caused further flattening of the circadian heart rate curve in this patient group. The circadian heart rate rhythms of neurotic depressives are more normal than those of the endogenously depressive at baseline and were unaffected by a 24-hour sleep loss.[253]

Levi[158] observed that one quarter of his subjects showed S–T segment depression during 75 hours of total sleep deprivation. In some cases, depression was pronounced and resembled a cardiac infarction in the apical area. The depression gradually disappeared after several days of sleep and rest.

Johnson et al.[127] reported that resting-finger pulse volume became very small due to peripheral circulatory constriction during a prolonged total sleep deprivation. Finger pulse volume showed a marked vasodilation, tripling in volume, during recovery sleep. Mirsky and Cardon[183] observed increased finger pulse volume near the end of their total sleep deprivation study during a complex vigilance task. Such transient increases may be attributable to periods of microsleep.

Generally, total sleep deprivation does not change respiratory rate,[95] although variability of rate was reported to increase over 60 hours of sleep loss.[116]

Skin conductance probably reflects sympathetic nervous activity. Different studies have reported equivocal and conflicting results as to sleep deprivation effects on skin conductance.[116] We conclude that total sleep loss has no consistent effect on skin conductance.[203] Strausbaugh and Roessler[280] reported that tonic skin conductance was higher—that is, subjects were more alert and activated—in the sleep-deprived subjects who had high "ego strength" than in those whose ego strength was low.

Briefly, no major autonomic changes are expected in resting subjects during total sleep loss of 2 days or less, although amplitudes of circadian curves may be blunted and general variability may be increased.

SLEEP LOSS AND EPILEPTIFORM DISCHARGES

Total sleep deprivation initially increases cerebral irritability, which may result in epileptiform discharges in predisposed individuals.[3,16,22,27–29,36–38,41,71–76,87,104,177,184,201,236,248,267–269,318] Because of this, sleep deprivation has been used to provoke abnormal paroxysmal electroencephalographic discharges in individuals with suspected epilepsy.[87] One night of total sleep loss is combined with other techniques of activation in clinical practice.[201] However, increased irritability appears to be limited to the first 2 days of total sleep deprivation; after that, extreme sleepiness reduces cerebral electrical excitability.

Because total sleep deprivation of 2 days or less under clinical laboratory conditions does not induce epileptiform discharges in normal healthy individuals, false positives rarely occur.[28,29,202,318] Only one child (8%) of a group of 12 normal children showed an abnormal electroencephalogram after a short period of total sleep deprivation.[104]

However, prolonged total sleep deprivation combined with other stressors may induce abnormal cerebral discharges in healthy individuals.[3,111] On continuous recordings of brain waves over 90 hours, a third of healthy subjects exhibited paroxysmal activity lasting for only a few seconds at a time. One subject showed, however, a total of 2.5 hours of spike-and-wave activity in one day. None of the subjects experienced grand mal seizures, but some exhibited "absence" or psychomotor seizures. Especially for the individuals with a pre-existing susceptibility, sleep deprivation sets the stage for epileptic seizures resembling short periods of inattention and battle shock.[111]

Briefly, all of us could develop psychomotor-type epileptiform discharges under the combined influence of sleep loss and other stressors. Some individuals are more susceptible than others.

SLEEP LOSS AND PHYSICAL WORKING CAPACITY

Maximal oxygen consumption is a measure of cardiovascular fitness or overall aerobic work capacity. Oxygen consumption increases with increasing physical workload. As physical workload continues to increase, we eventually reach a point where the pulmonary/cardiovascular system becomes incapable of supplying additional oxygen to the working skeleton and muscles, and oxygen consumption plateaus despite increasing physical workload. This plateau represents the maximal rate of oxygen consumption—that is, maximal aerobic capacity, VO_2 max.[334] A psychological factor of willingness to endure acute discomfort enters into a VO_2 max testing because the test is terminated by subjects. Aerobic working capacity can also be measured indirectly by the increase in heart rate and the speed of return to resting heart rate following standardized physical work regimens, such as the Harvard Step Test.[52,66]

In 1970, Vogel and Glaser studied three male subjects who underwent maximal and submaximal working capacity tests on a bicycle ergonometer before and after sleep deprivation. Reviewing their data, Harris and O'Hanlon reported that after 72 hours of total sleep deprivation, the VO_2 max values of the three subjects were reduced by 3.2%, 6.0%, and 3.8% against the baseline.[110] Plyley et al. observed a 6.9% decrease of VO_2 max during 64 hours of sleep deprivation.[233] Martin and Chen[175] reported a decline in physical performance after 50 hours of sleep derivation. The endurance-run time to exhaustion was reduced by 20% among the sleep-deprived. Takeuchi et al.[284] found that vertical jump performance decreased after 64 hours of sleep deprivation. Yeager et al., however, observed that 45 hours of sleep deprivation did not change maximal aerobic capacity.[334] Martin showed no change in VO_2 max after 30 hours of sleep deprivation.[173] Symons et al. found that sleep loss of up to 60 hours did not impair the capability for physical work.[283]

Pickett and Morris[231] found that cardiovascular endurance was not affected by total sleep deprivation of 30 hours, but it was affected by food and water deprivation of the same duration. Brodan and Kuhn,[52] using the Harvard Step Test, found that young men showed about a 5% drop in cardiovascular fitness during the first 48 hours of total sleep deprivation. Their cardiovascular fitness began to recover, however, and even increased, after continued sleep deprivation; after 5 days of total sleep loss, the mean score exceeded the baseline mean by 5%. The most surprising finding was a sharp drop of nearly 15% in cardiovascular fitness on the first day after the recovery sleep. In much younger subjects (ninth-graders), Copes and Rosentsweig[66] found a decline of cardiovascular fitness as measured by the Harvard Step Test during total sleep loss.

Orlee et al. reported that men lost their top physical conditioning quickly after one night of total sleep deprivation.[216] For physically conditioned men, however, the loss was limited to fitness gained by hard training. The degradation brought the fitness level down to the pretraining baseline but not below.

Total sleep deprivation of 24–30 hours slowed reaction time as well as speed of movement.[56,231] Resting electromyographic activity was reported to be reduced during total sleep deprivation.[116] Summarizing the results of past studies, Wilkinson commented, however, that electromyographic changes are unrelated to hours of sleep loss.[324]

It has been well established that continuous muscular activity, such as walking, can help sleep-deprived subjects remain awake.[138] Naitoh et al. observed that all subjects kept themselves physically active to stay awake; for example, a subject was willing to keep moving on his feet, walking 8.3 times more during the 165–191 hours of total sleep deprivation, compared with the 26-hour period at the start of the study.

Briefly, physical work capacity appears not to show major deterioration as a result of total sleep deprivation of 3 days or less. Movement speed, however, is slowed down. Willingness and ability to remain physically active (e.g., by walking) are severely tested by the increasing desire to rest.

ANTIDEPRESSIVE EFFECTS OF SLEEP LOSS

Health effects of sleep deprivation are not always negative. The antidepressant effects of total sleep deprivation have been well established. This is an area that is still actively researched. The bibliography of this chapter cites more than 30 references on it. Total sleep deprivation provides temporary relief from depression in one-third to one-half of endogenously depressed patients, but it is less effective in patients with involutional depression. With respect to the other major category of depression, reactively depressed patients benefit from sleep loss more if they have more somatic complaints (such as disturbed sleep and poor appetite) and large diurnal fluctuation in moods, as compared with few somatic complaints and poor circadian rhythm. Typically, a single night of total sleep deprivation is repeated over several weeks until the desired amelioration of depression is achieved. The patients must remain awake between 0400 and 0600 to get full antidepressant benefit from sleep deprivation. Cole and Muller[63] reported that when elderly depressives (57–79 years old, average age 69) were given repeated (once or twice a week) 36-hour periods of total sleep deprivation therapy, 9 (60%) of 15 patients responded to the therapy and 6 (40%) had a good outcome. However, total sleep deprivation therapy may trigger a manic phase.[316,317]

Post et al.[235] sampled lumbar cerebrospinal fluid from depressive patients to study central amine metabolism as reflected by levels of 5-hydroxyindoleacetic acid (5-HIAA), homovanillic acid, and 3-methoxy-4-hydroxyphenylglycol. Total sleep deprivation changed the central amine metabolism of the depressed patients, causing a decrease in 3-methoxy-4-hydroxyphenylglycol. The other parameters increased. In a study by Livrea et al.,[163] lumbar cerebrospinal fluid was examined for homovanillic acid and 5-HIAA before and after total or REM sleep deprivation. Cerebrospinal fluid levels of homovanillic acid and 5-HIAA were not affected by 30 hours of total sleep deprivation, but 5-HIAA increased after 2 nights of REM sleep deprivation.

Two hypotheses attempting to explain the antidepressant effects of total sleep deprivation are:

(1) total sleep deprivation assists in resynchronization of disordered circadian rhythms and re-entrainment to the 24-hour societal rhythm

(2) total sleep deprivation lowers an abnormally high arousal level in depressives.

REM sleep deprivation also has antidepressant effects.[304,305] The REM sleep deprivation procedure consists of awakening subjects every time they go into REM sleep. This is continued for six nights or until 30 awakenings per night are reached (REM frequency increases as deprivation accumulates), whichever comes first. Subsequently patients are permitted a single night of uninterrupted sleep. The REM sleep deprivation procedure is repeated until the desired amelioration of depressive symptoms is obtained.

In brief, total or REM sleep deprivation helps to temporarily reduce depression in some depressive patients. Mood effects of total or REM sleep deprivation in normal individuals are discussed in the following section.

SLEEP LOSS AND QUALITY OF LIFE

The most serious health cost in its broadest sense is a lowered quality of life during sleep deprivation. Sleep loss results in chronic excessive fatigue and sleepiness, sagging motivation for work, and poor job performance leading to frustrations and conflicts with other workers. The quality of life will be discussed in terms of (1) mood and motivation to work, (2) excessive daytime sleepiness and fatigue, and (3) mental health.

Mood and Motivation to Work

In the *Handbook on Human Engineering Data* (second edition) published by Tufts College for the Office of Naval Research in 1952, 17 papers on sleep deprivation are reviewed. The editors were surprised to see that "there are no significant physiological changes with up to 200 hours of sleeplessness" and that "subjective attitude (appearance, mood and behavior) is the only factor severely affected by sleep reduction." This conclusion is still valid.[116,118,119]

One night of total sleep deprivation was found to influence six factors: sleep/wakefulness, stress, euphoria, energy, irritation, and concentration, in a complex, but highly predictable, manner. For example, one night of total sleep deprivation lowered wakefulness and energy ratings, but did not significantly change stress and euphoria.[44] Simple negative mood changes, such as feeling tired, are consistently reported after total sleep deprivation and can be used to gauge the extent of accumulated sleep debt. Subjects felt progressively more negative and less positive during total sleep deprivation, and these mood changes showed strong circadian rhythm.[199,200] Thus, unlike depressives, normal subjects do not experience large positive mood changes or feelings of well-being after sleep deprivation.[44,69]

In the first scientific study of partial sleep deprivation, Mary Smith studied herself. She shortened the usual period of sleep over three consecutive nights by 1.5, 3.5, and 5.5 hours.[273] She experienced a double feeling tone—unpleasant muscular weariness that became pain at times, and pleasant sensations of exhaltation and power. For the most part, the pleasant aspect was dominant. Johnson and MacLeod[125] reduced the sleep of two subjects by 30 minutes, every two weeks, form their customary 7.5 hours to a minimum of 4 hours per 24 hours. Using the Profile of Mood States, they found that the subjects were less "happy," less "friendly," more "fatigued," and increasingly irritable. The subjects experienced difficulties maintaining concentration when the sleep period was reduced to 5.5 hours or less.

In another gradual sleep reduction study,[100] two young couples reduced their sleep by 30 minutes every two weeks until total sleep time reached 6.5 hours. They continued to reduce sleep at a rate of 30 minutes every three weeks. When total sleep time was down to 5 hours, the rate of sleep reduction became 30 minutes every four weeks to give the subjects more opportunity to adapt to the shorter sleep and longer day. Eventually, the subjects felt that they found the minimum sleep they needed, the point where their sleep was maximally reduced without jeopardizing their jobs and schoolwork. Over a 7-month period, one couple reduced their sleep time from 8 hours to 5 hours. The other couple reduced their sleep from 8 hours to 4.5 hours over an 8-month period. Both couples slept for a month at these low levels. Subsequently, the sleep period was lengthened by 30 minutes for a 2-week period, after which they were allowed ad lib sleep regimens.

The couples reported that they decided to stop reducing their sleep because they were overwhelmingly tired, they were falling asleep in class, playing cards, or visiting friends, and they had difficulty remaining alert while driving. However, objective school and job performances did not suffer during the partial sleep deprivation.

Webb and Agnew[315] examined 15 subjects who reduced sleep to 5.5 hours and maintained that amount for 60 days. The moods of these subjects showed initial dips but generally returned to baseline as partial sleep deprivation continued. During the study period, the subjects showed performance degradation that appeared to be due to boredom and lowered motivation.

In brief, mood deteriorates and motivation to work hard is lowered during total and partial sleep deprivation. Although controlled studies of regular gradual reduction in nightly sleep have demonstrated that we have a potential to adjust to partial sleep deprivation, these results are not directly applicable to the shiftworker. In shiftwork, partial sleep deprivation occurs acutely when nightshift work begins and, unlike strictly controlled studies, the amount of sleep loss may vary from day to day. Greater experience on a shiftwork schedule has not been shown to be associated with reduced complaints about sleep loss.

Excessive Daytime Sleepiness and Fatigue

Naitoh[199] reported that the levels of fatigue and sleepiness increase and decrease in a circadian manner and that total sleep deprivation of 2 nights increased subjectively rated fatigue and sleepiness without destroying these circadian rhythms. Sleepiness, as measured by the Stanford Sleepiness Scale,[114] peaks around 0200–0600 of the first night of total sleep deprivation. Once subjects pass this critically sleepy period, they feel much less sleepy even though they remain awake. However, Carskadon and Dement[58] found that objective sleepiness, as measured by the Multiple Sleep Latency Test, lost its normal circadian rhythm during the first night of total sleep deprivation; sleepiness peaked around 0600 the next morning and remained at peak level throughout the 2 nights of total sleep deprivation.

As shown in the studies of Friedman et al.[100] and Johnson and MacLeod[125] discussed in the preceding section, subjective feelings of tiredness and sleepiness provide an early warning of excessive sleep debt. Impairment of job performance appears much later than daytime feelings of excessive tiredness and sleepiness. In real workplace situations, worker motivation is an important variable with respect to how closely performance decrements follow sleep loss.

In brief, increased feelings of tiredness and sleepiness reliably follow total or partial sleep deprivation, reducing quality of life. These feelings constitute an early warning that serious deterioration in job performance will follow unless more sleep is obtained.

Mental Health

As mentioned previously, the most obvious and consistent changes due to total and partial sleep deprivation are psychological. When investigators lived with sleep-deprived subjects, they often observed frequent, but transient, psychotic behavior.[32] These behavioral pathologies are easily missed because of their transience. Whether a subject shows transient psychopathology during total sleep deprivation depends on age, physical health, psychological stability, and the environment of the study.

Total sleep deprivation experiments represent a complicated social psychological arrangement.[191–193] An illustration of the impact of experimental environments is found in the differences between the results of Tyler's study[293–295] and those from the Walter Reed Army Medical Institute of Research.[192,327]

Tyler's study involved 350 volunteers under military discipline during the period of 1942–1946. Under the stringent, stressful military exercise environment, 112 hours of total sleep deprivation caused more than 70% of the subjects to complain of auditory and visual illusions. Seventy-six of these men dropped out before the conclusion of the study for a variety of psychosomatic complaints. Seven men had to be removed from the study because they developed hallucinations and bizarre "psychotic" behaviors. The high attrition occurred despite excellent morale at the start and a considerable incentive offered for completing the study.

The Walter Reed study was conducted in a laboratory environment. The staff maintained a friendly and egalitarian atmosphere in order to keep frustration and aggression at a minimum. Gentle methods such as walking, playing games, holding conversations, and encouragement from staff were used to help 74 soldiers stay awake for 72–98 hours. No subjects dropped out, and no "psychotic" breakdowns were observed although visual hallucinations were reported.

Thus, the sociology of total sleep deprivation or the psychological characteristics of the environment play a critical role in determining mental health during total sleep loss.

Prior mental stability is also a determinant of a subject's psychological responses to total sleep deprivation.[134,167,168] Pasnau et al. reported a study involving 205 hours of total sleep deprivation.[224] One of the volunteer subjects experienced a panic response and all subjects had psychological problems, but they found no evidence of psychosis. In 1968, an editorial in the *Journal of the American Medical Association*[272] stated, on the basis of data later published by Kollar et al.[142] and Pasnau et al.,[224] that sleep deprivation does not cause mentally healthy people to become psychotic. Dement[79] similarly pointed out that REM sleep deprivation does not lead to psychosis. REM sleep deprivation does not cause intensification of thought disturbances, perceptual and motor disorganization, or increased withdrawal.[301,305,306]

In brief, total sleep deprivation does not cause permanent psychosis. Bizarre visual illusions, hallucinations, paranoid mentations, and other behavioral pathologies may be seen, but they are limited to the period of sleep deprivation and disappear after recovery sleep. Hostile or stressful work environments are more prone to produce abnormal responses than friendly supportive environments.

DISCUSSION AND SUMMARY

On the whole, the health consequences of total, partial, or selective sleep deprivation appear to be much smaller than might have been anticipated from the overwhelming sense of sleepiness, tiredness, and sluggishness it can cause. We can conclude that the only substantial and potentially serious effect of sleep deprivation is a reduction in the quality of life as defined by a person's feeling of well-being, willingness to work hard, and feeling of being efficient, wide awake, fresh, and in control. This does not mean that sleep deprivation fails to cause small changes in human biochemistry and physiology.

The belief that sleep should be 7–8 hours long, should offer a refreshed feeling upon awakening, and is needed for physical and mental recuperation appears to have resulted in unwarranted anxiety about sleep loss. This anxiety can affect how a person interprets minor, but perceptible, changes during sleep loss, such as tiredness, sleepiness, lapses of attention, inability to concentrate, and an overall feeling of not being well. With anxiety, these minor psychological changes may be interpreted as representing serious mental harm. The emotional reaction following such an interpretation can cause a person to urgently seek sleep in hopes of avoiding further harm, even to resort to the use of ethanol, sedatives, tranquilizers, and hypnotics.

Schachter[261] and Schachter and Singer[262] have proposed that the nature of emotional response is determined by two components: some perceptible physiological changes and the individual's appraisal of these physiological changes. For example, an increase in heart rate and facial flushing after drinking alcoholic beverages may be implicitly interpreted as a warm satisfying alcohol effect by a habitual drinker, but as a dangerous or uncomfortable effect by someone who rarely drinks.

Carskadon et al.[60] reported that a group of 109 chronic insomniacs actually differed very little, in terms of total sleep time and sleep latency, from a group of 87 normal sleepers. They did differ in the number of awakenings during sleep. The chronic insomniacs may have physiological or biochemical problems that cause their sleep to be fragmented. It could be argued that, since these insomniacs have normal total sleep time, they may only be suffering psychologically from the awakenings because they interpret them as life or health threatening. Their chronic fear of getting nothing but poor sleep may cause them to suffer much more than a normal sleeper would from a nocturnal awakening. Perhaps an overlay of fear can aggravate what is basically a physiological variation on the norm into a significant psychological problem.

How has the popular belief that poor sleep is dangerous to health come about? Anxiety about the effects of poor sleep or total lack of sleep may have an origin in experiments conducted near the turn of the century and reported by Pieron in 1913[232] and later by Kleitman.[138] They reported physical harm and even death among animals that had been subjected to total sleep deprivation. We have shown that, at least in humans, total sleep deprivation of up to 205 hours does not pose serious health problems.[130,141,142,202,203,224,252] Similarly, chronic reduction of sleep time does not produce any physical harm.[100,125,315]

In addition to supposedly producing physical harm, sleep deprivation is also believed to result in mental harm, i.e., psychosis or intensification of psychopathology.[319] The belief that psychosis of sleep deprivation occurs in normal individuals developed many years ago and is based on dramatic examples reported by Katz and Landis[133] and others. Katz and Landis described a 24-year-old man who was convinced that sleep was a habit and could be broken without any ill effects. He remained awake for 231 hours before developing delusions of persecution, at which time the study was terminated. In another study, a large number of young soldiers, marines, and civilians underwent paratrooper-like training that included a 35-mile night march; some subjects suffered a transient psychosis with paranoid mentation.[293,294]

Careful evaluation of these and other studies shows that psychosis was not caused by sleep deprivation itself, but by a combination of sleep loss with other stressors. The previously mentioned 1968 editorial in the *Journal of the American Medical Association* made a clear effort to correct the view that sleep deprivation causes mental harm. The editorial stated that sleep loss would not produce psychopathological reactions extending beyond the period of sleep deprivation and that "patients who suffer from periods of insomnia can be reassured as to the transiency and safety of a brief sleepless period"; it also said that no medication is necessary to protect patients against the psychosis of sleeplessness. The editorial cited the studies that found total sleep deprivation to be beneficial for temporarily relieving depression in some depressive patients.

In the 1960s and 1970s, REM sleep deprivation was also thought to cause mental harm.[61,79,88,119,160] However, it has since been shown to provide safe and effective, although temporary, relief from endogenous depression.

Thus, fear that total sleep and REM sleep deprivation directly cause physical and mental harm is groundless.

This report has attempted to provide information about health consequences of total sleep deprivation. We are surprised to learn from the surveyed literature that sleep deprivation produces only very small biomedical effects. However, some caveats are necessary.

For workers needing maximum alertness and uninterrupted concentration, such as air traffic controllers, heavy equipment operators, power plant operators, and blood bank technicians, anxiety about the effects of chronic partial sleep deprivation is warranted, particularly insofar as it may cause lapses of attention and inability to concentrate. Many physiological changes have the potential to cause major catastrophes. These workers' appropriate anxiety about their sleep loss may increase the likelihood of errors and may also produce health complaints associated with chronic anxiety.

Almost all of the past and current research on sleep deprivation is based on highly controlled laboratory studies using short-term data collection. Such studies are not able to assess the complex patterns of sleep deprivation combined with various stressors seen in working environments. Thus, the surveyed literature may be biased by protocols designed more to be simple, clean, and easy to interpret than to answer questions about the biomedical consequences of sleep loss in real life circumstances. Hence, the surveyed literature may have underestimated the true biomedical impact of sleep loss.

For example, most research reports are based on responses to a single exposure to sleep deprivation. Since real life experience more often involves repeated exposures to sleep loss, the findings in the literature may not be directly applicable. Health problems in shiftworkers, who are more apt than other workers to endure chronic sleep deprivation, have been extensively investigated (see Chapter 7). Gastrointestinal disorders, cardiovascular disease, and numerous other medical conditions occur more frequently or are aggravated in this group. These effects may be due wholly to disruption of biological rhythms, but the possibility that chronic sleep deprivation contributes to them cannot be dismissed.

Another caveat is that the findings of these studies cannot be generalized to the middle-aged or older population, especially not to people with less than ideal physical and mental fitness. Most of the studies have been conducted on young, physically and mentally fit people, usually students at universities. Worst of all, only a few (e.g., a series of fascinating studies on 5-day military training courses by Opstad, Palmblad, and others at the Norwegian Defense Research Establishment[1,2,209–215,219–222,249–251]) measured the interaction of physical and psychological stressors with sleeplessness. Since sleeplessness in daily experience often occurs concurrently with job-related, and other, stressors, results of these single-factor studies cannot be generalized to determine health consequences of sleep deprivation in daily life. If combining sleep loss with various stressors is still found to lead to no lasting physical or mental harm, it must be kept in mind that even a transient psychotic episode can be detrimental to health if it happens during dangerous military or industrial activity.

It has been said in jest that all sleep deprivation does is make us sleepy. However, sleepiness is a mystery of life worth careful investigation. Understanding it would help us gain a full appreciation of the nature of sleep and the impact of sleep loss on our bodies.

REFERENCES

1. Aakvaag A, Bentdal O, Quistad K, et al: Testosterone and testosterone binding globulin (TeBG) in young men during prolonged stress. Int J Androl 1:22–31, 1978.
2. Aakvaag A, Sand T, Opstad PK, Fonnum F: Hormonal changes in young men during prolonged physical strain. Eur J Appl Physiol 46:9–19, 1981.

3. Abraham P, Docherty TB, Haslam DR: Ambulatory EEG recording for extended periods under adverse conditions. In Acott FD, Raferty EB, Sleight P, Goulding (eds): ISAMM 77. London, Academic Press, 1978, pp 85–91.
4. Adam K, Oswald I: Sleep is for tissue restoration. J R Coll Physicians Lond 11:376–388, 1977.
5. Agnew H Jr, Webb W, Williams R: The effects of stage four sleep deprivation. Electroencephalogr Clin Neurophysiol 17:68–70, 1964.
6. Agnew HW Jr, Webb WB, Williams RL: Comparison of stage four and 1-REM sleep deprivation. Percept Mot Skills 24:851–858, 1967.
7. Ahnve S, Theorell T, Akerstedt T, et al: Circadian variations in cardiovascular parameters during sleep deprivation: A noninvasive study of young healthy men. Eur J Appl Physiol 46:9–19, 1981.
8. Akerstedt T, Froberg JE: Psychophysiological circadian rhythms in women during 72 h of sleep deprivation. Waking and Sleeping 1:387–394, 1977.
9. Akerstedt T, Froberg J: Sleep and sleep deprivation in relation to circadian rhythms in catecholamine excretion. Biol Psychol 8:69–80, 1979.
10. Akerstedt T, Froberg JE, Friberg Y, Wettenberg L: Melatonin excretion, body temperature and subjective arousal during 64 hours of sleep deprivation. Psychoneuroendocrinology 4:219–225, 1979.
11. Akerstedt T, Palmblad J, de la Torre MR, Gillberg M: Adrenocortical and gonadal steroids during sleep deprivation. Sleep 3:23–40, 1980.
12. Akindele MO, Evans JI, Oswald I: Mono-oxidate inhibitors, sleep and mood. Electroencephalogr Clin Neurophysiol 29:47–56, 1970.
13. Anders TF, Roffwarg HP: The effects of selective sleep state deprivation in the human newborn. Psychophysiology 6:264–265, 1969.
14. Anders TF, Roffwarg HP: The effects of total sleep deprivation on the human newborn. Psychophysiology 6:265, 1969.
15. Amin MM, Khalid R, Khan P: Relationship between sleep deprivation and urinary MPGH levels. Int Pharmacopsychiatry 15:81–85.
16. Armington JC, Mitnick LL: Electroencephalogram and sleep deprivation. J Appl Physiol 14:247–250, 1959.
17. Aschoff J: Features of circadian rhythms relevant for the design of shift schedules. Ergonomics 21:739–754, 1978.
18. Aschoff J, Giedke H, Poppel E, Wever R: The influence of sleep-interruption and of sleep-deprivation on circadian rhythms in human performance. In Colquhoun WP (ed): Aspects of Human Efficiency. London, English Universities Press, 1959, pp 135–150.
19. Ax A, Luby ED: Autonomic responses to sleep deprivation. Arch Gen Psychiatry 4:55–59, 1976.
20. Azumi K, Jinnai S: The effects of REM deprivation on electrodermal-activity in human sleep. In Weitzman ED (ed): Adv Sleep Res 2:164–176, 1976.
21. Baust W, Moppeney H, Schlosser A: The influence of REM sleep deprivation on heart rate and respiration. Arztl Forsch 26:302–308, 1972.
22. Bechinger D, Kriebel J, Schlager M: The EEG following sleep deprivation: An important tool for diagnosis of epileptic seizures. Z Neurol 205:193–206, 1973.
23. Beck U, Wenzel D, Sauer M: Selective deprivation of sleep in narcoleptic children. Arch Psychiatr Nervenk 223:107–115, 1977.
24. Beersma DGM, van den Hoffdakker RH: Depressive mood and physiology during sleep deprivation. Sleep Res 12:321, 1983.
25. Benca RM, Everson C, Kushida C, et al: Effect of sleep deprivation on immune function in rats. Sleep Res 15:8, 1986.
26. Benca RM, Kushida CA, Everson CA, et al: Sleep deprivation in the rat: VII. Immune function. Sleep 12:47–52, 1989.
27. Bennett DR: Sleep deprivation and major motor convulsions. Neurology 13:953–958, 1963.
28. Bennett DR, Mattson RH, Ziter FA, et al: Sleep deprivation: Neurological and electroencephalographic effects. Aerospace Med 35:888–890, 1964.
29. Bennett DR, Ziter FA, Liske EA: Electroencephalographic study of sleep deprivation in flying personnel. Neurology 19:375–377, 1969.
30. Benoit O, Foret J, Merle B, Bouard G: Diurnal rhythm of axillary temperature in long and short sleepers: Effect of sleep deprivation and sleep displacement. Sleep 4:359–365, 1981.
31. Bergamasco B, Brignoli F, Doriguzzi T, et al: Longitudinal polygraphic study of sleep in 11 patients with delirium tremens: Physiopathological considerations of "sleep deprivation." Acta Neurol (Napoli) 23:289–299, 1968.

32. Berger RJ, Oswald I: Effects of sleep deprivation on behaviour, subsequent sleep and dreaming. J Ment Sci 108:457–465, 1962.
33. Bergmann BM, Everson CA, Kushida CA, et al: Sleep deprivation in the rat: V. Energy use and mediation. Sleep 12:31–41, 1989.
34. Bergmann B, Fang VS, Kushida C, Everson C: Hypothalamic-adrenal variables in paradoxical and total sleep deprivation of rats. Sleep Res 15:212, 1986.
35. Bergmann B, Kushida C, Hennessy C, Winter J, Rechtschaffen A: Paradoxical sleep deprivation in the rat: II. Energy consumption. Sleep Res 13:185, 1984.
36. Berti-Ceroni G: Clinical and EEG effects of sleep deprivation in epileptics. Electroencephalogr Clin Neurophysiol 23:188, 1967.
37. Berti-Ceroni G, Pazzaglia P, Mantovani M, Sabatinni L: Effects of total deprivation of sleep in the narcoleptics. Rev Neurol (Paris) 123:263–265, 1970.
38. Berti-Ceroni G, Sabatinni L, Gambi D, Lugaresi E: Effects of sleep deprivation in epileptics. Riv Neurol 37:305–320, 1967.
39. Bhanji S, Roy GA: The treatment of depression by sleep deprivation: A replication study. Br J Psychiatry 127:222–226, 1975.
40. Billiard M: Competition between the two types of sleep and the recuperative function of REM sleep versus NREM sleep in narcoleptics. In Guilleminault C, et al (eds): Adv Sleep Res 3:77–96, 1976.
41. Billiard M, Echenne B, Besset A, et al: Comparative activating effects of sleep, sleep deprivation and sleep after sleep deprivation in children with suspected epileptic seizures. Sleep Res 12:302, 1983.
42. Bjerner B: Alpha depression and lowered pulse rate during delayed actions in a serial reaction test: A study of sleep deprivation. Acta Physiol Scand 19(suppl):65, 1949.
43. Bliss EL, Clark LD, West CD: Studies of sleep deprivation: Relationship to schizophrenia. Arch Neurol Psychiatry 81:348–359, 1959.
44. Bohlin G, Kjellberg A: Self-reported arousal during sleep deprivation and its relation to performance and physiological variables. Scand J Psychol 14:78–86, 1973.
45. Bol'shakova TD, Meshcheryakova SA, Tyabenkova VF, et al: Effect of 24-hour sleep deprivation on biogenic amine turnover. Hum Physiol 11:291–295, 1985.
46. Bond V, Balkisoon B, Franks BD, et al: Effects of sleep deprivation on performance during submaximal and maximal exercise. J Sports Med Phys Fitness 26:169–174, 1986.
47. Borbely AA, Wirz-Justice A: Sleep, sleep deprivation and depression. A hypothesis derived from a model of sleep regulation. Hum Neurol 1:205–210, 1982.
48. Brezinova V, Hort V, Vojtechofsky M: Sleep deprivation with respect to age: An EEG study. Act Nerv Super (Praha) 11:182–187, 1969.
49. Brezinova V, Hort V, Vojtechovsky M: The effect of centrophenoxine on EEG vigilance in the course of sleep deprivation and on the EEG pattern of all-night sleep. Act Nerv Super (Praha) 12:54–56, 1970.
50. Brezinova V, Oswald I, Loudon J: Two types of insomnia: Too much waking or not enough sleep. Br J Psychiatry 126:439–445, 1975.
51. Broadbent DE: Variations in performance arising from continuous work. Conference on Individual Efficiency in Industry. Cambridge, England, Medical Research Council, 1955, pp 1–5.
52. Brodan V, Kuhn E: Physical performance in man during sleep deprivation. J Sports Med Phys Fitness 7:28–30, 1967.
53. Brodan V, Vojtechovsky M, Kuhn E, Cepelak J: Changes of mental and physical performance in sleep deprived healthy volunteers. Act Nerv Super (Praha) 11:175–181, 1969.
54. Bruce LC: Some observations upon the general blood pressures in sleeplessness and sleep. Scott Med Surg J 7:109–117, 1900.
55. Buchsbaum MS, Gerner R, Post RM: The effect of sleep deprivation on average evoked response in depressed patients and in normals. Biol Psychiatry 16:351–363, 1981.
56. Buck L: Sleep loss effects on movement time. Ergonomics 18:415–425, 1975.
57. Bugge JF, Opstad PK, Magnus PM: Changes in circadian rhythm of performance and mood in healthy young men exposed to prolonged heavy physical work, sleep deprivation and caloric deficit. Aviat Space Environ Med 50:663–668, 1979.
58. Carskadon MA, Dement WC: Effects of total sleep loss on sleep tendency. Percept Mot Skills 48:495–506, 1979.
59. Carskadon MA, Dement WC: Sleep deprivation in insomniacs: Effects on daytime alertness and recovery sleep. Sleep Res 14:148, 1985.
60. Carskadon MA, Dement WC, Mitler MM, et al: Self-rated versus sleep laboratory findings in 122 drug-free subjects with complaints of chronic insomnia. Am J Psychiatry 133:1382–1388, 1976.

61. Cartwright RD, Ratzel RW: Effects of dream loss on waking behaviors. Arch Gen Psychiatry 27:277–280, 1972.
62. Clark RE, Warren N: The effect of loss of sleep on visual tests. Am J Opthalmol 16:80–95, 1939.
63. Cole MG, Miller HF: Sleep deprivation in the treatment of elderly depressed patients. J Am Geriatr Soc 243:308–313, 1976.
64. Collins WE: Some effects of sleep loss on vestibular responses. Aviat Space Environ Med 59:523–529, 1988.
65. Cooperman NR, Mullin FJ, Kleitman N: Studies on the physiology of sleep. XI. Further observations on the effects of prolonged sleeplessness. Am J Physiol 107:589–593, 1934.
66. Copes K, Rosentswieg J: The effects of sleep deprivation upon motor performance of ninth-grade students. J Sports Med Phys Fitness 12:47–53, 1972.
67. Corcoran DWJ: Changes in heart rate and performance as a result of loss of sleep. Br J Psychol 55:307–315, 1964.
68. Cortes-Gallegos V, Castaneda G, Alonso R, et al: Sleep deprivation reduces circulating androgens in healthy men. Arch Androl 10:33–37, 1983.
69. Cutler NR, Cohen HB: The effect of one night's sleep loss on mood and memory in normal subjects. Compr Psychiatry 20:61–66, 1979.
70. Davies B, Shapiro CM, Daggett A, et al: Physiological changes and sleep responses during and following a world record continuous walking record. Br J Sports Med 18:173–180, 1984.
71. Declerck AC, Martens WL, Wauquier A: Evaluation of the effects of antiepileptic drugs on sleep-wakefulness patterns following 1 night total sleep deprivation in epileptic patients. Neuropsychobiology 13:201–205, 1985.
72. Degen R: The diagnostic significance of sleep after sleep deprivation under antiepileptic-therapy. Nervenarzt 48:314–320, 1977.
73. Degen R, Degen HE: A comparative study of the diagnostic value of drug-induced sleep EEGs and sleep EEGs following sleep deprivation in patients with complex partial seizure. J Neurol 225:85–93, 1981.
74. Degen R, Degen HE: The diagnostic value of sleep. EEG with and without sleep deprivation in patients with atypicalabsende. Epilepsia 24:557–566, 1983.
75. Degen R, Degen HE, Reker M: Sleep EEG with or without sleep deprivation? Does sleep deprivation activate more epileptic activity in patients suffering from different type of epilepsy? Eur Neurol 26:51–59, 1987.
76. Degen R, Niedermeyer R (eds): Epilepsy, Sleep, and Sleep Deprivation. Amsterdam, Elsevier, 1984.
77. Dement W: The effect of dream deprivation. Science 131:1705–1707, 1960.
78. Dement WC: Sleep deprivation and the organization of the behavioral states. In Clemente CD, et al (eds): Sleep and the Maturing Nervous System. New York, Academic Press, 1972, pp 319–355.
79. Dement WC: Commentary to "The biological role of REM sleep (circa 1968"). In Webb WB (ed): Sleep: An Active Process. Glenview, IL, Scott, Foresman, 1973, pp 48–58.
80. Dement WC: The relevance of sleep pathologies to the function of sleep. In Drucker-Colin R, et al (eds): The Functions of Sleep. New York: Academic Press, 1979, pp 273–293.
81. Dessauer M, Goetze U, Tolle R: Periodic sleep deprivation in drug-refractory depression. Neuropsychology 13:111–116, 1985.
82. Dowd PJ: Sleep deprivation effects on the vestibular habituation process. J Apply Psychol 59:748–752, 1974.
83. Drucker-Colin RR: Sleep deprivation: Effects on the EEG and on the blood of anticoagulant treated rats. Unpublished Doctoral Dissertation, University of Saskatchewan, 1971.
84. Drucker-Colin RR, Jaques LB, Winocur G: Anemia in sleep-deprived rats receiving anticoagulant. Science 174:505–507, 1971.
85. Duncan WC Jr, Gillin JC, Post RM, et al: Relationship between EEG sleep patterns and clinical improvement in depressed patients treated with sleep deprivation. Biol Psychiatry 15:879–889, 1980.
86. Edwards AS: Effects of the loss of one hundred hours of sleep. Am J Psychol 54:80–91, 1941.
87. Ellingson RJ, Wilken K, Bennett DR: Efficacy of sleep deprivation as an activation procedure in epilepsy patients. J Clin Neurophysiol 1:83–101, 1984.
88. Ellman SJ, Spielman AJ, Luck D, et al: REM deprivation: A review. In Arkin AM, et al (eds): The Mind in Sleep: Psychology and Psychophysiology. Hillsdale, NJ, Lawrence Erlbaum, 1978, pp 419–457.
89. Elsenga S, van den Hoofdakker RH: Clinical effects of several sleep/wake manipulations on endogenous depression. Sleep Res 12:326, 1983.

90. Elsenga S, Zulley J: Rectal temperature and depression during total sleep deprivation. Sleep Res 15:520, 1987.
91. Everson CA, Kushida CA, Bergmann BM, et al: Recovery from chronic sleep deprivation in the rat. Sleep Res 16:521, 1986.
92. Fahndrich E: Effects of sleep deprivation on depressed patients of different nosological groups. Psychiatry Res 5:277–285, 1981.
93. Fahndrich E: Effect of sleep deprivation as a predictor of treatment response to antidepressant medication. Acta Psychiatr Scand 68:341–344, 1983.
94. Fenz WD, Craig JG: Autonomic arousal and performance during sixty hours of sleep deprivation. Percept Mot Skills 34:543–553, 1972.
95. Fiorica V, Higgins EA, Iampietro PF, et al: Physiological responses of men during sleep deprivation. J Appl Physiol 24:167–176, 1968.
96. Fort A, Mills JM: Influence of sleep, lack of sleep, and circadian rhythms on short psychometric test. In Colquhoun WP (ed): Aspects of Human Efficiency. London, English Universities Press, 1972, pp 115–127.
97. Fortune RF: Sleep and muscular work. Aust J Psychol 4:36–40, 1926.
98. Frank G, Halberg F, Harner R, et al: Circadian periodicity, adrenal corticosteroids, and the EEG of normal man. J Psychiatr Res 4:73–86, 1966.
99. Friedman RC, Kornfeld DS, Bigger TJ: Psychological problems associated with sleep deprivation in interns. J Med Ed 48:436–441, 1973.
100. Friedmann J, Globus GG, Huntley A, et al: Performance and mood during and after gradual sleep reduction. Psychophysiology 14:245–250, 1977.
101. Froberg JE: Psychophysiological circadian rhythms: A literature review. WHO Tech Rep Ser 9:6, 1975.
102. Froberg JE: Twenty-four-hour patterns in human performance, subjective and physiological variables and differences between morning and evening active subjects. Biol Psychol 5:119–134, 1977.
103. Froberg J, Karlsson C-G, Levi L, Lidberg L: Circadian variations in performance, psychological ratings, catecholamine excretion, and diuresis during prolonged sleep deprivation. Int J Psychobiol 2:23–36, 1972.
104. Geller MR, Gourdji N, Christoff N, Fox E: The effects of sleep deprivation on the EEGs of epileptic children. Dev Med Child Neurol 11:771–776, 1969.
105. Gerner RH, Post RM, Gillin C, Bunney W Jr: Biological and behavioral effects of one night's sleep deprivation in depressed patients and normals. J Psychiatr Res 15:21–40, 1979.
106. Gillberg M, Akerstedt T: Sleep deprivation in normals: Some psychological and biochemical data from three studies. In Koella WP (ed): Sleep. Basel, Karger, 1980, pp 16–22.
107. Glaubman H, Orbach I: How healthy is "healthy insomnia"? Waking and Sleeping 1:395–399, 1977.
108. Hamilton P, Wilkinson RT, Edwards RS: A study of four days partial sleep deprivation. In Colquhoun WP (ed): Aspects of Human Efficiency. London, English Universities Press, 1972, pp 101–113.
109. Handbook of Human Engineering Data. Medford, MA, Tufts College, 1952.
110. Harris W, O'Hanlon JF: A study of recovery function in man. Technical Memorandum No. 10-72. U.S. Army Human Engineering Laboratories, MD, Aberdeen Proving Ground, April, 1972.
111. Haslam DR, Abraham P: Sleep loss and military performance. In Belenky G (ed): Contemporary Studies in Combat Psychiatry. Contributions in Military Studies Number 62, Westport, CT, Greenwood Press, 1987.
112. Hasselman M, Schaff G, Metz B: Respective influences of work, ambient temperature and sleep deprivation on urinary excretion of catecholamines of normal man. C R Soc Biol (Paris) 154:197–201, 1960.
113. Hendrick C, Lilly RS: The structure of mood: A comparison between sleep deprivation and normal wakefulness conditions. J Pers 38:453–465, 1970.
114. Hoddes E, Zarcone V, Smythe H, et al: Quantification of sleepiness: A new approach. Psychophysiology 10:431–436, 1973.
115. Holmboe J, Bell H, Norman N: Urinary excretion of catecholamines and steroids in military cadets exposed to prolonged stress. Swed J Def Med 11:183–191, 1975.
116. Horne JA: A review of the biological effects of total sleep deprivation in man. Biol Psychol 7:55–102, 1979.
117. Horne JA: Restitution and human sleep: A critical review. Physiol Psychol 7:115–125, 1979.
118. Horne JA: Why we sleep: The functions of sleep in humans and other mammals. Oxford, Oxford University Press, 1988.

119. Hoyt MF, Singer JL: Psychological effects of REM ("Dream") deprivation upon waking mentation. In Arkin AM, et al (eds): The Mind in Sleep: Psychology and Psychophysiology. Hillsdale, NJ, Lawrence Erlbaum, 1978, pp 487–510.
120. Husband RW: The comparative value of continuous versus interrupted sleep. J Exp Psychol 18:792–796, 1935.
121. Jimerson DC, Lynch HJ, Post RM, et al: Urinary melationin rhythms during sleep deprivation in depressed patients and normals. Life Sci 20:1501–1508, 1977.
122. Joffe R, Brown P: Clinical and biological correlates of sleep deprivation in depression. Can J Psychiatry 29:530–536, 1984.
123. Joffe R, Brown P, Bienenstock A, Mitton J: Neuroendocrine predictors of the antidepressant effect of partial sleep deprivation. Biol Psychiatry 19:347–352, 1984.
124. John MW: Factor analysis of subjectively reported sleep habit, and the nature of insomnia. Psychol Med 5:83–88, 1975.
125. Johnson LC, MacLeod WL: Sleep and awake behavior during gradual sleep reduction. Percept Mot Skills 36:87–97, 1973.
126. Johnson LC, Naitoh P, Lubin A, Moses J: Sleep stages and performance. In Colquhoun WP (ed): Aspects of Human Efficiency. London, English Universities Press, 1972, pp 81–100.
127. Johnson LC, Slye ES, Dement W: Electroencephalographic and atuonomic activity after prolonged sleep deprivation. Psychosom Med 27:415–423, 1965.
128. Jones HS, Oswald I: Two cases of healthy insomnia. Electroencephalogr Clin Neurophysiol 24:378–380, 1968.
129. Jovanovic UJ, Liebaldt GP, Muhl M, et al: Sleep deprivation and its symptoms. Arch Psychiatr Nervenkr 214:183–202, 1971.
130. Kales A, Tan T-L, Kollar EJ, et al: Sleep patterns following 205 hours of sleep deprivation. Psychosom Med 32:189–200, 1970.
131. Kamiya J: Behavioral, subjective and physiological aspects of drowsiness and sleep. In Fiske DW, Maddi SP (eds): Functions of Varied Experience. Homewood, IL, Dorsey, 1961, pp 145–174.
132. Kant GJ, Genser SG, Throne DR, et al: Effects of 72 hour sleep deprivation on urinary cortisol and indices of metabolism. Sleep 7:142–146, 1984.
133. Katz SE, Landis C: Psychological and physiologic phenomena during a prolonged vigil. Arch Neurol Psychiatry 34:307–316, 1935.
134. King D: Pathological and therapeutic consequences of sleep loss: A review. Dis Nerv Sys 38:873–879, 1977.
135. King D: Sleep deprivation therapy in depression syndromes. Psychosomatics 21:404–407, 1980.
136. King D, Dowdy S, Jack R, et al: The dexamethasone suppression test as a predictor of sleep deprivation antidepressant effect. Psychiatr Res 7:93–99, 1982.
137. Klein KE, Wegmann HM, Bruner H: Circadian rhythm in indices of human performance, physical fitness and stress reistance. Aerospace Med 39:512–518, 1968.
138. Kleitman N: Sleep and Wakefulness, 2nd ed. Chicago, University of Chicago Press, 1963.
139. Knowles J, Southmayd S, Delva N, et al: Sleep deprivation: Outcome of controlled single case studies of depressed patients. Can J Psychiatry 26:330–333, 1981.
140. Kolka MA, Stephenson LA: Exercise thermoregulation after prolonged wakefulness. J Appl Physiol 64:1575–1579, 1988.
141. Kollar EJ, Namerow N, Pasnau RO, Naitoh P: Neurological findings during prolonged sleep deprivation. Neurology 18:836–840, 1968.
142. Kollar EJ, Pasnau RO, Rubin RT, et al: Psychological, psychophysiological and biochemical correlates of prolonged sleep deprivation. Am J Psychiatry 126:488–497, 1969.
143. Kollar EJ, Slater GR, Palmer JO, et al: Stress in subjects undergoing sleep deprivation. Psychosom Med 28:101–113, 1966.
144. Koranyi EK, Lehmann HE: Experimental sleep deprivation in schizophrenic patients. Arch Gen Psychiatry 2:534–544, 1960.
145. Kripke DF, Simons RN, Garfinkel L, Hammond EC: Short and long sleep and sleeping pills. Is increased mortality associated? Arch Gen Psychiatry 36:103–116, 1979.
146. Kuhn E, Brodan V: Changes in the circadian rhythm of serum iron induced by a 5-day sleep deprivation. Eur J Appl Physiol 49:215–222, 1982.
147. Kuhn E, Brodan V, Brodanova M, Friedman B: Influence of sleep deprivation on iron metabolism. Science 213:1041–1042, 1967.
148. Kuhn E, Brodan V, Brodanova M, Rysanek K: Metabolic reflection on sleep deprivation. Act Nerv Super (Praha) 11:165–174, 1969.
149. Kuhn E, Brodan V, Valek J: Changes in the white blood cell count due to deprivation of sleep. Cas Lek Cesk 106:513–514, 1967.

150. Kuhn E, Rysanek K, Brodan V, Spankova H: Changes in blood tryptophan level during sleep deprivation. Experientia 32:1117, 1976.
151. Kuhn E, Rysanek K, Spankova H, et al: Changes in cyclic AMP and dopamine-beta-hydroxylase during sleep deprivation. Act Nerv Super (Praha) 17:257–259, 1975.
152. Kushida C, Bergmann B, Everson C, et al: Paradoxical sleep deprivation in the rat. I. Physiological effects. Sleep Res 13:191, 1984.
153. Kushida C, Bergmann B, Fang VS, et al: Physiological and biochemical effects of paradoxical sleep deprivation in the rat. Sleep Res 15:219, 1986.
154. Larsen JK, Lindberg ML, Skovaard B: Sleep deprivation as treatment for endogenous depression. Acta Psychiatr Scand 54:167–173, 1976.
155. Lebedun A, Bootzin RR: Differential effects of sleep deprivation on the recovery sleep of insomniacs and good sleepers. Sleep Res 15:142, 1986.
156. Legg SJ, Haslam DR: Effect of sleep deprivation on self-selected workload. Ergonomics 27:389–396, 1984.
157. Legg SJ, Patton JF: Effects of sustained manual work and partial sleep deprivation on muscular strength and endurance. Eur J Appl Physiol 56:64–68, 1987.
158. Levi L: Emotional stress and biochemical reactions as modified by psychotrophic drugs with particular reference to cardiovascular pathology. Proceedings of an International Symposium on Psychotropic Drugs in Internal Medicine. Excerpta Medica International Congress Series, No. 182, pp 206–220, 1968.
159. Levi L: Psychological and physiological reaction to and psychomotor performance during prolonged and complex stressor exposure. In Levi L (ed): Stress and Distress in Response to Psychosocial Stimuli. Oxford, Pergamon, 1972, pp 119–139.
160. Lewin I, Glaubman H: The effect of REM deprivation: Is it detrimental, beneficial, or neutral? Psychophysiology 12:349–353, 1975.
161. Lindemann R, Ekanger R, Opstad PK, et al: Hematological changes in normal men during prolonged severe exercise. Am Correct Ther J 37:107–111, 1978.
162. Lisper H-O, Kjellberg A: Effects of 24-hour sleep deprivation in rate of decrement in a 10-minute auditory reaction time task. J Exp Psychol 96:287–290, 1972.
163. Livrea P, di Reda L, Puca FM, et al: Homovanillic acid and 5-hydroxyindoleacetic acids in lumbar cerebrospinal fluid after total and REM sleep deprivation in humans. Eur Neurol 16:280–285, 1977.
164. Loveland NT, Williams HL: Adding, sleep loss, and body temperature. Percept Mot Skills 16:923–929, 1963.
165. Lovett-Doust JW, Christie H: Repeated sleep deprivation as a therapeutic zeitgeber for circular type manic depressive disturbance. Chronobiologia 7:505–511, 1980.
166. Luby ED, Frohman CE, Grisell JL, et al: Sleep deprivation: Effects on behavior, thinking, motor performance, and biological energy transfer systems. Psychosom Med 22:182–192, 1960.
167. Luby ED, Gottlieb JS: Sleep deprivation. In Arieti S (ed): American Handbook of Psychiatry, Vol. 3. New York, Basic Books, 1966, pp 406–419.
168. Luby ED, Grisell JL, Frohman CE, et al: Biochemical, psychological, and behavioral responses to sleep deprivation. Ann NY Acad Sci 96:71–79, 1962.
169. Lund PM: Marathon volleyball: Changes after 61 hours play. Br J Sports Med 19:228–229, 1985.
170. Malmo RB, Surwillo WW: Sleep deprivation changes in performances and physiological indicants of activation. Psychol Monogr 74(15), Whole No. 502, 1960.
171. Mangold R, Sokoloff L, Conner E, et al: The effects of sleep and lack of sleep on the cerebral circulation and metabolism of normal young men. J Clin Invest 34:1092–1100, 1955.
172. Martin BJ: Effect of sleep deprivation on tolerance of prolonged exercise. Eur J Appl Physiol 47:345–354, 1981.
173. Martin BJ: Sleep deprivation and exercise. Exerc Sport Sci Rev 14:213–229, 1986.
174. Martin BJ, Bender PR, Chen H: Stress hormonal response to exercise after sleep loss. Eur J Appl Physiol 55:210–214, 1986.
175. Martin BJ, Chen HI: Sleep loss and the sympathoadrenal response to exercise. Med Sci Sports Exerc 16:56–59, 1984.
176. Martin BJ, Haney R: Self-selected exercise intensity is unchanged by sleep loss. Eur J Appl Physiol 49:79–86, 1982.
177. Mattson RH, Pratt KL, Calverley JR: Electroencephalograms of epileptics following sleep deprivation. Arch Neurol 13:310–315, 1965.
178. Matussek N, Ackenheil M, Athen D, et al: Catecholamine metabolism under sleep deprivation therapy of improved and not improved depressed patients. Pharmakopsychiatrie 7:108–114, 1974.

179. McMurray RG, Brown CF: The effect of sleep loss on high intensity exercise and recovery. Aviat Space Environ Med 55:1031–1035, 1984.
180. Meddis R: The Sleep Instinct. London, Routledge and Kegan Paul, 1977.
181. Meddis R, Pearson AJS, Langford G: An extreme case of healthy insomnia. Electroencephalogr Clin Neurophysiol 35:213–214, 1973.
182. Miles WR, Laslett HR: Eye movement and visual fixation during profound sleepiness. Psychol Rev 38:1–13, 1931.
183. Mirsky AF, Cardon P: A comparison of the behavioral and physiological changes accompanying sleep deprivation and chlorpromazine administration in man. Electroencephalogr Clin Neurophysiol 14:1–10, 1962.
184. Molaie M, Cruz A: The effect of sleep deprivation on the rate of focal interictal epileptiform discharges. Electroencephalogr Clin Neurophysiol 70:288–292, 1988.
185. Moldofsky H, Davidson JR, Lue FA: Sleep-related patterns of plasma growth hormone and cortisol following 40 hours of wakefulness. Sleep Res 17:69, 1988.
186. Moldofsky H, Lue FA, Davidson JR, Gorczynski R: The effect of 40 hours of wakefulness on immune functions in humans. II. Interleukins-1 & -2-like activities. Sleep Res 17:34, 1988.
187. Moldofsky H, Lue FA, Saskin P, et al: The effect of sleep deprivation on immune functions in humans. I. Mitogen and natural killer cell activities. Sleep Res 16:531, 1987.
188. Morgan BB Jr: Effects of continuous work and sleep loss in the reduction and recovery of work efficiency. Am Ind Hyg Assoc J 35:13–20, 1974.
189. Morris GO, Williams HL, Lubin A: Misperception and disorientation during sleep deprivation. Arch Gen Psychiatry 2:247–254, 1960.
190. Murawski BJ, Grabbe J: Effect of sleep deprivation on plasma 17-hydroxycortocoids. J Appl Physiol 15:280–282, 1960.
191. Murray EJ: Conflict and repression during sleep deprivation. J Abnorm Soc Psychol 59:95–101, 1959.
192. Murray EJ: Sleep, Dreams, and Arousal. New York, Appleton-Century-Crofts, 1965.
193. Murray EJ: Sleep deprivation and personality adjustment. In Abt LE, Riess BF (eds): Progress in Clinical Psychology, Vol. 8. New York, Grune and Stratton, 1968, pp 44–62.
194. Murray EJ, Schein EH, Erikson KJ, et al: The effects of sleep on social behavior. J Soc Psychol 49:229–236, 1959.
195. Murray EJ, Williams HL, Lubin A: Body temperature and psychological ratings during sleep deprivation. J Exp Psychol 56:271–273, 1958.
196. Myles WS: Sleep deprivation, physical fatigue and the perception of exercise intensity. Med Sci Sports Exerc 17:580–584, 1985.
197. Naitoh P: Sleep deprivation in humans. In Venables PE, Christie MJ (eds): Research Psychophysiology. New York, John Wiley, 1975, pp 153–180.
198. Naitoh P: Sleep deprivation in human subjects: A reappraisal. Waking and Sleeping 1:53–60, 1976.
199. Naitoh P: Circadian cycles and restorative powers of naps. In Johnson LC, Tepas DI, Colquhoun WP, Colligan MJ (eds): Biological Rhythms, Sleep and Shiftwork. Advances in Sleep Research, Vol. 7. New York, Spectrum, 1981, pp 553–580.
200. Naitoh P: Chronopsychological approach for optimizing human performance. In Brown FM, Graeber RC (eds): Rhythmic Aspects of Behavior. Hillsdale, NJ, Lawrence Erlbaum, 1982.
201. Naitoh P, Dement WC: Sleep deprivation in humans. In Remond A (ed-in-chief): Handbook of Electroencephalography and Clinical Neurophysiology, Vol. 7. Amsterdam, Elsevier, 1975, pp 7A46–7A51.
202. Naitoh P, Kales A, Kollar EJ, et al: Electroencephalographic changes after prolonged sleep loss. Electroencephalogr Clin Neurophysiol 27:2–11, 1969.
203. Naitoh P, Pasnau RO, Kollar EJ: Psychophysiological changes after prolonged deprivation of sleep. Biol Psychiatry 3:309–320, 1971.
204. Naitoh P, Townsend RE: The role of sleep deprivation research in human factors. Hum Factors 12:575–585, 1970.
205. Nakazawa Y, Kotorii M, Ohshima M, Haruzawa H: Changes in sleep pattern after sleep deprivation. Folia Psychiatr Neurol Jpn 32:85–93, 1978.
206. Nowlis V: Research with the mood adjective checklist. In Tomkins SS, Izard CE (eds): Affect, Cognition and Personality. New York, Springer, 1965, pp 352–389.
207. Oektedalen O, Flaten O, Opstad PK, Myren J: hPP and gastrin response to a liquid meal and oral glucose during prolonged severe exercise, caloric deficit, and sleep deprivation. Scand J Gastroenterol 17:619–624, 1982.

208. Oektedalen O, Opstad PK, Fahrenkrug J, Fonnum F: Plasma concentration of vasoactive intestinal polypeptide during prolonged physical exercise, calorie supply deficiency, and sleep deprivation. Scand J Gastroenterol 18:1957–1062, 1983.
209. Opstad PK, Aakvaag A: The effect of a high calorie diet on hormonal changes in young men during prolonged physical strain and sleep deprivation. Eur J Appl Physiol 46:31–39, 1981.
210. Opstad PK, Aakvaag A: Decreased serum levels of oestradiol, testosterone and prolactin during prolonged physical strain and sleep deprivation and the influence of high calorie diet. Eur J Appl Physiol 49:343–348, 1982.
211. Opstad PK, Aakvaag A: The effect of sleep deprivation on the plasma levels of hormones during prolonged physical strain and calorie deficiency. Eur J Appl Physiol 51:97–107, 1983.
212. Opstad PK, Aakvaag A, Rognum TO: Altered hormonal response to short-term bicycle exercise in young men after prolonged physical strain, caloric deficit, and sleep deprivation. Eur J Appl Physiol 45:51–62, 1980.
213. Opstad PK, Ekanger R, Nummestad M, Raabe N: Performance, mood and clinical symptoms in men exposed to prolonged, severe physical work and sleep deprivation. Aviat Space Environ Med 49:1065–1073, 1978.
214. Opstad PK, Falch D, Oektedalen O, et al: The thyroid function in young men during prolonged exercise and the effect of energy and sleep deprivation. Clin Endocrinol 20:657–669, 1984.
215. Opstad PK, Oektedalen O, Aakvaag A, et al: Plasma renin activity and serum aldosterone during prolonged physical strain: The significance of sleep and energy deprivation. Eur J Appl Physiol 54:1–6, 1985.
216. Orlee HD, Corbin B, Dugger G, Smith C: An evaluation of the effects of bed rest, sleep deprivation and discontinuing of training on the physical fitness of highly trained young men. NASA-CR-134044.N73-32008. Washington, D.C., NASA, 1973.
217. Oswald I: Human brain protein, drugs and dreams. Nature 223:893–897, 1969.
218. Pai MN: Searchlight on sleep disorders. London, Literary Services and Production, 1969.
219. Palmblad JEW: Stress-related modulation of immunity: A review of human studies. Cancer Detect Prev 1(suppl):57–64, 1987.
220. Palmblad J, Akerstedt T, Froberg J, et al: Thyroid and adrenomedullary reaction during sleep deprivation. Acta Endocrinol (Copenh) 90:233–239, 1979.
221. Palmblad J, Cantell K, Strander H, et al: Stressor exposure and immunological response in man: Interferon producing capacity and phagocytosis. J Psychosom Res 20:193–199, 1976.
222. Palmblad J, Petrini B, Wasserman J, Akerstedt T: Lymphocyte and granulocyte reactions during sleep deprivation. Psychosom Med 41:273–278, 1979.
223. Parker DC, Rossman LG, Pekary AE, Hershman JM: Effect of 64-hour sleep deprivation on the circadian waveform of thyrotropin (TSH): Further evidence of sleep-related inhibition of TSH release. J Clin Endocrinol Metab 64:157–161, 1987.
224. Pasnau RO, Naitoh P, Stier S, Kollar EJ: The psychological effects of 205 hours of sleep deprivation. Arch Gen Psychiatry 18:496–505, 1968.
225. Patrick GTW, Gilbert JA: on the effects of loss of sleep. Psychol Rev 3:469–483, 1986.
226. Paul A: Effects of sleep deprivation on visual function. Aerospace Med 36:617–620, 1965.
227. Pearson RG, Byars GE: The development of validation of a checklist for measuring subjective fatigue. Report No. 56–115. San Antonio, U.S. Air Force School of Aerospace Medicine, 1956.
228. Pflug B: Therapeutic aspects of sleep deprivation. In Koella WP, Levin P (eds): Sleep. Basel, Karger, 1973, pp 185–191.
229. Pflug B, Tolle R: Disturbance of the 24-hour rhythm in endogenous depression and the treatment of endogenous depression by sleep deprivation. Int Pharmacopsychiatry 6:187–196, 1971.
230. Phillips B, Cooper KR, Newsome HH, Dewey WL: Effect of sleep loss on beta-endorphin activity, epinephrine levels, and ventilatory responsiveness. South Med J 80:16–20, 1987.
231. Pickett G, Morris A: Effects of acute sleep and food deprivation on total body response time and cardiovascular performance. J Sports Med Phys Fitness 15:49–56, 1975.
232. Pieron G: The Physiological Problem of Sleep. Paris, Masson, 1913.
233. Plyley MJ, Shephard RJ, Davis GM, Goode RC: Sleep deprivation and cardiorespiratory function: Influence of intermittent submaximal exercise. Eur J Appl Physiol 56:338–344, 1987.
234. Poley GE, Shively CA, Vesell ES: Diurnal rhythms of aminopyrine metabolism: Failure of sleep deprivation to affect them. Clin Pharmacol Ther 24:726–732, 1978.
235. Post RM, Kotin J, Goodwin FK: Effects of sleep deprivation on mood and central amine metabolism in depressed patients. Arch Gen Psychiatry 33:627–632, 1976.

236. Pratt KL, Mattson RH, Weikers NJ, Williams R: EEG activation of epileptics following sleep deprivation: A prospective study of 114 cases. Electroencephalogr Clin Neurophysiol 24:11–15, 1967.
237. Rakestraw NW, Whittier FO: The effect of loss of sleep on the composition of the blood and urine. Proc Soc Exp Biol Med 21:5–6, 1923.
238. Rechtschaffen A: The control of sleep. In Hunt WA (ed): Human Behavior and Its Control. Cambridge, MA, Schenkman, 1971, pp 75–92.
239. Rechtschaffen A, Bergmann BM, Everson CA, et al: Sleep deprivation in the rat. X. Integration and discussion of the findings. Sleep 12:68–87, 1989.
240. Rechtshaffen A, Gilliland MA, Bergmann BM, Winter JB: Physiological correlates of prolonged sleep deprivation in rats. Science 221:182–184, 1983.
241. Rechtschaffen A, Kales A: A manual of standardized terminology, techniques and scoring system for sleep stages of human subjects. Public Health Service, National Institutes of Health publication no. 204, 1968.
242. Remes K, Kuoppasalmi K, Adlercreutz H: Effect of physical exercise and sleep deprivation on plasma androgen levels: Modifying effect of physical fitness. Int J Sports Med 6:131–135, 1985.
243. Reynolds CF III, Kupfer DJ, Hoch CC, et al: Sleep deprivation effects in older endogenous depressed patients. Psychiatr Res 21:95–109, 1987.
244. Richardson GS, Carskadon MA, Flagg W, et al: Excessive daytime sleepiness in man: Multiple sleep latency measurement in narcoleptic and control subjects. Electroencephalogr Clin Neurophysiol 45:621–627, 1978.
245. Ringer C: Psychological and physiological parameters of circadian periodicity in sleep deprivation. Medical dissertation, Ludwig Maximillians-Universitat zu Munchen, 1972.
246. Robinson ES, Herman SO: Effects of loss of sleep. I. J Exp Psychol 5:19–32, 1922.
247. Robinson ES, Richardson-Robinson F: Effects of loss of sleep. II. J Exp Psychol 5:93–100, 1922.
248. Rodin EA, Luby ED, Gottlieb JS: The electroencephalogram during prolonged experimental sleep deprivation. Electroencephalogr Clin Neurophysiol 14:544–551, 1962.
249. Rognum TO, Rodahl K, Opstad PK: Regional differences in the lipolytic response of the subcutaneous fat deposits to prolonged exercise and severe energy deficiency. Eur J Appl Physiol 4:401–408, 1982.
250. Rognum TO, Vaage O, Hostmark A, Opstad PK: Metabolic responses to bicycle exercise after several days of physical work and energy deficiency. Scand J Lab Invest 41:565–571, 1981.
251. Rognum TO, Vartdal F, Rodahl K, et al: Physical and mental performance of soldiers on high- and low-energy diets during prolonged heavy exercise combined with sleep deprivation. Ergonomics 29:859–867, 1986.
252. Rubin RT, Kollar E, Slater GG, Clark BR: Excretion of 17-hydroxycorticosteroids an vanillylmandelic acid during 205 hours of sleep deprivation in man. Psychosom Med 31:68–79, 1969.
253. Rudolf GA, Tolle R: Circadian rhythm of circulatory function in depressives and on sleep deprivation. Int Pharmacopsychiatry 12:174–183, 1977.
254. Rudolf GA, Tolle R: Sleep deprivation and circadian rhythm in depression. Psychiatr Clin (Basel) 11:198–212, 1978.
255. Rutenfranz J, Aschoff J, Mann H: The effects of a cumulative sleep deficit, duration of preceding sleep period and body-temperature on multiple choice reaction time task. In Colquhoun WP (ed): Aspects of Human Efficiency. London, English Universities Press, 1972, pp 217–229.
256. Safer DJ: The effect of LSD on sleep-deprived men. Psychopharmacology (Berlin) 17:414–424, 1970.
257. Safer DJ: the concomitant effects of mild sleep loss and an anticholinergic drug. Psychopharmacology (Berlin) 17:425–433, 1970.
258. Saito Y: Specification of variation patterns of physiological and performance measurements in sleep loss. J Hum Ergol (Tokyo) 1:207–216, 1972.
259. Salin-Pascual RJ, Ortega-Soto H, Huerto-Delgadillo L, et al: The effect of total sleep deprivation on plasma melatonin and cortisol in healthy human volunteers. Sleep 11:362–369, 1988.
260. Sawka MN, Gonzales RR, Pandolf KB: Effects of sleep deprivation on thermoregulation during exercise. Am J Physiol 246:R72–R77, 1984.
261. Schachter S: The interaction of cognitive and physiological determinants of emotional state. In Berkowitz L (ed): Advances in Experimental Social Psychology. New York, Academic Press, 1964, pp 49–80.

262. Schachter S, Singer JE: Cognitive, social and physiological determinants of emotional state. Psychol Rev 69:379–399, 1962.
263. Schiffman PL, Trontell MC, Mazar MF, Endelman NH: Sleep deprivation decreases ventilatory response to CO_2 but not load compensation. Chest 84:695–698, 1983.
264. Schilgen B, Tolle R: Partial sleep deprivation as therapy for depression. Arch Gen Psychiatry 37:267–271, 1980.
265. Schmocker M, Baumann P, Reyero F, Heinemann H: Sleep deprivation: A clinical, psychophysiological and biochemical study. Arch Psychiatr Nervenkr 221:111–122, 1975.
266. Scholander I: The effects of moderate sleep deprivation on the habituation of autonomic response elements. Acta Physiol Scand 51:325–342, 1961.
267. Schwarz JR, Zangemeister WH: The diagnostic value of the short sleep and other provocative methods following sleep deprivation. J Neurol 218:179–186, 1978.
268. Scollo-Lavizzari G, Pralle W, de la Cruz N: Activation effects of sleep deprivation and sleep in seizure patients. Eur Neurol 13:1–5, 1975.
269. Scollo-Lavizzari G, Scollo-Lavizzsari GR: Sleep, sleep deprivation, photosensitivity and epilepsy. Eur Neurol 11:1–21, 1974.
270. Scrimshaw NS, Habicht JP, Pellet P, et al: Effects of sleep deprivation and reversal of diurnal activity on protein metabolism of young men. Am J Clin Nutr 19:313–319, 1966.
271. Shapiro CM, Trinder J: Hormone release after sleep deprivation. J Physiol (Lond) 325:54P–55P, 1982.
272. Sleep deprivation and mental health. Editorial. JAMA 204:166, 1968.
273. Smith M: A contribution to the study of fatigue. Br J Psychol 8:327–350, 1916.
274. Soule RG, Goldman RF: Pacing of intermittent work during 31 hours. Med Sci Sports 5:128–131, 1973.
275. Southmayd SE, Cairns J, Brunet DG: Antidepressant response to sleep deprivation in relation to psychophysiologically defined wakefulness. Sleep Res 16:538, 1987.
276. Southmayd SE, Cairns J, Brunet D, Delva N: Spectral analysis of baseline sleep in depressed patients: Relation to outcome of sleep deprivation and the "S-deficiency hypothesis." Sleep Res 16:537, 1987.
277. Spadetta V: Deprivation of sleep in the electroencephalographic diagnosis of epilepsy. Acta Neurol (Napoli) 26:7–13, 1971.
278. Stack JA, Reynolds CF, Hoch CC, et al: Effects of sleep deprivation in the treatment of elderly endogenous depressives. Sleep Res 15:221, 1986.
279. Steinberg H, Guggenheim F, Baer L, Snyder F: Catecholamines and their metabolites in various states of "arousal." J Psychosom Res 13:103–108, 1969.
280. Strausbaugh LJ, Roessler R: Ego strength, skin conductance, sleep deprivation, and performance. Percept Mot Skills 31:671–677, 1970.
281. Stuss D, Broughton R: Extreme short sleep: Personality profiles and a case study of sleep requirement. Waking and Sleeping 2:101–105, 1978.
282. Svendsen K: Sleep deprivation therapy in depression. Acta Psychiatr Scand 54:184–192, 1976.
283. Symons JD, Vanhelder T, Myles WS: Physical performance and physiological responses following 60 hours of sleep deprivation. Med Sci Sports Exerc 20:374–380, 1988.
284. Takeuchi L, Davis GM, Plyley M, et al: Sleep deprivation, chronic exercise and muscular performance. Ergonomics 28:591–601, 1985.
285. Taub JM: Effects of habitual variations in napping on psychomotor performance, memory and subjective states. Int J Neurosci 9:97–112, 1979.
286. Taub JM, Berger RJ: Performance and mood following variations in the length and timing of sleep. Psychophysiology 10:559–570, 1973.
287. Teichner WH: Interaction of behavioral and physiological stress reactions. Psychol Rev 75:271–291, 1968.
288. Thayer RE: Measurement of activation through self-report. Psychol Rep 20:663–678, 1967.
289. Todor JI: Changes in depth perception during a non-stop walk of 302¼ miles. Percept Mot Skills 40:762, 1975.
290. Torsvall L, Akerstedt T: Extreme sleepiness: Quantification of EOG and spectral EEG parameters. Int J Neurosci 38:435–441, 1988.
291. Toru M, Shibuya H, Shimazono Y: Monoamine metabolism in rat brain after total sleep deprivation. In Weitzman ED (ed): Advances in Sleep Research, Vol. 2. New York, Spectrum, 1976, pp 116–130.
292. Tyler DB: The effect of amphetamine sulphate and some barbiturates on the fatigue produced by prolonged wakefulness. Am J Physiol 149:253–262, 1947.

293. Tyler DB: Psychological changes during experimental sleep deprivation. Dis Nerv Sys 16:293–299, 1955.
294. Tyler DB, Goodman J, Rothman T: The effect of experimental insomnia on the rate of potential changes in the brain. Am J Physiol 149:185–193, 1947.
295. Tyler DB, Marx W, Goodman T: Effect of prolonged wakefulness on the rate of urinary excretion of 17-ketosteroids. Proc Soc Exp Biol Med 62:38–40, 1946.
296. Van den Burg W, van den Hoofdakker RH: Total sleep deprivation on endogenous depression. Arch Gen Psychiatry 32:1121–1125, 1975.
297. Van Helder T, Symons JD, Radomski MW: Effects of sleep deprivation and exercise on glucose tolerance and insulin sensitivity. Submitted for publication.
298. Vein AM, Dallakyan IG, Levin YAI, Shakun KE: Physiological and psychological consequences of single sleep deprivation. Hum Physiol 8:392–396, 1983.
299. Vestergaard P, Bojer B, Kleist N: Prolactin response to sleep deprivation. In Schou M, Stromgren E (eds): Origin, Prevention and Treatment of Affective Disorders. London, Academic Press, 1979, pp 179–183.
300. Vidnes A, Opstad PK: Serum ferritin in young men during prolonged heavy physical exercise. Scand J Haematol 27:165–170, 1981.
301. Vogel GW: A review of REM sleep deprivation. Arch Gen Psychiatry 32:749–761, 1975.
302. Vogel GW: A motivational function of REM sleep. In Drucker-Colin R, et al (eds): The Functions of Sleep. New York, Academic Press, 1979, pp 233–250.
303. Vogel GW: Evidence for REM sleep deprivation as the mechanism of action of antidepressant drugs. Prog Neuro-Psychopharmacol Biol Psychiatry 7:343–349, 1983.
304. Vogel GW: REM sleep deprivation and depression. In Chase M, Weitzman ED (eds): Sleep Disorders: Basic and Clinical Research. New York: Spectrum, 1983, pp 393–400.
305. Vogel GW, Thompson F Jr, Thurmond A, Rivers B: The effect of REM deprivation on depression. Psychosomatics 14:104–107, 1973.
306. Vogel GW, Thurmond A, Gibbons P, et al: REM sleep reduction effects on depression syndromes. Arch Gen Psychiatry 32:765–777, 1975.
307. Vogel GW, Vogel F, McAbee RS, Thurmond AJ: Improvement of depression by REM sleep deprivation: New findings and a theory. Arch Gen Psychiatry 37:247–253, 1980.
308. Vojtechovsky M, Hort, V, Krus D, Simane Z, Brezinova V: The effect of centrophenoxine in sleep deprived subjects. Med Psicosom 13:1–12, 1968.
309. Vojtechovsky M, Hort V, Krus D, Skala J: Sleep deprivation in alcoholics. In Bertini M (ed): Psicofisiologia del sonno e del sogno. Milan, Editrice Vita e Pensiero, 1970, pp 232–240.
310. Vojtechovsky M, Hort V, Simane Z, et al: The influence of centrophenoxine (Lucidril) on the course of sleep deprivation in alcoholics. Act Nerv Super (Praha) 11:193–201, 1969.
311. Vondra K, Brodan V, Bass A, et al: Effects of sleep deprivation on the activity of selected metabolic enzymes in skeletal muscle. Eur J Appl Physiol 47:41–46, 1981.
312. Warren N, Clark B: Blocking in mental and motor tasks during a 65-hour vigil. J Exp Psychol 21:97–105, 1937.
313. Webb WB: Theories of sleep functions and some clinical implications. In Drucker-Colin R, et al (eds): The Functions of Sleep. New York, Academic Press, 1979, pp 19–35.
314. Webb WB, Agnew HW Jr: Sleep deprivation, age, and exhaustion time in the rat. Science 136:1122, 1962.
315. Webb WB, Agnew HW Jr: The effects of chronic limitation of sleep length. Psychophysiology 11:265–274, 1974.
316. Wehr TA, Rosenthal NE, Sack DA, Gillin JC: Antidepressant effects of sleep deprivation in bright and dim light. Acta Psychiatr Scand 72:161–165, 1985.
317. Wehr TA, Sack DA, Rosenthal NE: Antidepressant effects of sleep deprivation and phototherapy. Acta Psychiatr Belg 85:593–602, 1985.
318. Welch LK, Stevens JB: Clinical value of the electroencephalogram following sleep deprivation. Aerospace Med 61:349–351, 1971.
319. West LJ, Janszen HH, Lester BK, Cornelison FS: The psychosis of sleep deprivation. Ann NY Acad Sci 96:66–70, 1962.
320. White DP, Douglas NJ, Pickett CK, et al: Sleep deprivation and the control of ventilation. Am Rev Respir Dis 128:984–986, 1983.
321. White RM: The lengths of sleep. Abstr. JSAS Catalog of Selected Documents in Psychology, MS No. 1001, 5:274, 1975.
322. Wilkinson RT: Interaction of lack of sleep with knowledge of results, repeated testing, and individual differences. J Exp Psychol 62:263–271, 1961.

323. Wilkinson RT: Effect of up to 60 hours of sleep deprivation on different types of work. Ergonomics 7:175–186, 1964.
324. Wilkinson RT: Sleep deprivation. In Edholm OG, Bachrach AL (eds): The Physiology of Human Survival. New York, Academic Press, 1965, pp 399–430.
325. Wilkinson RT: Sleep deprivation: Performance tests for partial and selective sleep deprivation. In Abt LA, Riess BF (eds): Progress in Clinical Psychology. New York, Grune and Stratton, 1968, pp 28–43.
326. Wilkinson RT, Edwards RS, Haines E: Performance following a night of reduced sleep. Psychosom Sci 5:471–472, 1966.
327. Williams HL, Lubin A, Goodnow JJ: Impaired performance with acute sleep loss. Psychol Monogr 73(#14):1–26 (Whole No. 484), 1959.
328. Wolfe JW, Brown JH: Effects of sleep deprivation on the vestibulo-ocular reflex. Aerospace Med 39:947–949, 1968.
329. Wu JC, Buchsbaum MS, Gillin JC: Positron emission tomography study of sleep deprivation. Sleep Res 16:543, 1987.
330. Wu JC, Gillin C, Buchsbaum MS, et al: Regional cortical metabolism after sleep deprivation. Sleep Res 17:32, 1988.
331. Wyatt RJ, Fram DH, Kupfer DJ, Snyder F: Total prolonged drug-induced REM sleep suppression in anxious-depressed patients. Arch Gen Psychiatry 24:145–155, 1971.
332. Yamaguchi N, Maeda K, Kuromaru S: The effects of sleep deprivation on the circadian rhythm of plasma cortisol levels in depressive patients. Folia Psychiatr Neurol Jpn 32:479–487, 1978.
333. Yamasaki S: The effects of prolonged severe physical activities with food and water restriction and sleep deprivation on the total body water and psychological-physiological performance. Jpn J Aerospace Environ Med 24:47–57, 1987.
334. Yeager JE, Crisman RP, Sucec AA: The effect of sleep deprivation and moderate intermittent exercise on maximal aerobic capacity. Naval Health Research Center Report No. 86-36. San Diego, Naval Health Research Center, 1986.
335. Young DR, Pelligra R, Shapira J, et al: Glucose oxidation and replacement during prolonged exercise in man. J Am Physiol 23:734–741, 1967.
336. Zander KJ, Lorenz A, Wahllander B, et al: Biogenesis of the antidepressive effect of sleep deprivation. In Koella WP (ed): Sleep 1980. Basel, Karger, 1981, pp 9–15.

MICHAEL H. SMOLENSKY, PhD
ALAIN REINBERG, MD, PhD

CLINICAL CHRONOBIOLOGY: RELEVANCE AND APPLICATIONS TO THE PRACTICE OF OCCUPATIONAL MEDICINE

From the University of Texas
Health Science Center at Houston
School of Public Health
Graduate School of Biomedical Sciences
Medical School
and
Center for Medical and Public Health Chronobiology
Houston, Texas
and
Fondation A. de Rothschild
Paris, France

Reprint requests to:
Michael H. Smolensky, PhD
The University of Texas
Health Science Center at Houston
School of Public Health
P.O. Box 20186
Houston, TX 77225

Clinical medicine has developed in the tradition of homeostatic theory, which purports constancy of the *milieu interne*. In the United States and other countries of the world, the education of biologists and medical practitioners is based on this tenet. Even today, there is little or no time devoted to the teaching of chronobiology. This has many important ramifications on the philosophy and practice of clinical as well as occupational medicine. For example, in clinical medicine it is assumed that the time during the day or year when diagnostic procedures are conducted or when mechanisms underlying disease processes are researched is unimportant. Also, the time when medications are dosed, such as in the morning versus the evening, is viewed as an inconsequential influence on their pharmacokinetics and pharmacodynamics. In industrial medicine, it is assumed the biological time when exposure to workplace contaminants occurs is insignificant. Furthermore, investigations of the epidemiology and mechanisms of occupationally induced diseases are conducted without consideration of possible rhythm-dependencies.

The majority of our knowledge concerning medicine is based on the results of experiments conducted during the daytime, at the convenience of investigators. Typically, research is initiated by diurnally active scientists in the morning so their task can be completed by the end of the regular work day. Except for studies pertaining to the electrophysiology and/or disorders of sleep, very little is known about the biology of human beings during the nighttime hours. It has only been during the past two to three decades, in particular, that more comprehensive, around-the-clock investigations on laboratory animals and human beings have demonstrated that bodily processes and functions are precisely organized not only in *space* as a physical anatomy but in *time* as a biological time structure expressed as rhythms of specific cycle durations with precise stage relationships.

The purpose of this chapter is several-fold. One is to discuss the relevance of our biological time structure to clinical medicine. For example, the occurrence and/or exacerbation of human illnesses as well as the safety and efficacy of medications used in their treatment exhibit strong biological rhythm-dependencies. A second major concern of this writing is the application of chronobiologic methods to industrial medicine to achieve a better appreciation of the susceptibility/resistance of workers to potentially noxious contaminants as well as the epidemiology of occupationally related illnesses. As a foundation for addressing these as well as other important issues, however, it is necessary that the basic concepts and principles of human and medical chronobiology first be presented.

CHRONOBIOLOGY: DEFINITIONS AND CONCEPTS

Chronobiology is that branch of science dealing with the study of biological rhythms and their mechanisms.[1–3] Bioperiodicities are ubiquitous in nature. From an evolutionary perspective, they represent an aspect of the genetic adaptation of ancestral beings to predictable changes in time in the external environment resulting, for example, from the regular rotation of the earth about its axis once every 24 hours and also about the sun once each year.[1,4] Although human bioperiodicities have a genetic basis, their expression may be influenced by certain other factors, including health status, age, and environmental factors, among others.[5–8]

In plants, insects, lower animals, and human beings, the properties and features of bioperiodicities are quite similar.[1,2,9,10] All biological rhythms can be described by their oscillatory frequency. **Circadian** rhythms exhibit one cycle roughly *(circa)* per 24 hours *(dian).* Oscillations of shorter duration, such as the 60- to 90-minute temporal variability in the secretion of hormones from endocrine glands or in sleep-stage progression during rest, are termed **ultradian** (more than 1 cycle per 24-hour period) rhythms. Finally, oscillations that are longer than 24 hours, such as those of 7, 28 to 30, and 365 days are termed **infradian** (less than 1 cycle per 24 hours) rhythms. In actuality, ultradian, circadian, and infradian rhythms coexist at all levels of organization and constitute one aspect of the biological time structure of life forms.

A second feature of rhythms is **staging**, which refers to the occurrence of the peak and trough of bioperiodicities with respect to a given time scale, such as that of the 24 hours, month (menstrual cycle), or year. Within each biological time domain there exists a precise relationship between the staging of each and every one of the multitude of rhythmic processes and functions. This represents a second important attribute of our biological time structure.[1,11] The staging of circadian rhythms is organized efficiently to support the predictable-in-time variation in energy expenditure associated with the differential metabolic requirements of activity versus sleep. Although the temporal alternation of activity and rest during each 24 hours is not the origin of circadian rhythms, when according to clock time a person sleeps and is active does determine their staging.[12] Thus, individuals who consistently work dayshifts and sleep nights exhibit a nearly opposite staging, with reference to clock time, of their circadian functions as compared to those who consistently work nightshifts and sleep during the day.[11] In human beings, environmental light and social interaction during the activity span alternating with darkness and sleep during the rest span serve as powerful **synchronizers** of circadian bioclocks and the biological time structure.[1,11,13,14] With reference to this discussion, a synchronizer is a factor (or set of factors) that acts as a time cue, thereby influencing the staging and/or period length of biological rhythms and the biological time structure, per se.

The synchronization schedule of human beings may be ascertained from knowledge of the clock times of activity and sleep during the 24 hours and the nature of the work routine—regular day or rotating shiftwork. This information is critical for correctly applying findings from research in medical chronobiology. In the majority of human beings, the resetting of biological clocks following an abrupt change in the sleep-activity schedule is not immediate; instead several, as many as 4–10, days may be required for their complete resetting.[11,15] This fact is especially apparent to travelers rapidly transported by jet aircraft over several time zones as well as to rotating shiftworkers whose normal nocturnal sleep period is suddenly disrupted when changed from day to night work. In both situations, a "jet-lag" type of phenomenon is experienced.[16,17] The more formal term for jet lag is **desynchronosis.** It represents a transient disruption of the precise phase relationships between biological rhythms, especially circadian ones, as well as the biological time structure. Often, this condition results in some decrement of cognitive performance and loss of biological efficiency during the phase of the adjustment to the new or altered synchronizer schedule.[16,17]

A third feature of biological rhythms is **amplitude**. The amplitude refers to the extent of the predictable variability over a given time-scale that is ascribable to rhythmicity. It is numerically equal to the difference between the values found at the time of the peak and trough of a given bioperiodicity. Some rhythms are of relatively small amplitude. This is the case for the circadian variation in body temperature and heart rate in healthy persons. Other circadian rhythms are of quite high amplitude. This is exemplified by the 24-hour pattern in serum cortisol or adrenalin concentration and lymphocyte numbers. Finally, a fourth characteristic of rhythms is **level**, the baseline around which predictable-in-time variation occurs.

Changes in health status and aging may lead to alteration in the features of biological rhythms. For example, the amplitude and/or level of the circadian rhythm in airways patency typically differs between asthmatic and nonasthmatic persons and between young and elderly individuals.[7] In asthma patients, generally the amplitude of the 24-hour bioperiodicity is markedly enhanced and the mean level lowered in comparison to age- and gender-matched controls having normal lung function. In patients suffering from hypertension, both the 24-hour mean level and amplitude of the rhythm in blood pressure may be increased over the reference values of healthy persons.[18,19] Deterioration in environmental quality often results in an alteration in the level, amplitude, and peak time of circadian rhythms of airways status.[8,20] These points will be addressed in further detail later in this chapter.

BIOLOGICAL RHYTHMS AND DISEASE

Since bodily functions and processes are precisely organized in time as rhythms, it is not surprising that temporal patterns exist in which the symptoms

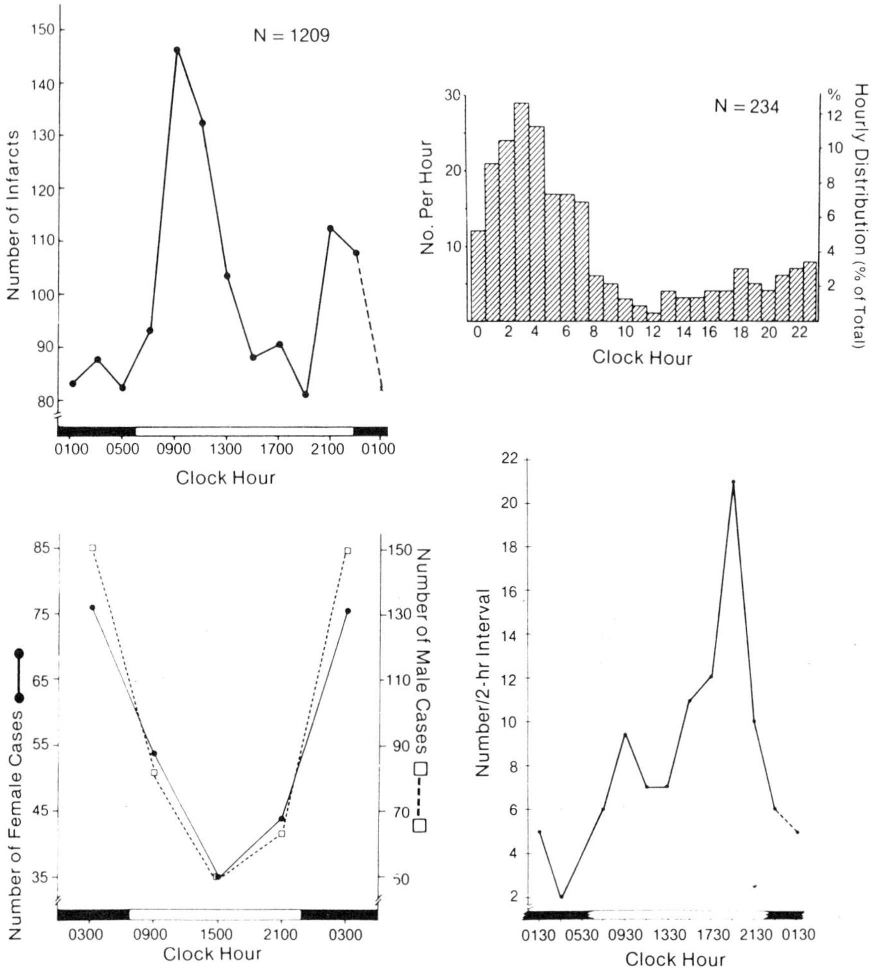

FIGURE 1. Examples of human circadian chronopathologies using diseases of the cardiovascular system: the occurrence of myocardial infarction (upper left), cerebral infarction (lower left), ST-segment anomaly of Prinzmetal's variant angina (upper right), and spontaneous intracerebral hemorrhage (lower right) is not random over the 24 hours. (From Smolensky and D'Alonzo, 1988,[22] with permission.)

of diseases worsen or morbid events are manifested. A branch of chronobiology, referred to as chronopathology, is concerned with the predictable-in-time alterations in the pathophysiology and the manifestations of illnesses and symptoms.[1] Certain chronopathologies can only be demonstrated through population studies. This is the case, for example, for myocardial and cerebrovascular infarction, as well as cerebral hemorrhage,[1,19,21,22] whose occurrence in a given individual may be limited, generally, to but one or two events per lifetime (Fig. 1). In contrast, the symptoms of chronic diseases tend to be recurrent in patients. Temporal patterns thus can be tracked by means of patient diaries or self-assessments done several times daily. In this manner, circadian patterns have been substantiated in the symptoms of rheumatoid arthritis (with pain and stiffness typically worse at the commencement of daily activity), osteoarthritis (with pain generally worse toward the end of daily activity), Prinzmetal's variant angina (with ST segment anomaly most frequent overnight and exercise capability most limited in the morning), allergic rhinitis (with stuffy and blocked nose worse typically upon awaking), and asthma (with exacerbation of wheezing or coughing during the usual sleep span), among others.[1,21-26] The occurrence and exacerbation of some illnesses may exhibit also, in women, menstrual rhythms (e.g., epilepsy and asthma) and, in both men and women, seasonal rhythms (e.g., asthma and cardiovascular disease).[1] Seasonal patterns in the incidence of disease, however, may represent changes in weather over the year rather than **circannual** (about 1-year) endogenous-in-origin rhythms in physiochemical status, although this remains to be substantiated.

When biological rhythms are exhibited in the occurrence or exacerbation of human illnesses, frequently the question arises as to whether they result from cyclic variation in ambient conditions and/or from rhythms in related biological processes. For example, asthmatic patients show a high-amplitude circadian rhythm in airways patency and dyspnea (Fig. 2). In such patients, the peak expiratory flow (PEF) may exhibit a circadian variation of 25% or more in airways status during the 24 hours.[7,27] This rhythm can be demonstrated even in

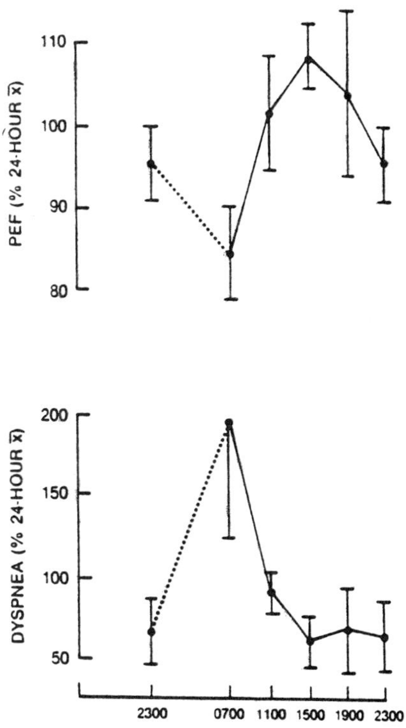

FIGURE 2. Circadian variation of PEF (peak expiratory flow—a measure of airways patency) and dyspnea in 13 diurnally active (sleep, ~ 11 p.m. to 7. a.m.) untreated asthmatics. Dyspnea is self-rated as greatest upon arising at 7 a.m. and least at 3 p.m. The 24-hour pattern of PEF is 12 hours out of phase with that of dyspnea. PEF is lowest at 7 a.m. and greatest at 3 p.m. The data of each graph were plotted as percentages (means and standard errors) from the 24-hour average set equal to 100%. (Redrawn from Reinberg et al.[27])

asthma patients housed in antigen and/or pollution-shielded environments.[28] In day-active patients, asthma tends to be a nocturnal event, with the symptoms most common between 11 p.m. and 5 a.m.[29] The nighttime susceptibility of patients to asthma arises from the staging of several key circadian functions and processes that influence or control airways caliber. For example, the urine and blood levels of anti-inflammatory hormones—adrenal corticosteroids (serum cortisol and urinary 17-hydroxycorticosteroids) and catecholamines (noradrenalin, adrenalin, and vanillylmandelic acid, VMA)—are at their minimum overnight.[7] Also the airways, as does the skin,[30] exhibit high-amplitude circadian rhythmicity in reactivity. Heightened susceptibility of the airways to antigens such as house dust and to the nonspecific chemical irritants of histamine and acetylcholine is manifested late in the evening and overnight.[7] This type of information helps explain why diurnally active asthma patients become worse overnight. It also indicates that rhythmic variations in one's physiology may sometimes be equally or even more important than aspects of the ambient environment in explaining the cyclic nature of certain human illnesses and also in defining their etiology.

The significance of the sleep-wake cycle as a synchronizer of the 24-hour patterns in illness has been particularly documented in studies on asthmatic as well as epileptic patients.[1,31–33] For the purpose of this discussion, the example of the temporal pattern in overt seizures by an epileptic individual engaged in shiftwork is cited (Fig. 3). When working during the daytime and active between 6 a.m. and 9 p.m., seizures were most commonly experienced after awakening, primarily between 7:30 a.m. and 7:30 p.m. After alteration of the sleep-activity routine to accommodate nighttime work, there was a change in the clock hours when symptoms were most frequent; symptoms then became most common between 12 p.m. and 7 p.m. However, with reference to the sleep-activity schedule of the individual, the occurrence of seizure activity was always most frequent during the hours immediately following the termination of the sleep span, whether scheduled at night or during the daytime.

Information pertaining to circadian and other rhythms in the symptoms of disease is important for several reasons. First, practitioners can better treat illness through an understanding of the chronopathology of each. Second, more appropriate steps may be taken to minimize or avert the occurrence of disease or the exacerbation of existing conditions. Third, such information can be utilized by physicians to determine if a disease might be occupationally induced. For example, a frequent difficulty of some workers employed in certain industries is occupationally induced recurrent nocturnal asthma.[34] Patients experiencing this disorder quite often exhibit marked circadian patterns in the status of their airway function. Figure 4 presents an example of circadian changes in airways patency of an individual suffering from occupationally induced nocturnal asthma.[35] It is readily apparent that in this day-active person a brief controlled exposure to the offending antigen during the morning around 10 a.m. of the test (T) day resulted initially in only a small immediate effect on airways patency as assessed by the $FEV_{1.0}$. About 12 hours later, around midnight, well after the single brief morning exposure, the effect was fully manifested. In fact, it was only at night, for several subsequent 24-hour spans, that the asthmatic condition severely worsened, even without any further exposure to the antigen. This so-called late or nonimmediate reaction, as it is commonly termed, most probably is dependent on the circadian organization of underlying bioprocesses, as well as on specific, nonrhythmic, but nonetheless time-related events.

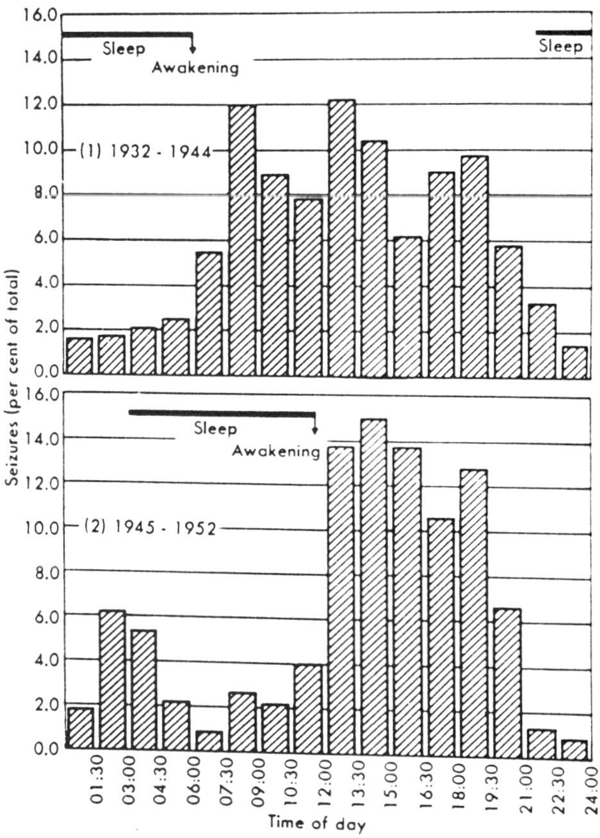

FIGURE 3. Circadian pattern in the initiation of epileptic seizures in one patient studied longitudinally over several years while residing in an institution. The temporal distribution with regard to the clock hour of the seizures changed following transfer to a different work-rest pattern when the sleep schedule was delayed from one of 9 p.m.–6 a.m. to 3 a.m.–11 a.m. Clock time along the horizontal axis is given in military fashion, for example, 1500 = 3 p.m.; 2100 = 9 p.m. (From Halberg and Howard, 1958,[33] with permission.)

Occupationally induced recurrent nocturnal asthma is not uncommon. It is often observed in day-working employees of several different industries, including those who work with wood, plastics, resins, grains, and pharmaceuticals.[34] The example cited in Figure 4 illustrates the fact that susceptible workers who are exposed to offending substances during daytime work need not manifest significant symptoms until much later (for example, in the case of dayworkers during the night). It illustrates also that the symptoms can reoccur again, not necessarily during the day while at work, but during the several consecutive nights even without further exposures. This example also serves to illustrate the fact that epidemiologic studies of occupationally induced disease need to take into account rhythmic variation in the manifestations or occurrences of disease. Quite often, patients and physicians do not associate the etiology of certain diseases with employment when complaints occur many hours after leaving the workplace. This appears to be especially true for occupationally induced asthma,

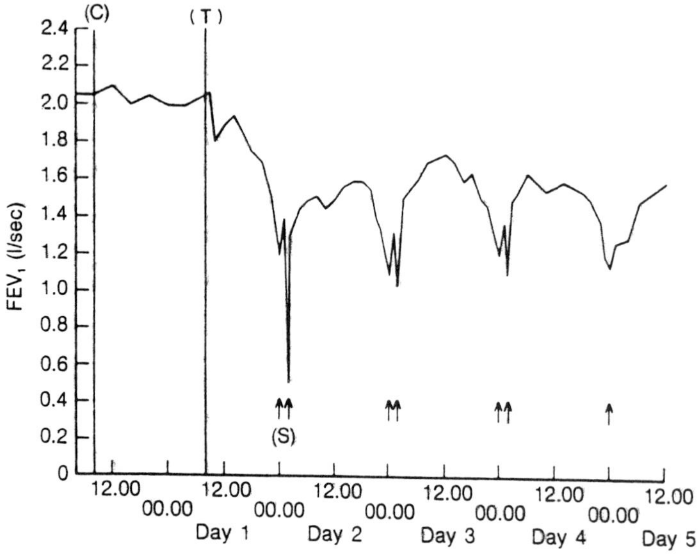

FIGURE 4. Recurrent nocturnal episodes of asthma in one person displaying hypersensitivity to budgerigar serum resulting from employment in pigeon breeding. Following a single morning (~ 10:30 a.m.) exposure to the antigen, severe nocturnal dyspnea recurred during four successive nights, always around midnight; during the daytime, the airway patency, measured by the FEV_1, was near normal. (S = salbuterol, a bronchodilator treatment to reverse airways obstruction). (From Taylor et al., 1979,[35] with permission.)

for which the interval between daytime exposure at work and the manifestation of the nighttime illness at home can be quite lengthy. It is possible that a similar phenomenon may exist for allergen-induced dermatoses. Late reactions have been demonstrated not only in clinical and research settings, but also in workers exposed to agents which provoke cutaneous reactions.[36]

Bioperiodicities in the symptom intensity and morbidity of human diseases define so-called **susceptibility-resistance rhythms** in individuals.[1,37] This means that with reference to the circadian time structure, there are spans during the 24 hours when there exists a heightened vulnerability to the expression of disease, whereas 12 hours earlier or later there exists reduced vulnerability or resistance to such. These susceptibility-resistance rhythms arise from bioperiodicities in contributory component processes and functions constituting the mechanisms of the given disease. The nocturnal exacerbation of asthma in day-active patients is but one example of a circadian susceptibility-resistance rhythm. The nighttime prevalence of symptoms is due to the specific staging of several 24-hour component bioperiodicities in biochemical and physiologic processes. These include rhythms in airways patency, adrenalin, and cortisol, in addition to an airways hyperreactivity to chemical mediators (histamine and acetylcholine) and antigens (house dust). Cyclic variation in environmental quality also has to be considered in the etiology of nocturnal asthma.[7] In industry, shift-related differences in the occurrence of medical complaints might represent the influence of susceptibility-resistance rhythms on the physiologic tolerance of workers exposed to specific agents. In the clinic, circadian and other temporal patterns in the susceptibility of predisposed persons to the breakthrough of disease and/or their exacerbation suggest varying-in-time requirements for medication, as discussed below.

THE CHRONOPHARMACOLOGY AND CHRONOTHERAPEUTICS OF MEDICATIONS

With consideration of homeostatic teachings, the kinetics and effects of medicines and other types of chemical agents are assumed to be the same, independent of the time of their dosing or exposure. However, numerous studies on laboratory animals and human beings dispute this assumption.[1,22,38] Spurred by findings from investigations on medications, a revised set of concepts concerning the kinetics and dynamics of chemical agents has been developed in recent years.[1,38,39] Indeed, a new field of science, **chronopharmacology**, has emerged. Chronopharmacology is defined as the study of biological rhythm-influences on medications and also the effect of medications on the features of biological time structure.[1,39] Several new concepts about the behavior of medications, for example, have been realized from chronopharmacologic studies. First, **chronopharmacokinetics** (or chronokinetics) refers to administration-time-dependent differences in the absorption, distribution, metabolism, and elimination of chemical agents due to rhythms in biological functions and processes.[1,39,40] Second, **chronesthesy** refers to rhythms in the susceptibility of target tissues to given medications.[1,39] Finally, **chronotherapeutics** is the dosing of medications with reference to biological rhythms to optimize their beneficial effects and/or control undesired ones.[1,22,39] Results of a very large number of investigations indicate that the pharmacokinetics and/or the effects of various classes of medications differ, sometimes markedly, as a function of their administration time, e.g., morning, midday, or evening.[1,40] This is the case for certain sustained-release theophyllines (especially in children),[41] and nonsteroidal anti-inflammatory,[42] antihistamine,[43] cardiovascular,[21] and synthetic corticosteroid[44] drugs, among others.[45] The chronokinetics of medications do not arise from meal-time and content effects on given dosage forms or from day-night alteration in one's posture. Instead, they result from bioperiodic (e.g., 24-hour) processes and functionings of specific organ-systems of the body.[46]

Chronopharmacology is concerned not only with biological rhythm-dependent influences on drug pharmacokinetics but on their pharmacodynamics as well, whether the effects be desired (in terms of chronoeffectiveness) or undesired (in terms of chronotoxicology) ones.[1,39] The ultimate goal of chronopharmacologic research is applied chronotherapeutics, the scheduling of medications in relation to biological rhythms to enhance desired effects and/or control or avert undesired ones. Chronotherapeutics is especially warranted under the following circumstances[22]:

1. when the risk of symptoms or disease is known to vary rhythmically;
2. when the therapeutic window for a given medication is narrow relative to the potential for drug-induced toxicity or if drug-induced toxicity is dose limiting;
3. when the drug kinetics and/or effects are administration-time-dependent;
4. when the goal of hormonal substitution therapy is to simulate the temporal patterns observed in normal persons; and
5. when the drug effect is achievable only by a time-modulated treatment program.

Thus far, in the United States and Europe, chronotherapies have been devised and practiced for several classes of medications. These include: (1) the suppertime or before-bedtime once-daily dosing of H_2-receptor antagonist medications to control the nocturnal surge of gastric acid secretion in ulcer patients,[47] (2) the once-a-day, evening dosing of controlled-release theophylline and beta-agonist formulations for patients suffering from nocturnal symptoms of asthma,[48] (3) the once-daily morning or alternate-day synthetic corticosteroid schedules for the treatment of inflammatory diseases,[49] (4) the evening administration of nonsteroid anti-inflammatory drugs (NSAIDs) for the control of morning symptoms of rheumatoid arthritis and midday/afternoon administration of NSAIDs for the clinical management of the manifestations of osteoarthritis,[42] and (5) the pulsatile (at 60–90-minute intervals) administration of gonadotrophin hormone analogues to treat hypothalamic amenorrhea,[50] to mention but a few.[38] Although the medical community may be aware of and use such schedules for the cited medications, the rationale for their timings (i.e., biological rhythm requirements) generally has not been widely advertised to practitioners.

BIOLOGICAL RHYTHMS AND THE RESPONSE TO TOXIC SUBSTANCES

As with medications, the response to workplace chemicals may be dependent not only upon dose, but the biological time (with regard to circadian rhythmic processes) of the exposure. Chronobiologic studies on rodents conducted primarily during the 1960s revealed that the effects of many chemical agents differ in the intensity of acute toxicity depending upon the time of exposure with respect to circadian and even circannual rhythms. F. Halberg[51] initially referred to this phenomenon as the "hours of diminished resistance." Chronobiologists term the study of temporal patterns in the response of life forms to toxic substances as **chronotoxicology.**

It has become quite clear that the acute and chronic toxicity of a variety of chemicals can be strongly influenced by the time of an animal's exposure, as shown by many investigators.[52] The results of the most common and fundamental test to evaluate toxicity, the LD_{50}, can be dramatically affected by rhythmic processes (Fig. 5). In certain instances, their effect may be so great that the LD_{50} may vary by one or two orders of magnitude. In addition, more subtle indicators of toxicity, such as the concentrations of serum liver enzymes as well as tests of behavioral toxicity, also may vary depending on the exposure or dosing time.[53] Other types of toxicity tests can be affected by biological rhythms as well. These include ones pertaining to teratogenicity, target organ toxicity, mutagenicity, and carcinogenicity.[52]

Clearly, circadian changes within the cells of the target organ and/or in the metabolism of chemical agents give rise to the observed circadian differences. For example, the duration of hexobarbital sodium-induced sleep in rodents (Fig. 6) is markedly influenced by circadian rhythms. The occurrence of longest hexobarbital-induced sleep duration at 2 p.m. coincides with the trough of the circadian rhythm of hepatic hexobarbital oxidase, the enzyme responsible for the metabolism of hexobarbital sodium. The occurrence of shortest hexobarbital sleep duration at 10 p.m. coincides with greatest liver levels of the enzyme.[54] It has been shown through a vast number of studies that the subcellular organelles that are responsible for the manufacture or elaboration of enzymes involved in metabolism and detoxification are circadian rhythmic.[53]

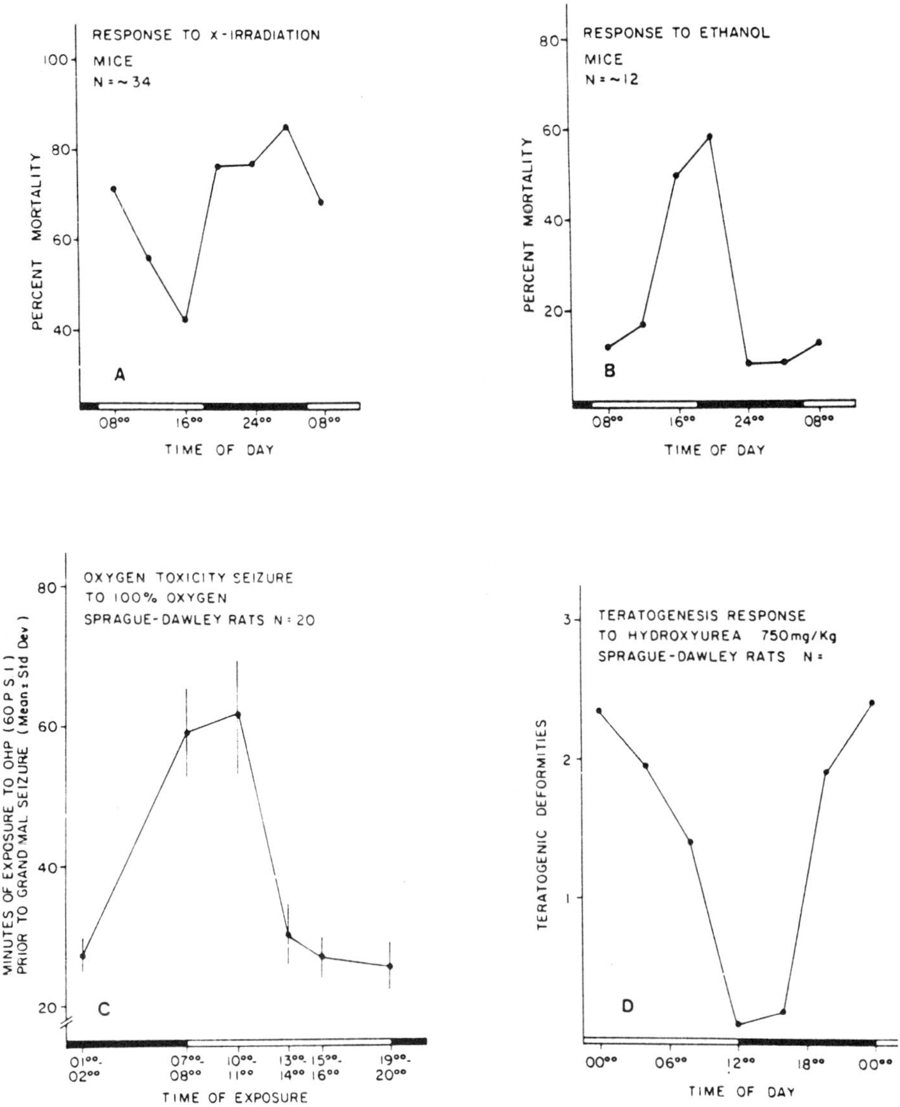

FIGURE 5. Circadian-susceptibility rhythm of rodents. *A,* mortality from whole body x-irradiation exposure; *B,* mortality from ethanol overdosing; *C,* seizures due to oxygen toxicity; and *D,* teratogenesis from hydroxyurea. The susceptibility to each type of exposure is markedly circadian rhythmic. Shaded portion of horizontal axis indicates the timing of darkness and activity for the nocturnally active rodents. (From Smolensky et al., 1985,[52] with permission.)

It is assumed that in the same person the effect produced by a given concentration of a chemical agent will be more or less the same independent of the time of its administration. This assumption may not be valid, as demonstrated by rodent studies. The differential effect of chemical toxicants as a function of their timing may result from bioperiodicities primarily related to receptor sites,

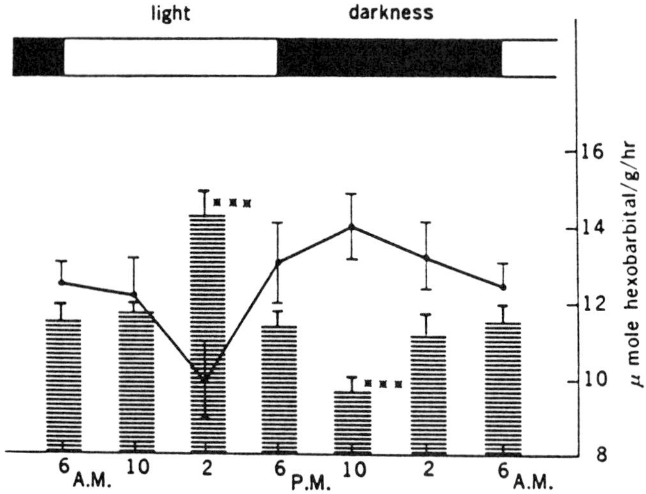

FIGURE 6. Circadian variation in the duration of hexobarbital-induced sleep (vertical bars) compared to the circadian changes in hepatic hexobarbital oxidase activity (solid line). The duration of induced sleep at each clock hour of study represents the average of 6 to 10 animals. Hexobarbital sodium (150 mg/kg) was given intraperitoneally. The enzyme activity is expressed as micromoles of hexobarbital metabolized per gram of tissue per hour; each datum represents the mean of six to eight animals. The shorter vertical lines represent the standard errors; the triple asterisks (***) = $p < 0.001$. The timing of highest and lowest hexobarbital oxidase activity at 10 and 2 p.m., respectively, coincides with shortest and longest hexobarbital-induced sleep. (Redrawn from Nair, 1974.[54])

enzyme activity, and metabolic processes.[1,38,39,52] One example of a circadian susceptibility-resistance rhythm in human beings is the response of the airways of asthmatic, emphysemic, or bronchitic persons to histamine at various times during the day or night. In these types of patients the airways exhibit a marked hyperreactivity to a variety of chemical agents, including histamine, resulting in an increased resistance to airflow in the airways. DeVries and his colleagues[55] demonstrated large variation during the 24 hours in the threshold concentration of histamine required to provoke a 20% alteration of airways status as assessed by the $FEV_{1.0}$. The airways of diurnally active persons are least susceptible around noontime and are most susceptible around midnight. The difference in the threshold concentration between the times of greatest and lowest reactivity can be as great as 100% or more. This phenomenon can be demonstrated also for other types of challenges to the airways, as shown in Figure 7.[56-58] The cutaneous response to histamine and specific antigens also exhibits rather marked circadian (Fig. 8) as well as menstrual cycle variability.[30,59] These findings suggest that persons with small or large airways disease or with cutaneous sensitivities who are employed in shiftwork involving exposure to irritant or antigenic matter may experience more reactivity and provocation during one shift (most likely the evening or night shift) in comparison to another. In other words, a given concentration of a chemical or irritant that may be rather well tolerated during the day shift may not be tolerated when encountered during the night shift.

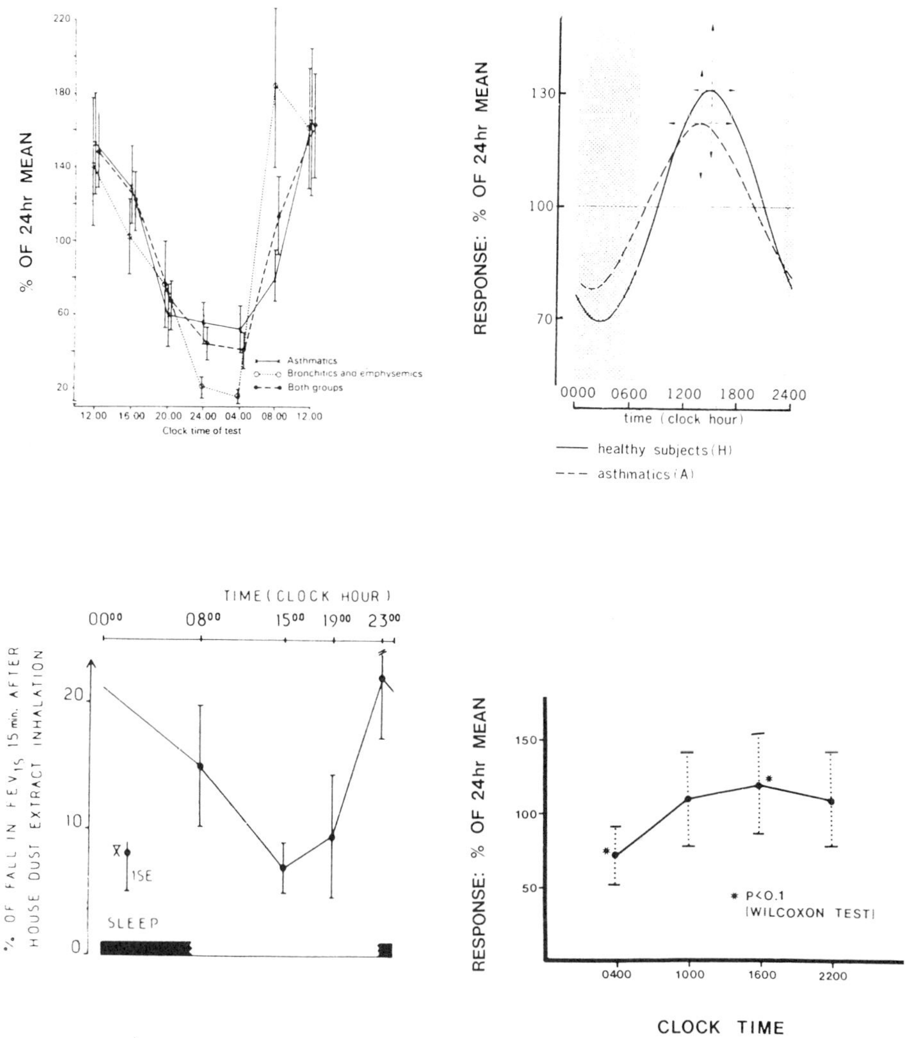

FIGURE 7. Circadian rhythm in airways reactivity to aerosols of histamine, acetylcholine, or house dust, and to hyperventilation of cold air in asthma or other day-active COPD patients. *A,* For histamine, the variation over the 24 hours in the threshold concentration required to induce 20% change in FEV_1 at each time of testing is plotted as relative values normalized to the group mean. *B,* For acetylcholine, the variation over the 24 hours in the threshold concentration required to induce 15% change in FEV_1 is plotted as relative values normalized to the group mean. *C,* For house dust, the data represent the before and after test-time change in FEV_1 from a standardized antigen challenge. *D,* For the cold air challenge, the 24-hour variation in the before-after change in the airways response to cold air is plotted. Except for the cold air challenge, when the airways were more affected by the 4 p.m. in comparison to the 4 a.m. test, the airways were most reactive (to acetylcholine, histamine, and house dust) during the evening and overnight. (Data from several reports.[55–58])

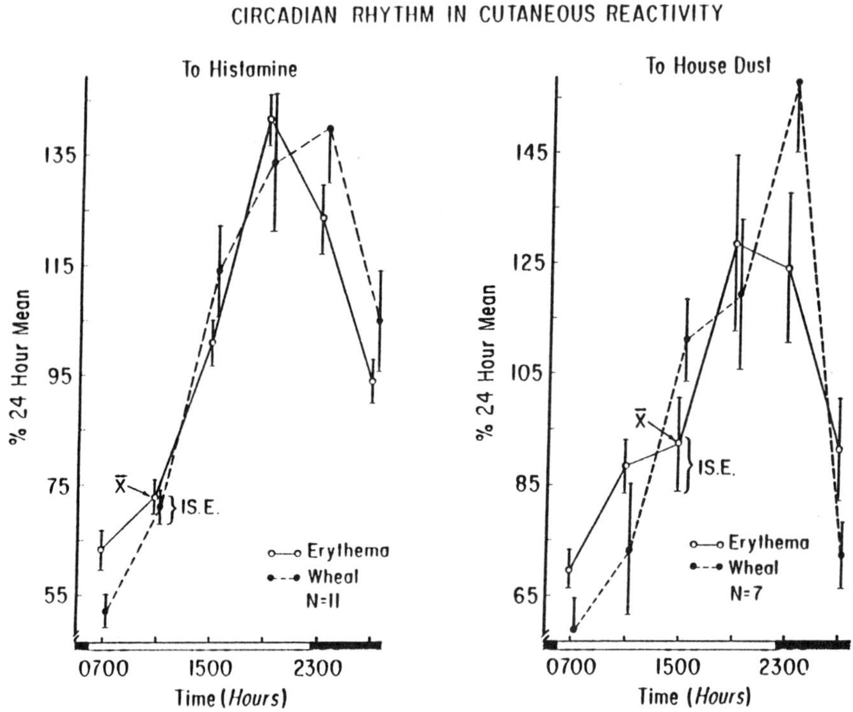

FIGURE 8. Cutaneous reactivity to histamine and house dust is markedly circadian rhythmic. The data are plotted as values expressed relative to the 24-hour mean set equal to 100%. Greatest cutaneous reactivity to histamine or house dust occurs between 7 p.m. (1900) and 11 p.m. (2300) and lowest in the morning at the start of the activity span. Light and shaded portions of the abscissa correspond to spans of activity and rest, respectively, for the individuals. (From McGovern et al., 1977,[30] with permission.)

In summary, based on results of chronobiologic studies conducted on laboratory animals, circadian and other period differences in the effects of toxic and tumor-inducing chemicals are to be expected. Although such rhythms have been rather well documented in laboratory animal studies, they have yet to be seriously evaluated in working populations.

CHRONOBIOLOGIC ASPECTS OF BIOLOGICAL MONITORING

The fact that all human functions are rhythmic (with respect to the 24-hour span, for example) has important implications for the manner in which biological monitoring is conducted and how findings are interpreted. Typically, biological assessments or samplings are done on employees immediately before and after the workshift or at nonspecific times during it. If measurements are gathered without respect to the influence of the circadian time structure, differences in values (e.g., before and after the workshift) may more represent the variation due to the amplitude of circadian rhythms than the effects of workplace exposures and activities, per se. It is possible that the data may be erroneously interpreted; the results of biological sampling can be not only indicative of the effect of exposure to workplace contaminants but the influence of bioperiodicities in the assessed variables. This is especially true when the monitored variable exhibits a large circadian amplitude. Even in clinical situations, circadian variation in certain blood and urinary variables can be so large that failure to take it into account may result in misleading findings and, perhaps, incorrect interpretations of laboratory tests.[52,60] In order to more effectively interpret findings and better conduct biological sampling, chronobiologists recommend the use of so-called time-qualified (with regard to biological rhythms) reference values as well as other techniques, such as repeated self-assessments of indicator variables.[60]

Time-Qualified Reference Values. Physicians and clinical pathologists have begun to realize that for certain functions the time *when* blood or urine samplings are done or *when* biological measurements are conducted can dramatically influence the findings of tests. In recognition of this, Haus and colleagues[60] have devised a large set of circadian time-qualified references for evaluating and interpreting hematological and other variables of clinical interest. Time-qualified references are very useful in clinical medicine (Fig. 9) and are potentially important in occupational medicine as well. They are useful for the interpretation of data obtained from preplacement as well as periodic medical re-examinations of employees and for the purpose of medical screenings and monitorings, for example in checking the status of white and red cell populations in workers at risk for such occupationally induced alterations.

Use of the time-qualified references requires knowledge of two critical pieces of information: (1) the synchronizing sleep-activity schedule of the person and (2) the timing, with regard to clock hours, of when the blood or other biological

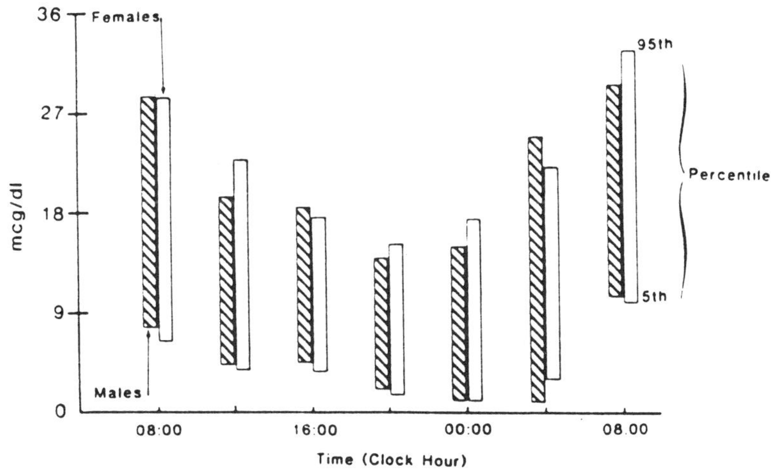

FIGURE 9. An example of time-qualified reference value system—the variable of plasma cortisol—for diurnally active healthy persons. Other such time-qualified references have been obtained for many other meaningful variables. A value of 3μg/dl from a sample of blood drawn at 0800 (8 a.m.) from a diurnally active worker is outside the appropriate time-qualified range of normal values at this time. The same value, however, found for a blood sample drawn at 8 p.m. (2000) is within this (8 p.m.) time-qualified normal range. (From Haus et al., 1988,[60] with permission.)

sample or measurement was obtained. In the case of urine samples, information on the time of its collection as well as the time of the previous voiding is needed in order to determine for what span the sampling is representative. Information on synchronizer schedule is easily obtainable by simply questioning the worker, for example, about the usual clock hour he or she goes to bed as well as awakening. Time-qualified references are directly useful for studies on permanent day as well as night workers, whose rhythms are not periodically subjected to shifts in their staging due to the alteration of their rest-activity routine. In the case of permanent night workers, however, the time-qualified ranges must be used in a special manner. Instead of referencing the time-qualified ranges according to clock hour time, they need to be referenced instead in terms of the hours after either the middle or end of the worker's usual sleep, whether it be scheduled during the night or daytime. Because the rhythms of rotating shiftworkers undergo shifts when moving from day to night work, time-qualified reference values are only useful when the circadian time structure has completed its adjustment to an alteration in the sleep-activity synchronizer schedule. This usually entails a span of several days for those involved in 7-day or longer rotas.

Biological Monitoring and Autorhythmometry. Biological monitoring has been a controversial topic in industry, to organized labor, and in occupational medicine. There are a myriad of difficulties associated with the accurate collection and assay of samples, the proper interpretation of findings, and thereafter selection and installation of interventions. Nonetheless, the advantages of biologic monitoring tend to outweigh the difficulties; thus, it is recommended for those situations wherein the health status of workers requires continued monitoring or intolerance needs to be identified in a quantitative manner.

Certain methods used in human chronobiology investigations appear to have application for the conduct of biological monitoring in industry. One of these is referred to as autorhythmometry. Autorhythmometry is the self-measurement of pertinent biological functions several times daily, usually at regular intervals, during waking for several consecutive days, with the data thus obtained analyzed and quantified for rhythms.[61] It can be used to investigate or monitor specific health functions or indicators on a more or less continuous basis or at set intervals, such as throughout the first and last days of each shift rotation. This methodology in the past has been used in many ways. Autorhythmometry has been used to study and screen blood pressure in children and adults, evaluate airways patency in asthmatic persons, quantitatively assay the irritant effects of air pollutants in the workplace and in the community, and to evaluate the biological rhythm-dependent effects of medications.[1,8,62–64] Autorhythmometry also has been used to intensively study various chronobiologic aspects of shiftwork in employees of certain industries. In particular, autorhythmometry has been extensively utilized to assess the changes in biological time structure of rotating shiftworkers in field as well as in laboratory settings.[11,65] It has been utilized recently, also, to investigate the chronobiology of shiftwork intolerance.[52,66,67]

In some industrial surveys, self-assessment of airways status has been achieved using portable peak flow meters; for example, in employees exposed to fumes of soldering fluxes and toluene diisocyanate. In particular, Gervais et al.[68] have used autorhythmometry to detect the occupationally induced airways hypersensitivity of one worker to CrO_3. Table 1 shows the findings for this worker, who monitored his peak expiratory flow (PEF) 4 to 5 times daily for

TABLE 1. Autorhythmometry Method. Changes in the 24-hour Mean PEF Related to CrO_3 Exposure of a Chromium-plating Worker*

Activity (Situation)	Autorhythmometry Month	(No. of Days)	PEF Circadian Mean in l/min ± 1 SE	P Value (Vacation vs. Work Each Span)
Work (1)	July	(5)	394 ± 20	< .02
Work (2)	July	(5)	396 ± 22	< .05
Vacation (3)	August	(9)	464 ± 15	—
Work (4)	September	(7)	394 ± 18	< .01

*A male (38-years-old) working in a chromium-plating industry (4 yrs), suffering from dyspnea and/or asthma for 3 yrs. Skin tests and bronchial challenge to Cr were inconclusive. PEF (peak expiratory flow—an indication of airways patency) self-measurements were done at fixed clock hours (8 a.m., 11 a.m., 3 p.m., 7 p.m. and 11 p.m.) for 5 to 9 days, both when working during the day (situations 1, 2 and 4) and when on vacation (situation 3) in a rural area. With reference to values obtained in the latter situation, a statistically significant fall in the 24-hour mean PEF occurred when this man was exposed to CrO_3. (From Gervais et al., 1979,[68] with permission.)

several consecutive days during specified spans of work or vacation. PEF is a direct measurement of airways patency; the lower the flow, the lower the patency. It is clear that values of the PEF measurements made during the work weeks were different from those made during vacation. The 24-hour PEF mean, which was consistent in value from one work span to another, was reduced in a statistically significant manner in comparison to that representative of the vacation time. In this example, the self-assessment of the PEF confirms for the employee in question that work in a CrO_3 environment is associated with a statistically significant reduction in airways status.

SHIFTWORK, SLEEP-WAKE SCHEDULES, AND CIRCADIAN-RHYTHM ADJUSTMENTS

Persons who work rotating shift schedules that necessitate nighttime hours must periodically alter their sleep-activity pattern in order to accommodate their job. Although the number of hours worked per week may remain unchanged, the clock-time of sleep and activities varies significantly. Similarly, travelers and airline crews who are rapidly transferred across several time zones face the same situation—a resulting alteration in the sleep-activity pattern relative to the clock time at home. A major alteration in the sleep-activity pattern lasting for at least 2 or 3 days represents a significant change in synchronizer schedule and necessitates compensatory adjustment of the circadian time structure.

The biological rhythms of most persons do not immediately adjust to an abrupt alteration of the sleep-activity synchronizer schedule.[3,11,15,16,65,69] The jet-lag syndrome experienced by vacationers after being rapidly transported across several time zones and the dull, lackluster feelings of lassitude and fatigue experienced by many shiftworkers for a few days after the commencement of night duty represent in large part a reduction in biological efficiency resulting from a disturbed circadian time structure.[17] This is not surprising, since a minimum of several days is usually required for circadian and other bioperiodicities to completely adjust to a new synchronizer schedule.[15,16] The exact duration of time needed, however, varies between individuals and biological functions (Table 2). It varies also with respect to the extent of the alteration in the synchronizer schedule and the direction of change in it. With reference to the usual routine,

TABLE 2. Rates of Acrophase Shift (Minutes/Day) in Selected Circadian Functions Following Either Westbound or Eastbound Flights Corresponding to Delays and Advances of Synchronizer Schedule*

Study Variable	Westbound (Delay)	Eastbound (Advance)
Urinary adrenalin	90	60
Urinary noradrenalin	180	120
Urinary 17-OHCS	47	32
Psychomotor performance	52	38
Reaction time	150	74
Heart rate	90	60
Body temperature	60	39

* From Klein and Wegmann, 1980, 1979,[15,16] with permission.

a **phase-delay** in the synchronizer schedule refers to a later timing of sleep and activity, as would be the case if rotating in sequence and direction from an afternoon to a nighttime shift or for a traveler going from Europe to the United States. A **phase-advance** in the synchronizer schedule refers to an earlier timing of the sleep-activity schedule, as would be the case in rotating in sequence and direction from a morning to a nighttime shift or for a traveler going from the United States to Europe. In general a phase-delay in the synchronization schedule is easier to adjust to biologically than a phase-advance; however, individual differences exist.[69–71]

To a large extent, the majority of our knowledge about the chronobiologic adjustments to 8-hour and other rotating shiftwork schedules comes from investigations on volunteers studied under simulated shiftwork conditions. While the findings from these are helpful in understanding the mechanisms of adjustment to shiftwork, their usefulness to the work situation is limited. Frequently, the volunteers of such investigations are studied under atypical conditions. Although they are subjected to simulated synchronizer shifts, they are not required to perform the same tasks found in an industrial setting. Furthermore, the social and experimental milieu of a simulated study is usually very different from that of the real situation. For these reasons, actual field evaluations of shiftworkers are mandatory.[11,65]

Field study of the chronobiologic adjustments of rotating shiftworkers has been conducted on selected groups of volunteering employees.[11,16,65,69,72] To investigate the biological rhythms of workers, several measurements separated by more or less equal intervals over the activity span are necessary. Recent developments have made available portable, light-weight instruments for conducting self-measurements on a variety of health-related functions.[63] Moreover, numerous questionnaires useful for studying aspects of shiftwork have been developed, field tested, and validated.

DIFFERENCES BETWEEN EMPLOYEES IN THE RATE OF BIOLOGICAL RHYTHM ADJUSTMENTS TO ROTATING SHIFTWORK

Aschoff[73] and Wever[74] conducted numerous studies on volunteers living in isolation under controlled conditions devoid of time cues. Their research suggested that persons exhibiting a high-amplitude oral temperature circadian rhythm, which represents evidence for a strong biological time structure, are less disturbed chronobiologically when exposed to conditions lacking synchronizers. Of interest to shiftwork researchers and chronobiologists is whether features of one's biological time structure are indicative of the innate capability to adjust to an alteration in synchronizer schedule as required by a rotating shiftwork routine. In order to examine this issue, field studies on shiftworkers have utilized autorhythmometry as a method of data collection and analysis. The resulting findings have served to address several theories concerning differences between workers in their biological capability for and tolerance to rotating shiftwork schedules. For example, it is of interest to know if the rate of change in the acrophase (designated as $\Delta\phi$) of a set of circadian rhythms is related to the strength (the amplitude) of the circadian time structure. In this respect, Reinberg et al.[75] found that the $\Delta\phi$ of the circadian rhythm of oral temperature and urinary 17-hydroxycorticosteroids is negatively related to the respective circadian amplitude. Specifically, the greater the amplitude exhibited by a worker, the slower the rate of the adjustment of the circadian time structure, as gauged by the change in acrophase ($\Delta\phi$) following the shift in the sleep-activity synchronizer schedule (Figs. 10 and 11).

Should these findings be validated in prospective investigations on large groups of shiftworkers, they have important implications. First, employees exhibiting large-amplitude circadian rhythms, such as in the rhythms of oral temperature and urinary 17-hydroxycorticosteroid concentration, should be considered as most suited for rapid, 2- to 3-day duration, rotating shiftwork routines.[75] This is because persons having high-amplitude rhythms tend to adjust

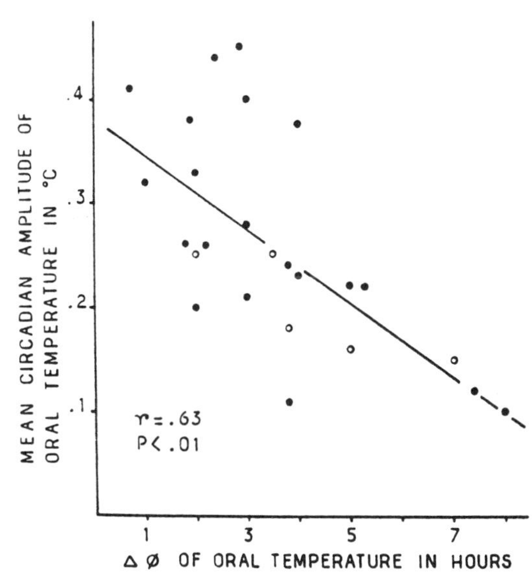

FIGURE 10. Correlation between the circadian amplitude of the oral temperature circadian rhythm and the rate of change in its acrophase ($\Delta\phi$) for 25 shiftworkers studied in two industrial plants. $\Delta\phi$ represents the difference between the clock time of the rhythm's peak on control days (day work) and after the first night shift (night work from 9 p.m. to 5 or 6 a.m. with daytime sleep). The $\Delta\phi$ of the rhythm is inversely related to the circadian amplitude ($p < 0.01$). (From Reinberg et al., 1979,[75] with permission.)

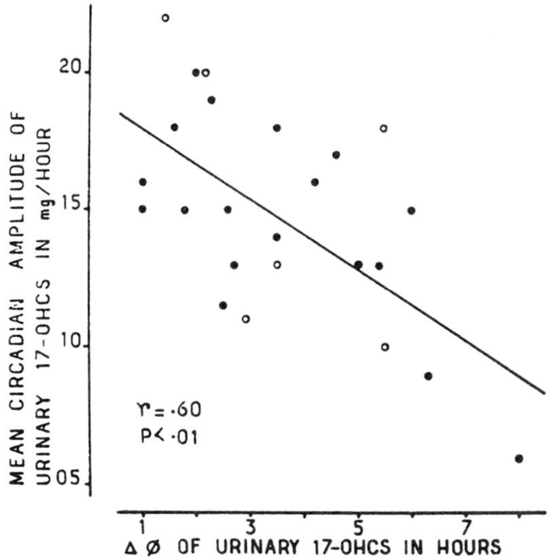

FIGURE 11. Correlation between the circadian amplitude of the rhythm in urinary 17-OHCS (chemical metabolite of cortisol in urine) and the shift in its acrophase ($\Delta\phi$) for 25 shiftworkers studied in two industrial plants. $\Delta\phi$ represents the difference between the clock time of the rhythm's peak on control days (day work) and after the first night shift (night work from 9 p.m. to 5 or 6 a.m. with daytime sleep). The $\Delta\phi$ of the rhythm is inversely related to the circadian amplitude ($p < 0.01$). (From Reinberg et al., 1979,[75] with permission.)

the acrophases of their circadian rhythms so slowly that by the last "day" of a regular nighttime shift, day 2 or 3 into the rota, the alteration of the circadian time structure is likely to be minimal. Thus, when rotating back to a pattern of nighttime sleep alternating with daytime work, the required chronobiologic reorganization of such employees is slight or nil. Second, persons exhibiting low-amplitude circadian rhythms, such as in oral temperature and 17-hydroxy-corticosteroid concentration, should be considered as most suited to 7-day or longer duration shifts before rotating to a new work schedule. Individuals who possess such a circadian time structure are likely to undergo a rather rapid shift in their circadian rhythms following a change to nighttime work necessitating daytime sleep. For these, the chronobiologic adjustment may be complete by the end of the first or second "day" of the nighttime shift. Thus, for this type of person, rapid, 2- to 3-day, rotational shiftwork is less appropriate than are the longer rotations.

CHRONOBIOTICS AND OTHER COUNTERMEASURES FOR HASTENING CHRONOBIOLOGIC ADJUSTMENT TO SHIFT CHANGES

Over the years, a number of medications or specific treatments have been proposed as a means of moderating or alleviating the undesired effects associated with an abrupt alteration in the rest-activity synchronizer schedule due to shiftwork or transmeridian travel. The goal of proposed countermeasures, in general, is the hastening of the adjustment of the circadian time structure to a newly imposed synchronizer schedule and/or facilitating daytime sleep such that there is minimal loss of performance capability, continued well being, and minimal sleep disturbance. Some have been investigated primarily through laboratory animal experimentation. Others have involved human beings. In human trials of chronobiotics (i.e., medications and other treatments to facilitate adjustment of the biological time structure), a variety of experimental methods have been utilized. In some, only one or a few biological rhythms have been monitored as a means of assessing the value of given interventions, whereas in others, sleep studies or logs and/or questionnaires of fatigue and arousal have been used. At this time, the investigation of various countermeasures is proceeding rather rapidly. In the sections that follow, the findings of trials involving popular interventions are reviewed as to their potential impact on the adjustment of employees to rotating shiftwork schedules.

Benzodiazepine Derivatives. A major problem commonly encountered by shiftworkers and travelers is securing sleep of needed quantity and quality at an atypical biological time, which is the case, for example, when trying to sleep during the daytime when assigned to the nightshift. The use of certain benzodiazepine derivatives (e.g., triazolam) for a few days in duration may be beneficial in aiding daytime sleep. In this manner sleep deprivation may be minimized and performance at work maintained at an acceptable level. However, it must be pointed out that although sleep-inducing medication such as triazolam and flurazepam enable daytime sleep, this does not constitute evidence that the circadian time structure is shifted by such an intervention.[76-81] Initially, investigations on laboratory animals, especially hamsters, suggested that triazolam might be capable of phase-shifting circadian rhythms.[81,82] However, subsequent trials have implied that the hamster model is not representative of the human.[81,84] Moreover, Bicokova-Rocher,[79] using a benzodiazepine, loflazepate, in studies on normal healthy human beings as well as patients suffering from anxiety, found no evidence of chronobiotic activities. Compared to the placebo period, loflazepate in a dose of 2 to 4 mg whether given once daily at 8 a.m. or 8 p.m. induced neither shifts in circadian staging of the several monitored variables nor alteration in the sleep-activity pattern itself. Thus, at the present time the benzodiazepine derivatives, while proven to be effective as anxiolytics and sleep aids, have yet to be shown to induce a more rapid adjustment of the circadian time structure following an alteration in synchronizer schedule. One must conclude that the role of benzodiazepines as chronobiotics in the case of human beings is not yet substantiated.

Theophylline. When theophylline is given to rodents in large doses and under special experimental conditions, it can induce phase-advances or delays in the biological time structure according to its administration time.[85] Based on the findings of animal studies, it was hypothesized that theophylline could be a chronobiotic to human beings. Theophylline is used by millions of asthmatics and other chronic obstructive pulmonary disease (COPD) patients routinely, either as a sustained-release formulation taken at 12-hour intervals or once daily, usually at night, in the case of the ultra-slow, controlled-release theophylline forms. A series of studies by the authors[86,87] on asthma patients routinely treated with such theophyllines, however, yielded no evidence that this medication affects the circadian time structure. On the other hand, Okudaira et al.[88] reported that a single 250-mg dose of theophylline induced a slight shift (of about 0.5 hours) in the sleep-wake rhythm of healthy persons never before treated with the drug. However, again there was no evidence in favor of an altered circadian time structure induced by the drug. The circadian acrophase of several rhythms—-self-assessed mood, vigor, sleepiness, heart rate, hunger, time estimation, and body temperature—was not changed.[88] Thus, while theophylline administered in quite large doses is capable of inducing alterations in the staging of the circadian time structure of *laboratory rodents* studied under very specific experimental conditions, it appears to possess no chronobiotic effect in human beings.[81]

Anti-Jet-Lag Diet. Ehret and colleagues, again based on laboratory rodent experiments, proposed an anti-jet-lag diet for aiding the adjustment of the time-keeping system of travelers to shifts in the sleep-activity regimen.[85,89-91] This "diet" consists of the programmed-in-time intake of methylxanthines (such as in the form of coffee), as well as carbohydrates or proteins, with spaced fasting spans. The incorporation of timed consumptions of carbohydrate and protein foodstuffs also is based on laboratory animal findings.[85,89] Although this anti-jet-lag diet has achieved popularity with the lay press, government officials, travelers, and even airline companies, there is as yet little scientific evidence that it is an effective countermeasure against the symptoms of jet lag in human beings.[72,92] The reported praise that the diet has received from its proponents and users may therefore represent the result of a placebo effect. Whatever the case, the anti-jet-lag diet has not yet been demonstrated to hasten the readjustment of circadian time structure of human beings.

Melatonin. Melatonin is an endogenously secreted pineal gland hormone. Plasma and urine concentrations of the hormone vary markedly as a circadian rhythm with high serum concentrations during the overnight span in human beings.[93,94] The pineal gland is considered by some to constitute a component of the biological time-keeping system in man and other animals.[93,94] Melatonin, even in human beings, produces a mild hypnotic effect and may be capable of inducing phasing shifts in the circadian time structure. In recently conducted studies,[95,96] melatonin was evaluated as a chronobiotic for minimizing the symptoms of jet-lag. In one trial, melatonin was tested using a double-blind, placebo-controlled study design. Participants were flown across 8 time zones, between San Francisco and London. For 3 days before flight, different groups of travelers took melatonin or placebo at 6 p.m. (equivalent to midnight, London time). On arrival at London, they continued to take their treatments between 10 p.m. and midnight local time for 4 additional days. Thereafter, each traveler was requested to rate the severity of their jet lag using a visual analog scale. By use of this scale, jet lag was considered problematic if scores of 50 or more were indicated. Two-thirds of the placebo group experienced significant jet lag as evidenced by very high scores. In comparison, none of the melatonin-treated travelers rated their jet-lag symptoms with more than a score of 17! This study did not directly address the effect of the timed melatonin adjustment on the *rate* of adjustment of the circadian time structure (individual biological rhythms) of the travelers; nonetheless, the results document the fact that melatonin does lessen the symptoms associated with rapid alteration of the sleep-activity synchronizer schedule. Although the data at this time are still preliminary, it may be that melatonin treatment does have an influence on the circadian time structure directly.[95] Further investigation of melatonin, however, is yet required on larger numbers of travelers as well as shiftworkers to fully evaluate its potential and its safety as a chronobiotic to facilitate the adjustment of persons to imposed alterations in their sleep-activity routine.

Bright Light Therapy. During the past decade, scientific and clinical interest in the effect of bright light on animal and, in particular, human biological time-keeping mechanisms has risen tremendously.[13,14,97-104] Early investigations on animals and thereafter human beings revealed bright light could phase-delay or phase-advance at least certain circadian variables.[97,98] In the past few years, bright light of 2500 to 5000 lux has been used in the treatment of seasonal affective disorder patients. It has been proven useful clinically in the management of a certain type of wintertime depressive illness.[97] It is believed that the beneficial effect of bright light is related, at least in part, to its influence on the pineal gland and melatonin, and on alterations in the circadian time-keeping mechanisms of the body.[99]

Of recent interest is the possible use of very bright light as a countermeasure against the problems arising from the required chronobiologic adjustments of rotating shiftworkers when doing night work. Although only a few such investigations have been completed as of this writing, the findings are worthy of discussion.[100-102] One of these examined the effect of a regimen of very bright light, 7,000–12,000 lux, timed between 1:15 a.m. and 7:45 a.m. and alternating with complete darkness between 9 a.m. and 5 p.m. on rotating shiftworkers. When this treatment was applied to a small group of shiftworkers while on the midnight to 8 a.m. rota, adjustment of the circadian time structure and cognitive performance were considerably better in comparison to the control situation when exposure was to normal light (150 lux) during night work.[100] It is of interest that bright light also is effective in enhancing cognitive performance and in reducing melatonin levels overnight in simulated work situations involving prolonged, continuous mental activity.[103,104]

The results of these studies are encouraging, in spite of the fact that they are representative of only a relatively small number of participants. Although it seems premature to endorse the installation of very bright lights in industrial settings for aiding the chronobiologic adjustment of nightworkers, the findings do reinforce the fact that bright light may have a significant influence on the human circadian time structure. Future research, if resulting in an exact understanding of the mechanisms underlying the effect of bright light on the circadian time-keeping system, may well lead to a convenient therapy for use by rotating shiftworkers to enhance their adjustment to night work. However, at the present time bright light therapy, itself, continues to be evaluated for its practical application in occupational medicine.

INTOLERANCE TO SHIFTWORK

Most occupational health professionals are aware of the fact that not all individuals are biologically capable of or tolerant to shiftwork. Some can adhere to rotating shift schedules, which include periodic nighttime duty, throughout their working life, for 35 years or more, without health problems or medical complaints of any kind. On the other hand, even some healthy young workers may exhibit medical intolerance to the rigors of shiftwork.

Both young as well as older workers may exhibit or develop a biological intolerance to rotating shiftwork schedules. Older workers around the age of 40 to 50 years in particular, after being successfully engaged in rotating shiftwork for several decades, may suddenly exhibit intolerance to shiftwork. This intolerance often is manifested by the onset or exacerbation of the typical shiftwork-associated medical complaints. Commonly, workers complain of problems in obtaining restful sleep.[52,105] The sleep, itself, may be disturbed; it may be shortened in duration and disrupted by frequent awakenings. Some even experience bouts of insomnia. Persisting fatigue, not necessarily the direct result of sleep difficulties, is another complaint. The intolerant shiftworker commonly feels unrested and tired immediately after awakening from sleep during the work week, during weekends away from work, and even during vacations. This type of persisting fatigue differs from the physiological fatigue resulting from physical and/or mental effort due to one's job, since the latter nearly always dissipates after an adequate night's rest. Intolerant shiftworkers also may exhibit an altered behavior. Often, there is an increase in irritability and excitability, with malaise and lowered performance both at work and at home. Digestive complaints such as dyspepsia, epigastric pain, and peptic ulcer are also common difficulties of the intolerant shiftworker.[52,105]

INTERNAL DESYNCHRONIZATION OF CIRCADIAN RHYTHMS AND SHIFTWORK INTOLERANCE

Internal desynchronization of biological rhythms is defined as an alteration in the circadian period and/or phase relationship between interdependent rhythmic functions.[16,52,65,69] Generally, circadian (and other) rhythms are synchronized such that a fixed phase relationship exists between interdependent bioperiodicities of a given frequency. Transient internal desynchronization of circadian rhythms, evidenced by an alteration of the phase relationship of biological functions, occurs during the chronobiologic adjustment of shiftworkers after changing from day to nighttime work involving daytime sleep. It is of interest that only certain workers develop a biological intolerance to rotating shiftwork. The question of why only certain, perhaps prone, employees develop intolerance to a rotating shiftwork schedule remains to be answered. It has been proposed by us previously[105] that some persons who are genetically endowed with a particular circadian time structure may be predisposed to an intolerance to internal desynchronization, such as the case when one is subjected to recurring, periodic alteration of the sleep-activity schedule.

Using special statistical analyses on data collected during field studies, Reinberg et al.[66,67,105–107] found differences in the circadian time structure between tolerant and intolerant shiftworkers. Individuals endowed with a large-amplitude oral temperature circadian rhythm (that is, a strong circadian time structure) exhibit a better long-term capability and biological tolerance for rotating shiftwork.[11,106] As shown in Table 3, senior shiftworkers with a large-amplitude oral temperature circadian rhythm, close to greater than 0.30° C, generally display a good tolerance to rotating shiftwork; they experience little difficulty working rotating schedules. On the other hand, senior employees who exhibit a small-amplitude oral temperature circadian rhythm, 0.23° C or less, are at elevated risk of biological intolerance to rotating shiftwork schedules.[106]

Another very important difference between the time structure of tolerant and nontolerant shiftworkers has been identified. In biologically intolerant shiftworkers, evidence of a persisting internal desynchronization of the circadian system has been documented repeatedly.[67,105–107] For example, the period duration of at least certain circadian rhythmic variables has been determined to be different than 24.0 hours. Table 4 shows exemplary findings for the oral temperature circadian rhythm in relatively young workers, who at the time of study reported good (subjects 1–11) or poor (subjects 12–15) biological tolerance

TABLE 3. Circadian Rhythm in Oral Temperature of Subjects with Good, Adequate or Poor Tolerance to Shiftwork: Single Cosinor Summary*

Group (Mean Age, years)	Tolerance to Shiftwork (No. of Subjects)	Rhythm Detection p = value	Mesor (24-hour-rhythm Adjusted Mean ± SE) (°C)	Circadian Amplitude (95% Confidence Limit)	Acrophase ϕ in h and min, Referenced to Midnight (95% Confidence Limit)
I (25.3)	Good (6)	<0.005	36.53 ± 0.08	0.37 (0.29–0.45)	1549 (1438 to 1700)
II (50.0)	Good (10)	<0.005	36.51 ± 0.07	0.35 (0.30–0.40)	1534 (1438 to 1627)
III (50.2)	Adeq. (6)	<0.005	36.53 ± 0.11	0.30 (0.24–0.36)	1657 (1541 to 1905)
IV (47.4)	Poor (7)	<0.005	36.52 ± 0.12	0.23 (0.17–0.29)	1711 (1607 to 1814)

* All subjects were shiftworkers at the same oil refinery. Groups differed mainly by a good (e.g., group II) versus a poor (group IV) tolerance to shiftwork as well as by a large (group II) versus a small (group IV) amplitude. Group II (good tolerance) involved 10 senior operators (no history of shiftwork difficulty; mean age = 50 years, range 44–57 years; and mean shiftwork duration = 25.1 years, range 15–32 years). Group IV involved 7 senior operators (who were to be discharged from shiftwork due to nontolerance; mean age = 47.4 years, range 30–56 years; mean shiftwork duration = 22.9 years, range 9–29).

Notes: In any group, amplitude differs from zero with p <0.005; mesor: no difference between groups; amplitude (½ of total peak to trough variability): large in groups I and II (good tolerance): small in group IV (poor tolerance to shiftwork); acrophase ϕ (crest time): no difference between groups. (From Reinberg et al., 1984, 1983,[66,106] with permission.)

TABLE 4. Characteristics of the Circadian Rhythm of Body Temperature in Tolerant and Nontolerant Shiftworkers*

Subject # (Age)	History of Rotating Shiftwork	Dominant Circadian Period[1] (in hours)	Circadian Amplitude[2] (°C)
Tolerant			
1 (20)†	1 month	25.1	0.21
2 (22)	2.5 years	24.0	0.23
3 (22)	2.5 months	24.0	0.27
4 (25)	3 years	24.0	0.31
5 (25)	4 years	24.0	0.25
6 (27)	1 month	24.0	0.35
7 (27)	3 months	24.0	0.19
8 (31)	1.5 years	24.0	0.21
9 (36)	2.5 years	24.0	0.27
10 (35)	4 years	24.0	0.36
11 (43)	2 years	24.0	0.42
Nontolerant			
12 (20)	1 month	25.7	0.04
13 (28)	3 months	25.1	0.04
14 (30)	3 months	24.9	0.13
15 (31)	3 years	25.2	0.09

* From Reinberg et al., 1984, 1983,[66,106] with permission.

[1] Estimated by power spectrum.

[2] Estimated by single cosinor method.

† Following publication of these data, subject No. 1 had to be transferred from rotating shiftwork to permanent daywork because of a developed intolerance to the former.

for rotating shiftwork. With the exception of subject No. 1, the circadian period of the oral temperature circadian rhythm in tolerant shiftwork employees was precisely 24.0 hours. Moreover, the amplitude of this rhythm in the tolerant workers was larger than it was for the nontolerant shiftworkers. In contrast, for the biologically intolerant workers of this sample, the circadian period for the oral temperature rhythm was longer, being between 24.9 and 25.7 hours, and the circadian amplitude was quite small, equal or less than 0.13°C. It is of interest that since the publication of these findings, it became necessary to transfer subject No. 1 from rotating shiftwork to permanent daywork because of a developed biological intolerance to shiftwork. Thus, it appears that the etiology of shiftwork tolerance includes (1) the strength of the circadian time structure, as best gauged at present by the magnitude of the amplitude of the oral temperature circadian rhythm, and (2) the maintenance of a precisely organized 24.0-hour time structure. According to Reinberg and his colleagues,[11,67] shiftworkers with a large-amplitude circadian time structure tend to be less prone to developing an internal desynchronization of circadian functions and intolerance to rotating shiftwork regimens.

The phenomenon of internal desynchronization as an aspect of intolerance to shiftwork is clearly apparent in Figure 12.[106] The upper left-hand portion of the figure shows the clock-hour timing of the circadian acrophase (indicated by closed circles) of the oral temperature rhythm for one subject (No. 3) who possessed good biological tolerance to shiftwork. The timing of the acrophase of this rhythm was quite stable from day-to-day, despite the regular rotation to night work (shown by the asterisked horizontal bars) during the weekdays. The bottom left-hand portion of this figure shows the so-called power spectrum of the oral temperature data for this worker. This method indicates the existence of prominent bioperiodicities through a partitioning of the variance of the data sets. It can be seen for subject No. 3 that the rhythm of oral temperature is exactly 24.0 hours in duration. The upper right-hand portion of Figure 12 gives an example of a desynchronized circadian oral temperature rhythm of an intolerant shiftworker (No. 13). It can be seen that the timing of the circadian acrophase (closed circles) of the oral temperature rhythm occurred progressively later day-by-day. Such a finding would be expected if the circadian period of the oral temperature rhythm is longer than 24.0 hours. In this biologically intolerant worker, the period of this rhythm as shown by the power spectrum analyses (lower right-hand portion of Figure 12) is 25.1, rather than the expected 24.0, hours in duration. Thus, the later timing of the circadian acrophase represents a prolongation of the period length of the oral temperature circadian rhythm.

In this and other presumably shiftwork-intolerant persons, internal desynchronization apparently results from recurring changes in the hours of sleep and activity associated with shiftwork schedules, which include work during the nighttime and sleep during the daytime. Although only reports dealing with desynchronization of the oral temperature circadian rhythm are cited here, other circadian functions appear to become internally desynchronized in shiftwork-intolerant employees as well.[67] Presumably, alteration in the circadian time structure, when manifested as a persisting internal desynchronization of the circadian rhythms, constitutes a significant feature of the biological intolerance to rotating shiftwork.

It has been suggested that in predisposed persons, internal desynchronization is associated with a set of symptoms that is common both to clinical depression

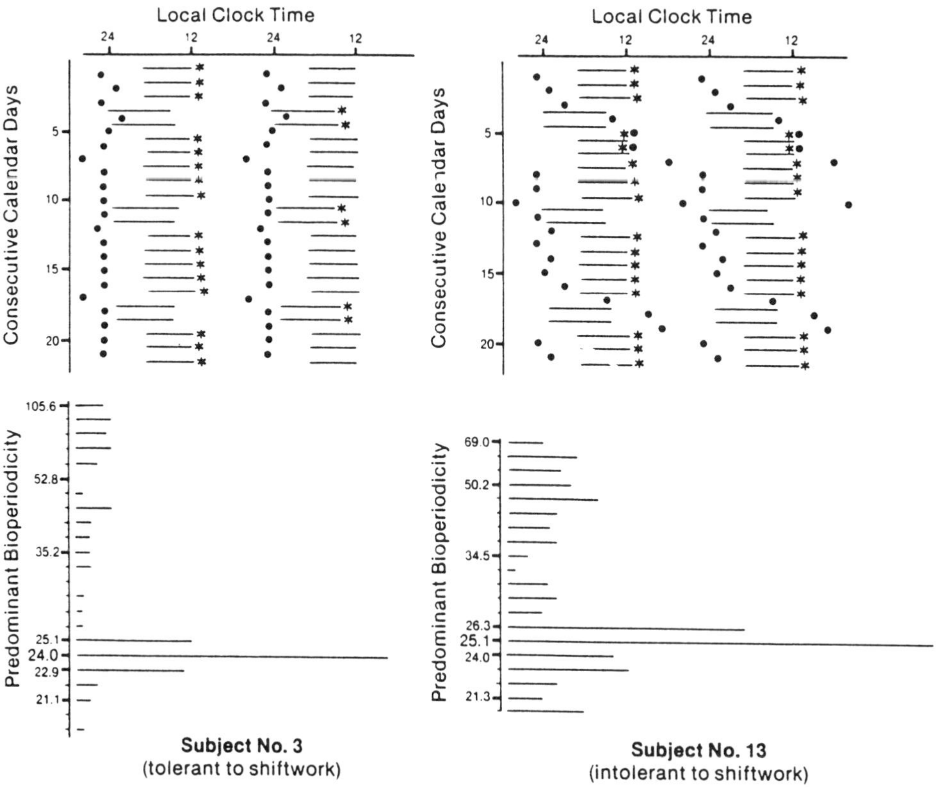

FIGURE 12. The plots at the top indicate the timing of the circadian acrophase (peak time) of the body temperature rhythm of a worker exhibiting either good tolerance (subject No. 3, left side) or poor tolerance (subject No. 13, right side) to rotating shiftwork. The acrophase of the rhythm is consistently timed from one day to the next in subject No. 3, even when sleeping during the day (shown by asterisks) for 5 of 7 days of each week. The acrophases for subject No. 13 exhibit a systemic delay with each consecutive day. This latter phenomenon suggests a period length for this rhythm greater than 24 hours. This is documented statistically by spectral analysis (bottom right). The most prevalent period for the body temperature of subject No. 13 was shown to be 25.1 hours rather than 24 hours as shown for subject No. 3 in the lower graph to left. (From Reinberg et al., 1983,[106] with permission.)

and shiftwork intolerance.[105] Michel-Briand et al.[108] reported a greater incidence of depression and affective illness in *retired shiftworkers* than in *retired dayworkers*, in whom cardiovascular and locomotor illnesses and disorders were most common. In patients suffering from depressive illness, effective treatment with specific medications, such as lithium and other antidepressants or with light therapy, which are known to influence the circadian period of specific rhythms, can moderate or correct the internal desynchronization. Often nontolerant shiftworkers resort to using medications of another type—sleep-inducing aids, such as barbiturates, tranquilizers, benzodiazepine derivatives, and antihistamines. These medications, which lack the capability of affecting the period length of circadian functions, frequently are overused, sometimes leading to addiction, although typically without effective resolution of the employee's sleep disorders or persisting fatigue.

It is important to note that persons intolerant to rotating shiftwork do recover from their untoward symptoms when they are returned to a regular pattern of activity and sleep. Permanent daywork with nighttime sleep leads to an eventual resynchronization of biological rhythms, with modulation or alleviation of the associated clinical symptoms of shiftwork intolerance. However, complete regression of the symptoms may require quite some time to resolve in certain cases. In this regard, the decision to discharge an employee from shift to permanent daytime work must be done early, when the signs and symptoms of biological intolerance first appear. This is important in order to increase the likelihood that the biological effects of shiftwork intolerance will be minimal and that recovery will be rapid.

SUMMARY

In this chapter, the topic of medical chronobiology has been presented. Emphasis has been placed on issues related to clinical and occupational medicine. Results of initial studies conducted primarily by clinical pathologists indicate that the results of several commonly ordered diagnostic tests are influenced in a significant way according to the circadian time when samplings or tests are conducted.[60] In addition, the pharmacokinetics and pharmacodynamics of medications can vary significantly according to their administration time.[40,45] Indeed, the safety as well as efficacy of certain medications or dosage forms are circadian time dependent.[38] A new thrust in the clinic is the application of chronotherapeutics to maximize the effectiveness and safety of medications.[22,38]

For the occupational health practitioner, the topic of medical chronobiology offers new perspectives to better address common problems experienced in clinical occupational medicine. First, the utilization of time-qualified (for circadian rhythmicity) reference values serves to differentiate with greater precision normal from unusual test findings; for example, among those arising during the pre-employment and scheduled follow-up physical examinations. Second, it provides better insight into the basis for the biological intolerance to rotating shiftwork. Too often, employee complaints of shiftwork intolerance are met with skepticism by members of the management and/or medical staff. The phenomenon of biological intolerance to rotating shiftwork is real. It has only been during the past decade that shiftwork intolerance has been demonstrated to have a chronobiologic basis. It seems that persons who possess a weak circadian time structure, that is, rather low-amplitude bioperiodicities, are more prone to develop biological intolerance to shiftwork later in life. Those endowed with a strong (high-amplitude) time structure are least prone. Thus, although persons with a weak circadian time structure might be at an advantage in tolerating rotating shiftwork schedules while young, they appear to be at a high risk of developing intolerance to it later in life. It is hypothesized that a weak circadian time structure predisposes one to desynchronization when subjected to work schedules entailing regular disruption of the activity-rest synchronizer schedule. The mechanisms underlying this biological intolerance to shiftwork require much additional investigation. However, if the initial findings which have been discussed herein are substantiated, future pre-employment examinations might well include tests to determine the strength/weakness of the circadian time structure in relationship to the projected long-term capability of workers to safely cope with the various rotating shiftwork schedules used in industry.

In this chapter, the issue of chronotoxicity was addressed. It is primarily in laboratory animal experiments that circadian rhythms in the effects of and responses to potentially noxious agents have been demonstrated. Thus far, evidence for the existence of chronotoxicities to contaminants commonly found in the workplace has yet to be established. Primarily, this is because no industrial studies have yet been conducted. The multitude of laboratory animal studies confirming such a phenomenon, however, must not be ignored. If there is evidence for a workshift differential in toxic reactions or occupationally related illness in employees, this may well implicate circadian susceptibility-resistance rhythms to workplace contaminants or activities. In this regard, the epidemiology of industrial health-related issues has assumed a homeostatic model. Whether implicitly stated or not, it is assumed that the effects of a potentially harmful workplace agent of a given concentration will be the same no matter what the circadian (shift) time of the exposure. A chronobiologic perspective (Fig. 13), on the other hand, entails a different philosophy. It considers the possibility that the effect of a potentially harmful agent may vary as a function of circadian time (or shift). Moreover, it considers the possibility that the dose-response relationship for chemical agents may differ according to the circadian time of exposure, as demonstrated in insects, laboratory animals, and even human beings.[37,109,110]

Finally, methods for the self-monitoring of selected endpoints of human functions that are indicative of health status were discussed. It is possible to easily accumulate meaningful data by self-assessments of workers, themselves, using portable, light-weight instrumentation. When the data are obtained frequently enough, then analyses can be done to contrast physiological status during work hours versus off-hours, and work days versus off-days. Moreover, such methods seem to be useful in documenting objectively an intolerance to rotating shiftwork, either through (1) an alteration in the circadian time structure such as illustrated in an earlier section of this chapter, (2) data contained in a home diary using an activity and sleep log, or (3) through the use of wrist actigraphy to substantiate sleep times and sleep continuity.[11] Autorhythmometry involving the self-assessment

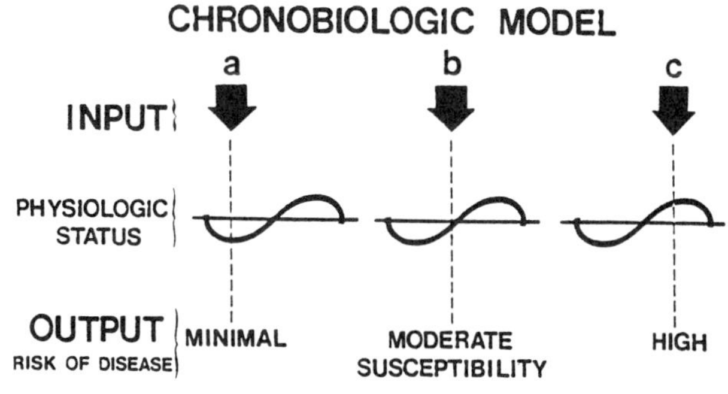

FIGURE 13. Depicted is a conceptualized circadian rhythm in physiological status indicative of 24-hour susceptibility-resistance to potentially noxious agents. Depending on the biological time of the postulated exposure (input to system), the effect (output) may be little or great in terms of medical complaints and/or industrially induced illness. Although circadian susceptibility-rhythms have been demonstrated in rodents in response to toxic substances and in human beings in terms of the morbidity of disease,[37] their importance in industrial medicine has yet to be demonstrated.

of airways status by PEF has already proven worthwhile in clinical, community, and industrial applications; for example, to monitor the beneficial response to antiasthma medications and to objectively quantify the effect of air pollutants on the airways.[8,27] In a sense, such autorhythmometric applications represent an extension of the common procedure of Holter monitoring of employees reassigned to different duties upon returning to work following myocardial infarction. Actually, self-assessment techniques and instrumentation have great potential for industrial applications.[63]

During the past couple of decades, the science of chronobiology has developed rapidly. Large strides have already begun to be realized in the clinic, especially with regard to the documentation of temporal patterns in the occurrence or exacerbation of disease and also the chronotherapeutics of diseased states. In occupational medicine, much has been learned about the chronobiologic mechanisms underlying acclimation to alterations in the sleep-activity synchronizer schedule, whether the result of rotating shiftwork or rapid geographic displacement by aircraft across several meridians. One challenge for the future is the definition of chronobiologic criteria for the selection of employees for rotating shiftwork and other unusual work schedules. In addition, the search for chronobiotics—drugs or other interventions that are capable of speeding the adjustment of the circadian time structure in response to alteration in the sleep-wake routine—must be intensified. Although bright light and selected chemical agents might act as chronobiotics, certain practical issues remain to be resolved before they can be broadly applied. Future investigations will continue to provide new insight and solutions to those chronobiologic problems commonly experienced by shift-workers. The contents of this entire issue, in particular, point to this.

REFERENCES

1. Reinberg A, Smolensky MH: Biological Rhythms and Medicine. New York, Springer Verlag, 1983.
2. Moore-Ede MC, Sulzman FM, Fuller CA: The Clocks That Time Us. Cambridge, Harvard University Press, 1982.
3. Arendt J, Minors DS, Waterhouse JM: Biological Rhythms in Clinical Practice. London, John Wright, 1989.
4. Assenmacher I, Farner DS: Environmental Endocrinology. Berlin, Springer-Verlag, 1978.
5. Reinberg A, Touitou Y, Restoin A, et al: The genetic background of circadian and ultradian rhythm patterns of 17-hydroxycorticosteroids: A cross-twin study. J Endocrinol 105:247–253, 1985.
6. Halberg F, Nelson W: Chronobiologic optimization of aging. In Samis HV Jr, Capobianco S (eds): Aging and Biological Rhythms. New York, Plenum Press, 1978, pp 5–56.
7. Smolensky MH, Barnes PJ, Reinberg A, McGovern JP: Chronobiology and asthma. I. Day-night differences in bronchial patency and dyspnea and circadian rhythm dependencies. J Asthma 23:321–343, 1986.
8. Smolensky MH, Reinberg A, Prevost RJ, et al: The application of chronobiological findings and methods to the epidemiological investigation of the health effects of air pollutants on sentinel patients. In Smolensky MH, Reinberg A, McGovern JP (eds): Recent Advances in the Chronobiology of Allergy and Immunology. New York, Pergamon Press, 1980, pp 211–236.
9. Edmunds LN Jr: Cellular and Molecular Bases of Biological Clocks. New York, Springer-Verlag, 1988.
10. Halberg F: Chronobiology. Ann Rev Physiol 31:675–725, 1975.
11. Reinberg A (ed): Chronobiological field studies of oil refinery shift workers. Chronobiologia 6(Suppl 1):1–119, 1979.
12. Halberg F, Simpson H: Circadian acrophase of human 17-hydroxycorticosteroid excretion referred to midsleep rather than midnight. Human Biol 39:405–413, 1967.
13. Czeisler CA, Richardson GS, Zimmerman JC, et al: Entrainment of human circadian rhythms by light-dark cycles: A reassessment. Photochem Photobiol 34:239–247, 1981.

14. Czeisler AC, Allan JS, Strogatz SH, et al: Bright light resets the human circadian pacemaker independent of the timing of the sleep-wake cycle. Science 233:667–671, 1986.
15. Klein KE, Wegmann HM: The effects of transmeridian and transequatorial air travel on psychological well-being and performance. Chronobiology: Principles and Applications to Shifts in Schedules, NATO Advanced Study Institutes Series D: Behavioral and Social Sciences, No. 3. The Netherlands, Sijthoff & Nordhoff, 1980, pp 339–352.
16. Klein KE, Wegmann HM: Circadian rhythms in air operations. In Nicholson AN (ed): Sleep, Wakefulness and Circadian Rhythm. NATO, AGARD Lecture Series No. 105, 1979, pp 2:1–2:9.
17. Arendt J, Marks V: Physiological changes underlying jet-lag. Br Med J 284:144–146, 1982.
18. Caradente F, Halberg F (eds): Chronobiology of blood pressure in 1985. Chronobiologia 11:189–310, 1984.
19. Smolensky MH, Tatar SE, Bergman SA, et al: Circadian rhythmic aspects of human cardiovascular function: A review by human chronobiologic statistical methods. Chronobiologia 3:337–371, 1976.
20. McKerrow CB, McDermott M, Gilson JC, Schilling RSF: Respiratory function during the day in cotton workers: A study in bysinosis. Br J Ind Med 15:75–83, 1958.
21. Lemmer B: Temporal aspects of the cardiovascular active drugs in humans. In Lemmer B (ed): Chronopharmacology. New York, Marcel Dekker, 1989, pp 525–541.
22. Smolensky MH, D'Alonzo GE: Biologic rhythms and medicine. Am J Med 85(Suppl 1B):34–46, 1988.
23. Kowanko IC, Pownall R, Knapp MS, et al: Circadian variations in the signs and symptoms of rheumatoid arthritis and in the therapeutic effectiveness of flurbiprofen at different times of the day. Br J Clin Pharmacol 11:477–484, 1981.
24. Levi F, LeLouarn C, Reinberg A: Timing optimizes sustained indomethacin treatment of osteoarthritis. Clin Pharmacol Ther 37:77–84, 1986.
25. Reinberg A, Gervais P, Levi F, et al: Circadian rhythms of allergic rhinitis: An epidemiologic study involving chronobiologic methods. J Allergy Immunol 81:51–62, 1988.
26. Turner-Warwick M: Epidemiology of nocturnal asthma. Am J Med 85(Suppl 1B):6–8, 1988.
27. Reinberg A, Guillet P, Gervais P, et al: One-month chronocorticotherapy (Dutimelan 8–15R mite). Control of the asthmatic condition without adrenal suppression and circadian rhythm alteration. Chronobiologia 4:295–312, 1977.
28. Reinberg A, Gervais P, Frambourg JC, et al: Rhythms circadiens de fonctions respiratoires et de la temperature d'asthmatiques sejournant en milieu hypoallergnique. Presse Med 78(42):1817–1831, 1970.
29. Dethlefsen U, Repges R: Ein neues Therapieprinzip Nachtlichem Asthma. Klin Med 80:44–47, 1985.
30. McGovern JP, Smolensky MH, Reinberg A: Circadian and circamensual rhythmicity and cutaneous reactivity to histamine and allergenic extracts. In McGovern JP, Smolensky MH, Reinberg A (eds): Chronobiology in Allergy and Immunology. Springfield, Ill, Charles C Thomas, 1977, pp 79–116.
31. Hetzle MR, Clark TJH: Does sleep cause nocturnal asthma? Thorax 34:749–754, 1979.
32. Halberg F, Reinberg A, Reinberg A: Chronobiologic serial sections gauge circadian rhythm adjustments following transmeridian flight and life in a novel environment. Waking and Sleeping 1:259–279, 1977.
33. Halberg F, Howard RB: 24-hour periodicity and experimental medicine; examples and interpretations. Postgrad Med 24:349–358, 1958.
34. Cockcroft DW: Modulation of airway hyperresponsiveness. Ann Allergy 60:465–475, 1988.
35. Taylor AN, Davies RJ, Hendrick DJ, Pepys J: Recurrent nocturnal asthmatic reaction to bronchial provocation tests. Clin Allergy 9:213–219, 1979.
36. Hannuksela M: Occupational dermatoses: Appropriate diagnosis and therapy. Allergologie, Jahrgang 12 Kongressausgabe Proceedings, 1989, pp 71–74.
37. Smolensky MH: Chronobiology and epidemiology. Path Biol (Paris) 3:991–1004, 1987.
38. Lemmer B (ed): Chronopharmacology. New York, Marcel Dekker, 1989.
39. Reinberg A, Smolensky MH, Labrecque G: New aspects in chronopharmacology. Ann Rev Chronopharmacol 2:1–26, 1986.
40. Reinberg A, Smolensky MH: Circadian changes of drug disposition in man. Clin Pharmacokinet 7:401–420, 1982.
41. Smolensky MH: Chronopharmacology of theophylline and beta-sympathomimetics. In Lemmer B (ed): Chronopharmacology. New York, Marcel Dekker, 1989, pp 65–113.
42. Labrecque G, Reinberg AE: Chronopharmacology of nonsteroid anti-inflammatory drugs. In Lemmer B (ed): Chronopharmacology. New York, Marcel Dekker, 1989, pp 545–579.

43. Reinberg AE: Chronopharmacology of H_1-antihistamines. In Lemmer B (ed): Chronopharmacology. New York, Marcel Dekker, 1989, pp 115–135.
44. Reinberg AE: Chronopharmacology of corticosteroids and ACTH. In Lemmer B (ed): Chronopharmacology. New York, Marcel Dekker, 1989, pp 137–167.
45. Bruguerolle B: Chronopharmacokinetics. Path Biol 35:925–934, 1987.
46. Vener KJ, Moore JG: Chronobiologic properties of the alimentary canal affecting xenobiotic absorption. Ann Rev Chronopharmacol 4:259–282, 1988.
47. Merki H, Witzel L, Harre K, et al: Single dose treatment with H_2-receptor antagonists: Is bedtime administration too late? Gut 28:451–454, 1987.
48. Smolensky MH, D'Alonzo GE, Kunkel G, Barnes PJ (eds): Circadian rhythm-adapted theophylline schedules for asthma. Chronobiol Internatl 4:301–466, 1987.
49. Harter JG, Reddy WJ, Thorn GW: Studies on an intermittent corticosteroid dosage regimen. N Engl J Med 296:591–595, 1963.
50. Reinberg A, Smolensky M, Labrecque G, Hallek M: Aspects of chronopharmacology and chronotherapy in children. Chronobiologia 14:303–325, 1987.
51. Halberg F: Temporal coordination of physiologic function. Cold Spring Harbor Symp on Quant Biol 25:289–310, 1960.
52. Smolensky MH, Scheving LE, Paustenbach D: Biological rhythms in shift work and occupational health. In Cralley LJ, Cralley L (eds): Patty's Theory and Practice of Industrial Hygiene; Vol 3B, Biological Responses, 2nd ed. New York, John Wiley, 1985, pp 175–311.
53. Feuers RJ, Scheving LE: Chronobiology of hepatic enzymes. Ann Rev Chronopharmacol 4:209–255, 1988.
54. Nair V: Circadian rhythm in drug action: A pharmacologic, biochemical and electromicroscopic study. In Scheving LE, Halberg F, Pauly JE (eds): Chronobiology. Tokyo, Igaku Shoin, 1974, pp 182–186.
55. DeVries K, Goei JT, Booy-Noord H, Orie NG: Changes during 24 hours in the lung function and histamine hyperreactivity of the bronchial tree in asthmatic and bronchitic patients. Intl Arch Allergy 20:93–101, 1962.
56. Reinberg A, Gervais P, Morin M, Abulker C: Rythme circadien humain du seuil de la response bronchique a l'acetylcholine. Comp-Rend, Acad Sci (Paris) 272:1879–1881, 1971.
57. Gervais P, Reinberg A, Gervais C, et al: Twenty-four-hour rhythm in the bronchial hyperreactivity to house dust in asthmatics. J Allergy Clin Immunol 59:207–213, 1977.
58. Sly PD, Landau LI: Diurnal variation in bronchial responsiveness in asthmatic children. Pediatr Pulmonol 2:344–352, 1986.
59. Smolensky MH, Reinberg A, Lee RE, McGovern JP: Secondary rhythms related to hormonal changes in the menstrual cycle: Special reference to allergology. In Ferim M, Halberg F, Richart RM, Vande Wiele RL (eds): Biorhythms and Human Reproduction. New York, John Wiley, 1974, pp 287–308.
60. Haus E, Nicolau GY, Lakatua D, Sackett-Lundeen L: Reference values for chronopharmacology. Ann Rev Chronopharmacol 4:333–424, 1988.
61. Halberg F, Johnson EA, Nelson W, et al: Autorhythmometry. Procedures for physiologic self-measurements and their analysis. Physiol Teacher 1:1–11, 1972.
62. Halberg F, Bakken E, Cornelissen G, et al: Blood pressure assessment in a broad chronobiologic perspective. In Refsum H, Sulg JA, Rasmussen K (eds): Heart and Brain, Brain and Heart. Berlin, Springer-Verlag, 1989, pp 142–162.
63. Scheving LE, Halberg F, Ehret CF (eds): Chronobiotechnology and Chronobiological Engineering. NATO ASI Series; Series E: Applied Sciences, No. 120. Dordrecht, Martinus Nijhoff Publishers, 1987.
64. Randem B, Smolensky MH, Hsi B, et al: Field survey of circadian rhythm in PEF of electronic workers suffering from colophony-induced asthma. Chronobiol Internatl 2:264–277, 1987.
65. Rutenfranz J, Knauth P, Angersbach D: Shift work research issues. In Johnson LC, Tepas DI, Colquhoun WP, Colligan MJ (eds): Biological Rhythms, Sleep and Shift Work. New York, SP Medical & Scientific Books, 1981, pp 165–196.
66. Reinberg A, Andlauer P, De Prins J, et al: Desynchronization of the oral temperature circadian rhythms and intolerance to shift work. Nature 308:272–274, 1984.
67. Reinberg A, Motohashi Y, Bourdeleau P, et al: Alteration of period and amplitude of circadian rhythms in shift workers. Eur J Appl Physiol 57:15–25, 1988.
68. Gervais P, Reinberg A, Fraboulet C, et al: Circadian changes in peak expiratory flow of subjects suffering from allergic asthma documented both in areas of high and low air pollution. In Reinberg A, Halberg F (eds): Chronopharmacology. Oxford, Pergamon Press, 1979, pp 203–212.

69. Johnson LC, Tepas DI, Colquhoun WP, Colligan MJ (eds): Biological Rhythms, Sleep and Shift Work. New York, SP Medical & Scientific Books, 1979.
70. Aschoff J: Circadian rhythms: Interference with and dependence on work-rest schedules. In Johnson LE, Tepas DI, Colquhoun WP, Colligan MJ (eds): Biological Rhythms, Sleep and Shift Work. New York, SP Medical & Scientific Books, 1981, pp 11–34.
71. Halberg F: Some aspects of chronobiology relating to the optimization of shift work. NIOSH Research Symposium, Shift-Work and Health. Cincinnati, 1976, pp 13–47.
72. Graeber C: Alterations in performance following rapid transmeridian flight. In Brown FM, Graeber RC (eds): Rhythmic Aspects of Behavior. New Jersey, LEA Publishers, 1982, pp 173–212.
73. Aschoff J: Features of circadian rhythms relevant for the design of shift schedules. Ergonomics 39:739–754, 1978.
74. Wever RA: The Circadian System of Man. New York, Springer-Verlag, 1979.
75. Reinberg A, Vieux N, Ghata J, et al: Consideration of the circadian amplitude in relation to the ability to phase shift circadian rhythms of shift workers. Chronobiologia 6(Suppl 1):57–63, 1979.
76. Fröberg E: Sleep deprivation and prolonged working hours. In Folkard S, Monk TH: Hours of Work: Temporal Factors in Work Scheduling. Chichester, John Wiley, 1985, pp 67–75.
77. Walsh JK, Muehlbach MJ, Sweitzer PK: Acute administration of triazolam for the daytime sleep of rotating shift workers. Sleep 7:223–229, 1984.
78. Seidel WF, Roth T, Roehrs T, et al: Treatment of a 12-hour shift of sleep schedule with benzodiazepines. Science 224:1262–1274, 1984.
79. Bicakova-Rocher A, Frowirth C, Gorceix A, Reinberg A: Once-a-day dosing (morning versus evening) of ethyl loflazepate in anxiety disorders. Changes in the circadian rhythm of self-rated symptoms. Ann Rev Chronopharmacol 3:433–436, 1986.
80. Nicholson AN, Stone BM: Hypnotics and shift work. In Johnson LC, Tepas DI, Colquhoun WP, Colligan MJ (eds): Biological Rhythms, Sleep and Shift Work. New York, SP Medical & Scientific Books, 1981, pp 383–398.
81. Reinberg A, Smolensky MH, Labrecque G: The hunting of a wonder pill for resetting all biological clocks. Ann Rev Chronopharmacol 4:171–208, 1988.
82. Turek FW, Losee-Olson S: A benzodiazepine used in the treatment of insomnia phase-shifts the mammalian circadian clock. Nature 321:167–168, 1986.
83. Van Reeth O, Turek FW: Adaptation of circadian rhythmicity to a shift in the light-dark cycle can be accelerated by a benzodiazepine. Am J Physiol 253:R204–R207, 1987.
84. Mrosovsky N, Salmon A: Triazolam and phase-shifting acceleration re-evaluated. Chronobiol Internatl 7:35–42, 1990.
85. Ehret CF, Potter VR, Dobra KW: Chronotypic action of theophylline and of pentobarbital as circadian zeitgebers in the rat. Science 188:1212–1215, 1975.
86. Reinberg A, Pauchet F, Ruff F, et al: The advantage of once-daily evening versus morning sustained release theophylline dosing for nocturnal asthma. Ann Rev Chronopharmacol 3:147–150, 1986.
87. Smolensky MH, Albright D, Hsi B, et al: Sustained-release theophylline at 12-hour intervals does not alter staging of circadian rhythms. Ann Rev Chronopharmacol 3:131–133, 1986.
88. Okudaira N, Kripke DF, Mullaney DJ: Theophylline delays human sleep phase. Life Sciences 34:933–938, 1984.
89. Ehret CF, Groh KR, Meinert JC: Considerations of diet in alleviating jet lag. In Scheving LE, Halberg F (eds): Chronobiology: Principles and Applications to Shifts in Schedules. NATO Advanced Study Institutes Series D: Behavioral and Social Sciences No. 3. The Netherlands, Sijthoff & Noordhoff, 1980, pp 393–402.
90. Ehret CF, Scanlon LW: Overcoming Jet Lag. New York, Berkley, 1983.
91. Wurtman JJ: Managing Your Mind and Mood Through Food. New York, Rawson, 1986.
92. Leathwood P: Circadian rhythms of plasma amino acids, brain neurotransmitters and behavior. In Arendt J, Minors DS, Waterhouse JM (eds): Biological Rhythms in Clinical Practice. London, John Wright, 1989, pp 136–159.
93. Arendt J: Melatonin and the pineal gland. In Arendt J, Minors DS, Waterhouse JM (eds): Biological Rhythms and Clinical Practice. London, John Wright, 1989, pp 184–205.
94. Reiter RJ: Intrinsic rhythms of the pineal gland and associated hormone cycles in body fluids. Ann Rev Chronopharmacol 4:77–105, 1988.
95. Armstrong SM, Cassone VM, Chesworth MJ, et al: Synchronization of mammalian circadian rhythms by melatonin. J Neural Transm 21(suppl):375–398, 1986.

96. Arendt J, Aldhous M, Marks V: Alleviation of jet lag by melatonin: Preliminary results of a controlled double-blind trial. Br Med J 292:1170, 1986.
97. Rosenthal NE, Blehar MC (eds): Seasonal Affective Disorder and Phototherapy. New York, Guilford Press, 1989.
98. Thompson C, Silverstone T (eds): Seasonal Affective Disorder. London, CRC Clinical Neuroscience Press, 1989.
99. Lewy AJ, Sack RL: Phase typing and bright light therapy of chronobiologic sleep and mood disorders. In Halaris A (ed): Chronobiologic and Psychiatric Disorders. Amsterdam, Elsevier, 1987, pp 181–206.
100. Czeisler CA, Johnson MP, Duffy JP, et al: Exposure to bright light and darkness treat physiologic maladaptation to night work. N Engl J Med 322:1253–1259, 1990.
101. Eastman CL: Bright light in work-sleep schedules for shift workers: Application of circadian rhythm principles. In Rensing L, An der Heiden U, Mackay MC (eds): Temporal Disorder in Human Oscillatory Systems. New York, Springer-Verlag, 1987, pp 176–185.
102. Powers LM, Terman M, Link MJ: Bright light treatment of night-shift workers. Abstract, Annual Meeting, Society for Light Treatment and Biological Rhythms, Bethesda, MD, June 1989.
103. French J, Hannon P, Brainard G: Illuminance and management of biological rhythms. Ann Rev Chronopharmacol 7: 1990 (in press).
104. Englund C, Loving R, Kripke D: Bright light amelioration of shift work. Ann Rev Chronopharmacol 7: 1990 (in press).
105. Reinberg A, Vieux N, Andlauer P, Smolensky MH: Tolerance to shift work: A chronobiologic approach. Adv Biol Psychiatry 11:35–47, 1983.
106. Reinberg A, Andlauer P, Teinturier P, De Prins J, et al: Desynchronisation du rythme circadien de la temperature orale chez des hommes jeunes tolerant mal le travail de nuit. CR Acad Sci 296:267–269, 1983.
107. Motohashi Y, Reinberg A, Levi F: Axillary temperature: A circadian marker rhythm for shift workers. Ergonomics 30:1235–1247, 1987.
108. Michel-Briand C, Chopard JL, Guiot A, et al: The pathological consequences of shift-work in retired workers. In Reinberg A, Vieux N, Andlauer P (eds): Night and Shiftwork Studies: Biological and Social Aspects. Oxford, Pergamon Press, 1981, pp 399–407.
109. Smolensky MH: The conceptual implications of chronotoxicology and chronopathology for occupational health and shift work. In Scheving LE, Halberg F (eds): Chronobiology: Principles and Applications to Shifts in Schedules. NATO Advanced Study Institutes Series D: Behavioral and Social Sciences No. 3. The Netherlands, Sijthoff & Noordhoff, 1980, pp 325–337.
110. Reinberg A, Levi F: Dose-response relationships in chronopharmacology. Ann Rev Chronopharmacol 6: 1990 (in press).
111. Brown AC, Smolensky MH, D'Alonzo GE: Actigraphy: A means of assessing circadian patterns in human activity. Chronobiol Internatl 7: 1990 (in press).

ALLENE J. SCOTT, MD, MPH
JOSEPH LADOU, MD

SHIFTWORK: EFFECTS ON SLEEP AND HEALTH WITH RECOMMENDATIONS FOR MEDICAL SURVEILLANCE AND SCREENING

Allene J. Scott, MD, MPH
LCDR, MC, USNR
Head, Occupational Medicine Division
Navy Environmental Health Center
Norfolk, Virginia

Joseph LaDou, MD
Clinical Professor and Chief
Division of Occupational and Environmental Medicine
University of California, San Francisco
San Francisco, California

The views expressed in this article are those of the authors and do not reflect the official policy or position of the Department of the Navy, Department of Defense, or the U.S. Government.

Reprint requests to:
Allene J. Scott, MD, MPH
Occupational Medicine Division
Navy Environmental Health Center
Norfolk, VA 23513-2617

Shiftwork, meaning work done at a time other than during the dayshift, is an occupational stressor.[23,32,83,136] At least 21 million people in the United States are shiftworkers (about 1 out of 4 employed men and 1 out of 6 employed women).[57] Up to 20% of workers are not able to tolerate working at night.[26,103] As the makeup of the work force in the United States changes, a larger percentage of shiftworkers will likely suffer some adverse effect from their work schedule. Predictions for the next century, based on current trends, anticipate that the U.S. work force will be older and more female.[69] With respect to shiftwork issues, two categories of workers at increased risk of sleep deprivation associated with nightwork are those in their late forties or older and single or married women with children.[26,52,58,84]

BIOLOGICAL RHYTHMS

Numerous human biological variables have been found to follow a 24-hour rhythm under normal nychthermal conditions—for example, body temperature, the sleep/wake cycle, cardiovascular parameters, psychomotor performance, endocrine and metabolic factors, responsiveness to various medications, as well as psychological variables of mood and anxiety. A summary of some of the relevant studies is given in Table 1.

That a biological "clock" exists in humans was first shown in temporal isolation studies in

TABLE 1. Human Variables Observed to Follow a Circadian Rhythm

Variable	Reference(s)
Temperature	11, 28, 44, 66, 72, 92, 94, 134
REM sleep	159
Heart rate	24, 28, 44, 63, 66
Blood pressure	28, 66, 134
Respiratory rate	59, 143
Respiratory functions: FEV1, tidal volume, minute ventilation	59, 143
Urinary parameters: volume, electrolytes, calcium, phosphates, 17-OHCS, 11-OHCS, 5-HIAA, catecholamines	11, 12, 31, 51, 55, 60, 80, 92, 94, 134
Melatonin	81, 5
Salivary secretions: rate, sodium, chloride, steroidal hormones	47, 156
Tear flow	157
Plasma or serum: 11-OHCS, electrolytes, total protein, albumin, alkaline phosphatase, SGOT, BUN, glucose, bilirubin, triglycerides	30, 134
Self-rated arousal, anxiety	44
Addition speed, finger tapping, counting	44
Short-term and long-term memory	44, 98
Digit summation, symbol cancellation, reaction time, psychomotor performance	71
Handgrip strength, neuromuscular control	66
Blood eosinophil and leukocyte count	61
Thermal and metabolic responses to heat exposure	79

FEV1, forced expiratory volume in one second; OHCS, hydroxycorticosteroids; HIAA, hydroxyindoleacetic acid; SGOT, serum glutamic oxaloacetic transaminase; BUN, blood urea nitrogen.

the cellar of a hospital in Munich.[15] In that classic study, three men and three women were isolated from the natural day/night cycle and other time cues for 8–19 days. All the subjects maintained a free-running activity/rest cycle with a non-24-hour period. The existence of endogenous rhythms in humans has been repeatedly demonstrated since Aschoff and Wever's classic experiment (see Fig. 1 and Table 2). Studies have consistently shown that these biological rhythms, when allowed to free-run in isolation studies, have a cycle of about 25 hours.[11] That is, the human biological clock runs slow with respect to the solar day. The term **circadian** (Latin *circa*, "about," *dies*, "a day") has been used to describe these rhythms.[62]

In order to keep in time with the solar day, the human clock must daily be set ahead about 1 hour. Following a normal day/night, wake/sleep cycle, the circadian rhythms are entrained to the 24-hour solar day by time cues referred to as **zeitgebers** (German "time givers"). Zeitgebers enable the biological clock, which runs with a periodicity of about 25 hours, to be reset to the shorter, 24-hour solar day. Thus the circadian system is synchronized or entrained to the 24-hour rotation of the earth.[11] Various factors have been shown to act as zeitgebers, including the light/dark cycle, natural noises, social factors, awareness of the time of day, and behavioral patterns such as eating schedules.[13,14,36,37,99,104,156,172] Even electromagnetic fields appear to be able to act as zeitgebers.[166] Zeitgebers are necessary to keep the human circadian rhythm in phase with the 24-hour solar day. For most people, physical and social zeitgebers are complementary

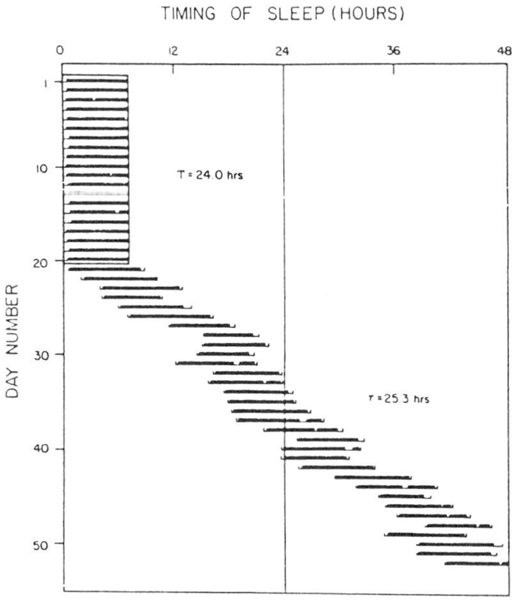

FIGURE 1. A typical response to temporal isolation is demonstrated in this sleep/wake pattern. The horizontal bars represent sleep periods. For the first 20 days, the subject was on a scheduled sleep time. The following 32 bars show the sleep time of the subject during isolation from time cues. Notice that the free-running sleep/wake pattern runs slow by about 1.3 hours with respect to the 24-hour-day sleep/wake pattern. Adapted with permission from Czeisler CA, Richardson GS, Coleman RM, et al: Chronotherapy: Resetting the circadian clocks of patients with delayed sleep phase insomnia. Sleep 4(1): 1–21, 1981.

and perhaps of insignificant relative importance. But for the shiftworker, physical and social zeitgebers conflict and thus oppose adjustment to the work schedule. The slow rate of adaptation by workers to a new shift may be, at least in part, due to competing influences of different zeitgebers.[96] Circadian rhythms are more easily re-entrained if all the important zeitgebers are synchronously shifted (such as happens in transmeridian flights) than when some change and others do not, as is the case in shiftwork.[14] It takes about a week for the circadian system to adjust to a 6-hour time change experienced in a transmeridian flight, and in that situation, all the new zeitgebers are synchronized.[71] But even after 21 consecutively worked nightshifts, the body temperature rhythm does not completely invert. Some researchers have concluded, therefore, that the circadian system never fully adapts to nightwork.[73] (Some studies[30] have found evidence of complete adjustment in permanent nightworkers who maintain a night schedule on their days off.)

Not only is there the problem of desynchronization between endogenous rhythms and external time cues (external desynchronization), but the biological rhythms, which are normally temporally linked to each other, also become uncoupled (internal desynchronization). Internal desynchronization suggests that more than one self-sustaining oscillator controls the body's circadian rhythms. Further discussion of studies and theories about the nature of these oscillators can be found elsewhere.[38,53,93,102,165] The significant point for shiftworkers and for

TABLE 2. Studies Demonstrating Endogenous Circadian Rhythms in Man

Type of Study	Findings	Reference
Data from several isolation studies, 156 subjects in several experiments, all studies without external influences or time cues	Free-running period of 25.00 + 0.5 hours for temperature and sleep/wake cycle	165, 171
29 male subjects, 72 hours sleep deprivation with no daylight exposure and no access to clocks, subjects were aware of 3-hour intervals between urine collections	Diurnal rhythm persisted in several psychological and physiological variables—e.g., urinary adrenaline and fatigue	51
3 men and 3 women studied in isolation from light/dark cycle and other time cues	All subjects maintained a free-running rhythm of rest/activity cycle	169
16 female subjects, 72 hours sleep deprivation, no daylight exposure, no access to clocks, subjects unaware that testing periodicity was at 3-hour intervals	Body temperature and subjective alertness showed circadian oscillation on a background of gradual decline over 72 hours; performance variables demonstrated circadian rhythms	50
23-year-old male subject in 2 weeks of temporal isolation choosing own sleep and meal times	Circadian rhythm of sleep/wake cycle free-ran at 24.7 hours	163
14 subjects in temporal isolation, subjects' estimation of 1-hour intervals recorded	Bimodal circadian rhythm demonstrated	12
10 subjects in temporal isolation, polygraphic measurements of sleep stages made, continuous temperature readings, blood cortisol and growth hormone every 20 minutes	During free-running conditions, timing and amount of sleep following sleep onset occurred preferentially at specific phase of temperature rhythm; 2 components of cortisol curve—one phase advanced with respect to sleep, the other following sleep onset; growth hormone related to the first 2 hours of sleep onset	162

those taking transmeridian flights is that different rhythms adjust at different rates to time shifts.

The disruption of biological rhythms is frequently associated with a variety of symptoms, both physical and emotional. The term **desynchronosis** refers to this situation. It cannot be said with certainty how often desynchronosis occurs with desynchronization, but the percentage of jet travelers with symptoms of jet lag suggests that most people experience at least some ill feelings after a time change of several hours. A survey of 784 frequent jet travelers in the *Washington Post* of May 10, 1988, reported that 90% indicated daytime sleepiness or fatigue, 78% difficulty sleeping at night, 69% impaired concentration, 66% slowed physical reflexes, 50% irritability, 47% abnormal digestion, 44% hunger at unusual times, and 31% depression.

SLEEP

In addition to, and partly as a result of, biological rhythm disruption, nightworkers, both rotating and permanent, are at risk of sleep deprivation. Both the quantity and quality of sleep are affected. The significance of the impact of shiftwork on sleep is reflected in Weitzman's observation[161] that "the most significant complaint when human beings are shifted in an industrial situation is a disturbance of their sleep patterns. It is the most universal complaint in their own daily lives as well as in their family and other social relationships" (p. 53).

Tepas discusses the impact of shiftwork on sleep in this volume (Chapter 3), and Naitoh et al. (Chapter 4) review studies dealing with sleep deprivation. Sleep issues are, therefore, only briefly mentioned in this chapter. However, the reader should keep in mind that distinguishing the health problems of shiftworkers related to desynchronization of biological rhythms from those due to chronic sleep deprivation is generally not possible because the majority of nightworkers complain of sleep disruption and sleep loss.[130] Also, the sleep problems of shiftworkers are due (in addition to daytime noise disturbance) to disruption of the normal sleep/wake rhythm, of the normal circadian rapid eye movement (REM) sleep/rhythm, and of the rhythm of REM/non-REM sleep patterns.[34,151,164] That is, the sleep problem of the nightworker is primarily a circadian one. The total duration of sleep has been shown to be correlated to the phase of the body temperature rhythm at bedtime, *not* to the length of prior wakefulness.[37,56,142] As stated by Reinberg et al., "there is a 'best time' to work and a 'best time' to sleep which are in agreement with the human temporal structure."[122] Because nightwork regularly shortens sleep length on workdays, chronic sleep deprivation ensues. Even employees who have worked nights for years continue to sleep less on workdays than dayworkers.[147,148]

Sleeping habits should be of concern to physicians because sleep disturbances and chronic sleep deprivation have been associated with poor health. In a survey of performance records of almost 3,000 U.S. Navy personnel, although school performance did not differ between poor and good sleepers, the number of promotions, the pay grade, and recommendations for re-enlistment were lower for poor sleepers, and a larger percentage of poor sleepers had two or more hospitalizations during their Navy career.[68] It has also been observed that for patients with sleep disturbances, the severity of the disturbance is positively correlated with the probability that the patient will have serious medical problems.[41] Insomnia has been associated with chronic illness and somatic complaints.[64] Finally, decreased sleep time has been associated with reduced life expectancy.[77]

PSYCHOSOCIAL STRESS

Besides causing (or perhaps because of) disruptions of circadian rhythms and disturbances of sleep, shiftwork has been shown to be a potential source of occupational stress.[23,32,83] One reason workers have given for leaving shiftwork is a health problem related to their shift schedule. Psychosomatic complaints and complaints of irritation and strain are among the problems mentioned. Freese and Okenek[49] found in their survey of former shiftworkers that over half had left shiftwork for primarily health reasons and that they generally had received medical counsel to leave shiftwork. The authors present a "vulnerability-stress model" to explain the situation. They suggest that people who leave shiftwork for health reasons continue to work nightshifts "up to their biological/psychological breaking point" because of the financial rewards of shiftwork.

Mott et al.[105] observed that, for some shiftworkers, difficulties in performing perceived roles in their families combined with complaints reflecting circadian rhythm disruption have a deleterious impact on psychological health. The complaints concerning body rhythmic functioning appear to aggravate problems of role performance. Interestingly, role performance difficulties due to shift schedules were found to be more psychologically damaging to the less neurotic worker than to the more neurotic worker. Overall, the personality type of the male worker did not seem to be as important as the degree of acceptance of his schedule by his wife with respect to the impact of a perceived role problem on self-esteem, anxiety, and conflict.

Verhaegen et al.[153] surveyed 104 male shiftworkers at the start of their work in a new wire mill and at 6 months (96 workers available), 4 years (64 workers available), and 7 years (51 workers available) later. In summarizing data from the 7-year follow-up, they found a continuous increase in subjective health complaints, neuroticism, and somatic/neurotic complaints. At the 4-year follow-up, 31 workers who left shiftwork were asked to give the reasons for their leaving. Of the 50 reasons given, one-third were related to disturbances of subjective well-being or of social relations; 25% of workers ranked these reasons as most important.[89]

In some studies, the disruption of social life was a more common complaint than sleep disturbances.[19,89,109,136,155,158] Of special concern is the impact of shiftwork on families. A husband may be more concerned about how his wife accepts his work schedule than about how he likes or dislikes it.[19] Mott et al.[105] point out that "the schedules of husbands and wives are so closely interwoven that it would be a serious mistake to consider the effects of shiftwork upon only one of the marriage partners" (p. 90). Both spouses may find it difficult to fulfill their perceived roles when one is on a shiftwork schedule. Nightworkers have blamed their shift schedule for broken or strained marriages, and higher divorce rates have been reported for both shiftworkers and "dropouts" from shiftwork.[22,76,74,174]

HEALTH EFFECTS

It can be seen that shiftwork-related stress results from three general problems—circadian rhythm desynchronization, disruption of social and family life, and sleep deprivation—that may interact to produce deleterious effects on the general psychological and physical well-being of the shiftworker. While there is little evidence that shiftwork *causes* a specific illness, shiftworkers (especially rotating shiftworkers) do have more health-related complaints such as digestive problems, chest pain, wheezing, nervousness, colds, and fatigue.[136] Studies comparing sickness absence rates of shiftworkers to those of dayworkers have produced conflicting results. For example, Taylor et al.[146] in a matched-pair study of several shift schedules, found shiftworkers to have a lower absence rate. However, in the United Kingdom, studies have found rotating shiftworkers to have higher sickness absence rates.[75,144] At least one study also suggests that rotating shiftworkers have more illness as reflected in the number of visits to work-site clinics and the number of and reasons for sick days taken.[144] Likely reasons for the discrepancies between these studies are that sickness absence is not synonymous with morbidity, and that the freedom of shiftworkers with schedule-related health complaints to change to the dayshift is variable. It would not be surprising for workers who are prevented by labor, management, or personal economic needs from leaving nightwork despite schedule-related complaints to have a higher absenteeism rate.

Other studies have found certain diseases to be aggravated by, and some possibly caused by, shiftwork. These are reviewed below.

Gastrointestinal Disorders

The health problem that has most clearly been shown to be associated with shiftwork is that of gastrointestinal (GI) disorders, including peptic ulcer disease.[9,34,95,96] An early study found that 30% of a group of shiftworkers who switched to regular daywork for health reasons complained of symptoms of gastritis.[150] In this same study, the incidence of peptic ulcers was found to be higher for shiftworkers than for dayworkers. In a study of textile workers, Costa et al.[33] found higher incidence rates of gastroduodenitis and peptic ulcer in nightworkers (both permanent and rotators) than in those working days or afternoons. Aanonsen[1] found 2.5 times as many cases of peptic ulcer disease and 2 times as many other GI disorders in dayworkers who had left shiftwork for health reasons than in dayworkers who had never done shiftwork. For both current and past shiftworkers, GI morbidity was increased by 34%. A NIOSH study of almost 900 workers found four health factors associated with nightwork or rotating shifts. The strongest association was found for constipation (especially in women) and the use of medication for stomach or digestive problems (more frequent in men).[26] Another NIOSH-sponsored study, which included a questionnaire survey of more than 2,400 workers, found rotating shiftworkers to have a significantly higher incidence of digestive problems.[136] Angersbach et al.[9] in a retrospective cohort study, found a higher incidence of GI disease in both current shiftworkers and "dropouts" than in dayworkers who had never worked shifts. It has also been observed that digestive symptoms arising during shiftwork may not completely resolve even after a normal schedule is resumed.[1,153]

One possible reason for GI complaints is the altered eating habits of shiftworkers, including changes in the timing of meals and the types of food eaten.[122,137,141,153] Nightworkers eat fewer meals, have poorer appetites, and are less satisfied with their eating habits. Since differences in eating habits have been observed in comparisons of nonworkdays with workdays for nightworkers and not for workers of different shifts, a causal relationship is likely.[147]

The role of excessive alcohol or caffeine consumption in shiftworker GI problems is unclear. Whereas some studies have found alcohol consumption to be higher in shiftworkers,[136] others have not.[147,148] Caffeine consumption is generally assumed to be greater on the nightshift, but in some plants it has been shown to be less for experienced nightworkers than for dayworkers.[147] Because worker demographics vary from plant to plant, it should not be surprising that the use of alcohol and caffeine is variable. Smoking habits of shiftworkers may also contribute to their higher rate of peptic ulcer disease, but consistent patterns have not been demonstrated.

Circadian rhythm disruption, of course, must also be considered in the etiology of shiftworker GI disease. A circadian rhythm has been demonstrated in gastric acidity and may be endogenous.[21,100] Endogenous circadian rhythms in the timing, quantity, and quality of meals have also been observed.[122]

Stress in general has long been associated with digestive disorders, and shiftwork, as pointed out earlier, contributes to physiological and psychological stress.

Cardiovascular Disorders

Shiftwork is less certainly associated with cardiovascular disease than with GI disorders, but evidence of an association is mounting. This is not surprising because heart disease has been associated with anxiety, work dissatisfaction, family conflicts, sleep disturbance, and fatigue.[67] Also, as shown in Table 1, heart rate and blood pressure have been shown to follow a circadian rhythm.

Angersbach et al.[9] found no significant excess of cardiovascular disease in people who worked shifts for 10 years but did find an increased incidence in shiftworkers who changed to daywork. Although Aanonsen[1] did not find angina or myocardial infarction (MI) to be more frequent in shiftworkers or in dayworkers who had left shiftwork for health reasons, a Swedish retrospective study of 334 cases and 882 controls found men with a history of MI significantly more likely to be shiftworkers than nonshiftworkers matched for sex and age.[6]

In another Swedish study, several cardiac risk factors were altered in policemen whose normal counterclockwise rotation of shifts was switched to a clockwise rotation.[110,111] Policemen on phase-advance schedules had significantly higher triglycerides (but not cholesterol) than those on a phase-delay schedule. Systolic (but not diastolic) blood pressure was significantly lower after phase-delay (clockwise) rotations than after phase advance (counterclockwise). Sleep was found to be better and longer with phase-delay rotation.

Michel-Briand et al.[90] studied two groups of retired workers—93 former dayworkers and 99 former shiftworkers. Alcohol and tobacco consumption were not significantly different between the groups, but the dayworkers were of a higher socioeconomic class and their diets were lower in lipids. Shiftworkers had more physically demanding off-the-job activities. The incidence of heart attacks and high blood pressure was greater in the former shiftworkers than in the former dayworkers.

In another study, irregular working hours were associated with significantly higher total and low density lipoprotein cholesterol and lower high density lipoprotein cholesterol. These differences were independent of smoking habits, obesity, diet, and physical activity.[40]

Recently male papermill workers in Sweden[74] were followed for 15 years, and the incidence of ischemic heart disease (IHD) was compared between shiftworkers and dayworkers. The shift schedule was a three-shift rota, generally with a phase-delay direction. The shiftworkers' total weekly hours were reduced from 40 to 38 in 1975 and to 36 in 1976. The 504 numbered cohort at the end of the study represented only a 5% loss from an original 528 workers. Shiftworkers were 394 of the total. Mean age was 39.3 years for the shiftworkers and 42.0 for dayworkers. A higher percentage of dayworkers were past 50 years of age, however (40% versus 23%). The relative risk of IHD was found to increase with increasing exposure to shiftwork. The trend, which continued for up to 20 years of exposure, was significant at the $p < 0.05$ level. Shiftworkers were noted to be more likely to be divorced and to smoke more, but the smoking difference decreased during the follow-up period. Multiple logistic regression analysis found age to be the main predictor of IHD and the duration of shiftwork the second predictor. Neither family status nor smoking had any significant independent predictive power. Thus an association between shiftwork and an increased risk of IHD was found to exist, at least for the first 20 years of shiftworking, and the association was independent of age and smoking habits.

Pregnancy

Although employment of expectant mothers in general does not appear to have an adverse effect on pregnancy outcome,[16,82,107,132] certain working conditions have, in recent studies, been associated with low birth weight (2500 g or less) or preterm birth (less than 37 weeks of gestation).[82,86]

Mamelle et al.[82] looked at sources of occupational fatigue that might be risk factors for premature birth in their survey of 3,437 women interviewed after giving birth. A fatigue index was constructed on the basis of five defined elements of fatigue determined by an analytical breakdown of jobs into their diverse components. The five elements included were standing posture, work on industrial machines, physical exertion, mental stress, and environmental exposures (heat, cold, chemicals, and noise). A significant relationship was found between high fatigue scores and prematurity. As scores varied from 0 to 5, the rate of preterm births increased from 2.3% to 11.1%. A significant association was also found between premature birth and weekly working times beyond 41 hours, with a rate of 8.8% found for long working hours compared to 5.6% for a work week of 40 hours or less and 3.6% for part-time work. Shiftwork was also found to be significantly associated with an increased risk of premature births (the risk ratio was 1.6). Also noted was a *combined* effect of occupational fatigue and working more than 40 hours (see Fig. 2).

McDonald and colleagues[86] conducted a large study in Montreal in which 22,761 live births were assessed for maternal employment risk factors for low birth weight and preterm birth. All the women included in the study worked 30 or more hours/week at conception and continued to work at least until the 28th week of pregnancy. Observed-to-expected (O/E) ratios were calculated for 60 occupational groups defined by work requirements. Six main industrial sectors were included. The O/E ratios for low birth weight and preterm birth were increased significantly for heavy lifting (1.25 and 1.26, $p < 0.01$). The ratio was also increased for long hours of work—46 hours/week or more—with ratios of 1.34, $p < 0.01$, and 1.24, $p = 0.03$. For preterm birth, the association with lifting was seen in five of the six occupational sectors, and the association with long hours was seen in all six. For low birth weight, the association with lifting was almost as consistent. Rotating shiftwork was strongly, but less consistently, associated with low birth weight, O/E 1.38, $p < 0.01$. A significant association

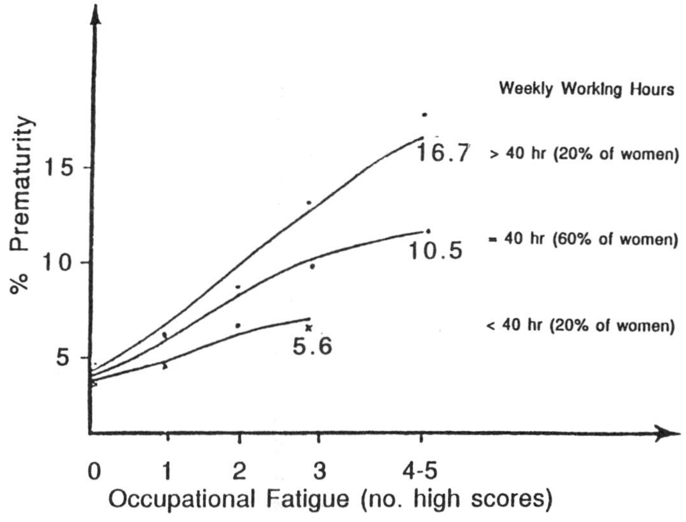

FIGURE 2. Prematurity rate according to number of high fatigue scores, after standardization for weekly working hours, in 1,928 women who gave birth to infants in Lyon and Haguenau, France, in 1977–1978. Adapted with permission from Mamelle M, Lauman B, Lazar P: Prematurity and occupational activity during pregnancy. Am J Epidemiol 119:309–322, 1984.

was found in the services sector between rotating shiftwork and preterm birth, O/E 1.88, $p < 0.01$.

Axelsson et al.[16] looked at the effect of nightwork, evening work, working irregular hours outside the period of 0645–1745, and rotating shiftwork (three shifts per 24 hours) compared to permanent daywork on pregnancy outcome. They found an association between irregular working hours and an increased risk of low birth weight. For nonsmoking mothers with infants of birth order 2 or more, an increased risk of low birth weight was associated with irregular hours ($p < 0.01$) and with rotating shiftwork ($p < 0.05$). The relative risk of miscarriage from irregular hours or rotating shiftwork compared to permanent daywork was 1.42 (95%, confidence interval 0.80–2.50) and 1.50 (95%, confidence interval 0.55–4.09), respectively. Although irregular working hours outside the normal dayshift time were looked at separately from "rotating" shiftwork, the difference seems to be of no consequence. The investigators also noted that "irregular time" and "rotating shift" both refer to hours of work that are not regular from day to day and calculated a combined relative risk of 1.44 for miscarriage (95%, confidence interval 0.83–2.51).

McDonald and co-workers[85,87] have also found an association between rotating shiftwork and an increased risk of spontaneous abortion. In their 1988 study, in which 22,613 previous pregnancies of the 56,067 Montreal women interviewed between 1982 and 1984 were further analyzed, a small but significant increased risk of spontaneous abortion was associated with working more than 46 hours per week (O/E 1.19, $p < 0.01$) and with rotating shiftwork (O/E 1.25, $p < 0.01$). Although recall bias was a possible confounder in this study (as it is in many retrospective studies), information about hours of work and the shift schedule is relatively objective, and when grouped analysis was done, the relative risk ratios remained significant, although they were decreased. Other factors found in this study to be associated with an increased risk of spontaneous abortion were job requirements such as heavy lifting (more than 15 times per day), other physical effort, standing posture (more than 8 hours per day), and exposure to vibration, noise, and cold.[87] Further analysis of the Montreal study suggested that shiftwork slowed fetal growth and increased risk of preterm delivery.[10]

With respect to permanent nightwork, few data are available. Saurel-Cubizolles and Kaminsky[133] did not find an association between nightwork and preterm delivery or low birth weight. However, only 4% of the female hospital employees interviewed were nightworkers, and some of them worked nights only occasionally. Another study found no increased pregnancy risks for permanent nightworkers, but 91% of the nightworkers questioned were part-time employees.[16]

It would be premature to state categorically that shiftwork is a risk factor for expectant mothers with respect to low birth weight, preterm delivery, or spontaneous abortion. Certainly no one of the above studies sufficiently establishes that conclusion. However, looking at the studies together, it would seem prudent, at least, to consider rotating shiftwork an added stressor during pregnancy. This conclusion also is reasonable in view of the increased incidence of sleep deprivation and fatigue observed in shiftworkers. The potential for adverse effects from stressors, such as heavy lifting, other strenuous work, mental stress, and so forth, may be increased if the pregnant woman is also a shiftworker. Recall that long hours of work were noted to increase the effect of occupational fatigue (see Fig. 2). Certainly overtime worked in conjunction with shiftwork should be avoided during pregnancy. Whether or not circadian disruption might directly influence the outcome of the pregnancy is not known, but desynchronosis has been associated with hormonal disruption. For instance, a high frequency of menstrual irregularities has been observed in airline stewardesses. A circadian rhythm of the luteinizing hormone level has been observed in women.[114] Despite this discussion, if shiftwork is a requirement of continued employment, caution is in order with respect to recommending removal of the pregnant worker from the job. In Newton and Hunt's study of the effect of major life events on pregnancy outcome, low birth weight and prematurity were associated with objective major life events. Unemployment and a decrease in income (as well as family illness) were the events most often recorded by the women in the low birth weight and preterm group.[108]

Shift Maladaptation Syndrome

From 5% to 20% of shiftworkers have disproportionate symptoms of illness when beginning on shiftwork, especially with rotating schedules.[26,103,104] Some symptoms resulting from circadian rhythm disruption are likely to occur in everyone when beginning shiftwork, but most workers adjust, at least partially, so that they have no, or only mild, symptoms. The worker with shift maladaptation syndrome (SMS), however, never adjusts or may decompensate with aging (see Fig. 3).

Manifestations of SMS include a combination of symptoms that have been mentioned in the preceding sections with respect to desynchronosis. In SMS these symptoms are pronounced, and instead of improving with time, they get worse. Thus the worker with SMS has a syndrome consisting of:[103,119]

1. Sleep disturbance and chronic tiredness
2. GI complaints such as heartburn, constipation, diarrhea
3. Alcohol or drug abuse usually related to self-treatment of insomnia
4. Higher rates of accidents or near misses
5. Depression, fatigue, mood disturbance, malaise, personality changes
6. Interpersonal relationship difficulties

Risk factors for SMS include age past 40 years, living with people who pursue a normal daytime routine, and poor tolerance of circadian rhythm disruption. The interaction of causal factors and outcomes is illustrated in Figure 4.

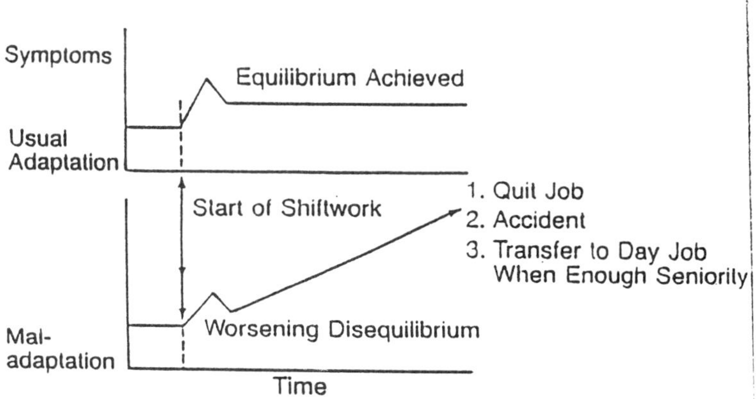

FIGURE 3. Expected mild circadian disruptions compared to shift maladaptation syndrome. Adapted with permission from Darlington AC: Shift maladaptation syndrome. Paper presented at Am Occup Med Assoc Postgrad Sem #12, April 27, 1987.

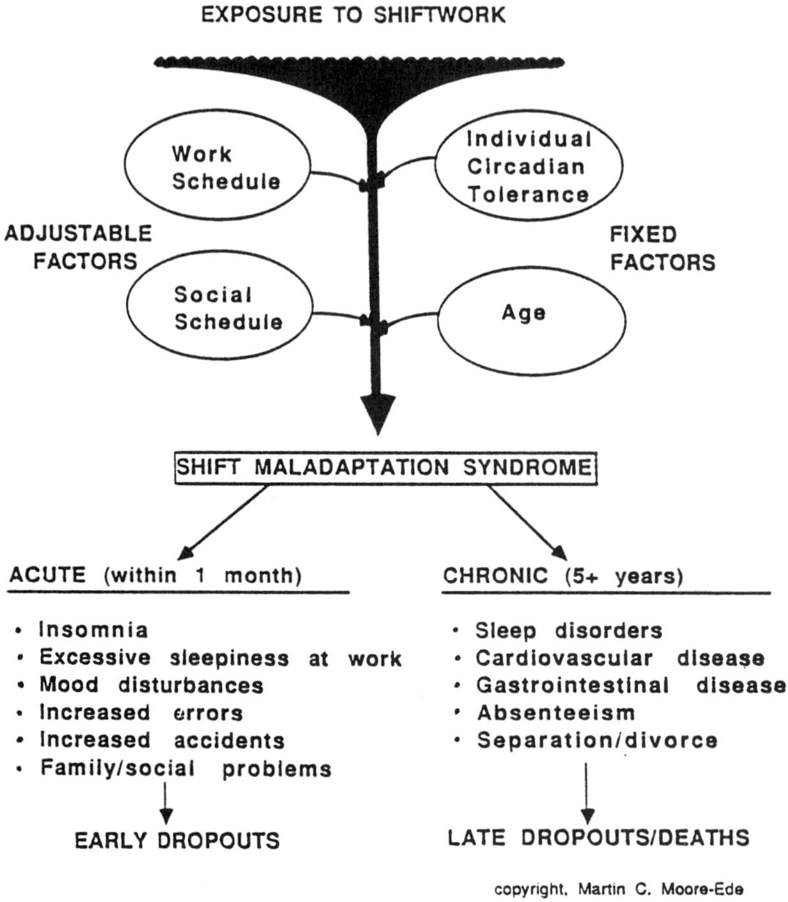

FIGURE 4. Variables affecting the development and outcome of shift maladaptation syndrome. Adapted with permission of MC Moore-Ede from Moore-Ede MC, Krieger GR, Darlington AC: Shiftwork maladaptation syndrome: Etiology, diagnosis, and management. Notes, Am Occup Med Assoc Postgrad Sem #12, April 27, 1987.

Individual symptoms are apt to be treated by a physician who is unaware of the entire picture and, therefore, can give only partial or temporary relief.

The worker with SMS is likely to get into a vicious cycle due to lack of recognition and understanding of his problem. His psychological symptoms make him unpleasant to be around and lead to poor job performance. Poor performance is apt to deprive the worker of promotions that would end nightwork. The longer the worker stays on shiftwork, the worse the symptoms become. Eventually, the worker may be fired or may quit or be involved in a serious accident.

In diagnosing SMS, other causes of the symptoms, such as endogenous depression, primary substance abuse, peptic ulcer disease, and irritable bowel syndrome, must be ruled out. The history and the *combination* of symptoms are most important. Once SMS is diagnosed, it may be difficult to convince management or a labor union that a medical reason exists for removing the worker from shiftwork without regard to seniority, but no other treatment is adequate.

Exacerbation of Existing Disorders

As pointed out in the discussion of biological rhythms, many physiological variables follow a circadian rhythm. Medical disorders involving these variables may be expected to be exacerbated by the desynchronization that accompanies shiftwork. Because the metabolism and effectiveness of certain medicinal drugs have been observed to follow a circadian rhythm, desynchronization can interfere with the pharmacological treatment of some diseases. Disorders associated with, or aggravated by, sleep disruption or deprivation also may be affected by shiftwork because sleep problems are frequently observed among shiftworkers.

Circadian rhythms of airway resistance have been demonstrated by respiratory function testing in both normal and asthmatic subjects.[59,121] In the Reinberg study,[121] asthmatics' dyspnea was shown to be greatest and their peak expiratory flow rates (PEFR) lowest in the morning (around 0700); the reverse occurred in the afternoon (around 1500). A three-fold difference in amplitude was found for dyspnea, and the amplitude for PEFR was found to be 20% of the mesor (the mean value of the sinusoidal curve describing the circadian rhythm). (In nonasthmatics, the 24-hour mean is higher, and the amplitude only about 5% of the mean.[138]) Smolensky[138] reviewed many studies on this subject and concluded that dyspnea in asthmatics is more frequent at night and during early morning hours. He also noted that nocturnal sensitivity is strongly related to circadian rhythms as demonstrated by: coincidently decreased circulating or urinary levels of adrenocortical hormones and catecholamines; decreased dynamic lung compliance; decreased airway patency; and increased bronchial reactivity to house dust, histamine, and acetylcholine.

The pharmacokinetics and effectiveness of bronchodilators also vary with the time of administration in a circadian fashion. For instance, theophylline levels reach higher peaks when given in the morning (0700–0800) than when given in the afternoon or evening, as shown in several studies reviewed by Reinberg.[116] Recently, chronobiological considerations have been used to optimize the effectiveness of bronchodilators and steroids in controlling asthma.[139] The time of day these drugs are given can be critical in achieving around-the-clock control of symptoms. But such schedules are based on regular diurnal activity by the patient. Maintaining consistent control of symptoms in someone engaged in rotating shiftwork can be exceedingly difficult. (Most workers who are on "permanent" nightshifts return to a diurnal activity pattern on their days off and are, thus, actually on a rotating schedule.)

Diabetes is another disease in which chronobiological considerations are important. Basal insulin secretion and glucose tolerance normally follow a circadian rhythm. The blood glucose level normally follows a shorter (ultradian) rhythm of 6–8 hours.[117] Plasma insulin response to intravenous tolbutamide has been shown to peak early in the morning (around 0400), but the resulting fall in blood sugar does not show a circadian rhythm.[135] The fall of blood glucose in nonobese, mild diabetics was also found to be higher in the morning in response to insulin, even though in these patients morning glucose values were higher than afternoon ones, suggesting that mild impairment of carbohydrate metabolism alters the circadian rhythm of basal blood glucose values and glucose tolerance.[42]

Ghata and Reinberg[54] found the circadian rhythm of urinary potassium to be delayed 2 hours in diabetics whose blood sugars were controlled with neutral protamine Hagedorn (NPH) insulin. Mirouse et al.[97] found a diurnal variation in the effect of the type of meal (simple versus carbohydrates) on blood glucose control in insulin-dependent diabetics. Thus, shiftwork not only interferes with the timing and type of meals eaten by the worker, but circadian rhythm disruption likely affects the blood glucose levels and pharmacological control of the disease.

Epileptics are another group of people at increased risk of ill effects from unusual work hours. Sleep deprivation of 24–26 hours can cause electroencephalograph (EEG) activation in epileptics, and in many patients in whom this has been observed the usual seizures are related to sleep loss.[113] Bergonzi et al.[17] found that REM stage deprivation activates EEG epileptic activity and sometimes clinical seizures in persons with generalized or focal epilepsy. Tharp,[149] in a review of several studies, stated that lack of sleep leads to an increased frequency of seizures in some epileptics. In view of these observations, and the association of shiftwork with sleep loss and sleep stage disruption, the possibility that shiftwork can trigger epileptic seizures must be seriously considered.

A relationship between circadian disruption and certain mental disorders has been demonstrated.[45,159] As noted previously, more than one circadian rhythm oscillator is thought to exist in humans. The body temperature rhythm, rhythms of the hypothalamic-pituitary-adrenal axis (particularly cortisol), and the REM sleep rhythm have been shown to be under control of a stronger group I circadian system oscillator, while the more labile sleep/wake cycle is under a weaker group II oscillator. Desynchronization of these oscillators is apparent in patients suffering from depression. The classic early morning awakening seen in endogenous depression suggests phase advancement of the circadian rhythm with respect to normal. The diurnal variation in mood also seen in this type of depression, with the deepest depression in the morning, may also be tied to a circadian rhythm. It is, therefore, not unlikely that depressed patients are suffering from a phase disruption of the sleep/wake and "awaking/readiness" rhythms, with the former being early and the latter being late.

Depressives also have been found to experience more REM sleep in the first third of the night than people studied as controls and less in the last third. They also have a shorter REM latency.[127,128] These findings are consistent with a phase advance in the circadian rhythm of REM sleep so that its maximum occurs at the beginning of sleep instead of the normal near-dawn time. Wehr and Goodwin[159] reviewed several studies that support a phase-advance hypothesis of endogenous depression including demonstrations of a phase advance of REM sleep, body temperature, cortisol secretion, and neurotransmitter metabolites such as urinary metabolites of serotonin, dopamine, and norepinephrine. Circadian rhythms in the postsynaptic responsiveness of hippocampal pyramidal cells to serotonin and norepinephrine have been demonstrated in rats, and it has been suggested that if this occurs in humans it could be related to the diurnal variation of mood seen in depressed patients.[20]

More directly related to shiftwork is the observation that phase-advancing the time of sleep with respect to the REM-temperature-cortisol circadian rhythm leads to a remission of symptoms in depressed patients.[131] The converse—that delaying the time of sleep would precipitate depression in susceptible persons—may have been observed. Two weeks after a study in which four subjects underwent a 12-hour sleep delay, one of the subjects committed suicide. It was observed, in retrospect, that that subject's circadian temperature rhythm was phase-advanced with respect to the other three and remained advanced relative to the schedule shift.[129] Rockwell et al.[128] observed, when studying responses of subjects assigned to groups of three in temporal and social isolation, that shifts in the light/dark cycle were associated with increased depression, verbal aggression, and physical complaints.

The possible effect of shiftwork on workers receiving medication for depression must also be considered because tricyclic antidepressants, monoamineoxidase inhibitors, and lithium have been shown in animal studies to cause a phase delay of several circadian rhythms.[159,173] Although sleep loss has been shown to cause remissions in some cases of depression, it also can cause a switch to mania in manic-depressives.[160] Another interesting observation is that bright light has been used successfully as an antidepressant; the timing of the light treatment, however, is critical.[78]

The propensity for shiftwork to cause irregular sleep schedules has already been discussed. This is important in discussing psychological problems related to shiftwork because changes in mood have been shown to be associated with chronic irregularity of sleep patterns.[145] Changes in attitude related to sleep deprivation[48] have already been mentioned in the preceding discussion of sleep deprivation. Overall, based on the above, the potential for shiftwork to exacerbate or to initiate symptoms of affective disorders should be taken seriously. (Cole et al. discuss psychological effects of shiftwork in Chapter 7.)

As has been alluded to in the discussions of asthma, diabetes, and epilepsy, the effectiveness of certain medications varies with a circadian rhythm due to the effects of metabolic and hormonal circadian rhythms. Thus, for any worker taking medications, beginning shiftwork may disrupt treatment. Medications, in addition to theophylline, insulin, and tolbutamide, which are discussed above, for which circadian variation in recipient response has been demonstrated include penicillin, sodium salicylate, halothane, indocin, glucagon, erythromycin, dexamethasone, triamcinalone, methylprednisolone, prednisone, lidocaine, hydrochlorothiazide, acetominophine, and digitalis.[96,115,116] (See Chapter 5 by Smolensky and Reinberg for a complete discussion of chronopharmacology as it relates to shiftwork.) The point that needs to be made for this discussion is that shiftwork may compromise the medicinal treatment of medical disorders. Furthermore, effective and safe control may be particularly difficult in shiftwork patients who take more than one medication.

PRE-EMPLOYMENT SCREENING AND MEDICAL SURVEILLANCE

Appropriate pre-employment screening and medical surveillance of workers applying for, or already engaged in, a job requiring shiftwork should be based on consideration of the worker's health status, the job performance requirements, and interindividual differences in adjustment to and tolerance of shiftwork. The general categories of factors influencing adjustment to shiftwork are shown in Figure 5. Medical problems associated with shiftwork or aggravated by it have already been discussed. Circadian rhythms and performance are discussed in Chapters 1 and 2 of this issue. An overview of individual differences is presented below. The reader is also referred to Chapter 5 for an in-depth look at this topic.

There is considerable variation among individuals with respect to the rate at which the circadian system adjusts to an acute time shift. As stated previously,

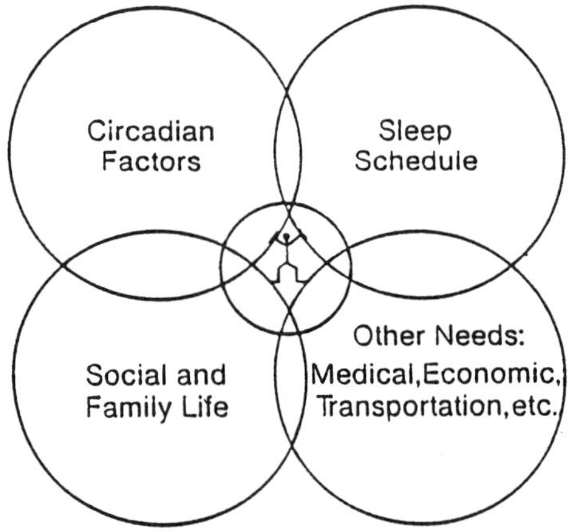

FIGURE 5. Interactions of factors influencing the adjustments of an individual to shiftwork.

the human biological "clock" runs with a period of about 25 hours; the range is about 24.5–25.5 hours. The amount of resetting of the "clock" to a time shift will be different for a person whose "clock" runs at 24.5 hours than for one whose clock runs at 25.5 hours. Adjustment to a transmeridian eastbound flight can take 3–18 days and for a westbound flight, 3–9 days.[103] The body temperature curve has been shown to take 2–3 weeks to completely adjust to sleep/wake reversal.[161]

Differences in adjustment to phase shifts are particularly evident when "morning"-type people (or "larks") are compared to "evening"-types (or "owls"). For instance, the rate of the biological "clock's" natural drift to 25 hours is faster in evening-types, evening-types reach a temperature maximum later than morning-types (Fig. 6), morning-types perform logical reasoning tests best around 0800 as opposed to 1100 for evening-types, and subjective alertness peaks about 2 hours later in evening-types.[3,70] Examples relating these differences to the shiftwork situation follow: evening-types tend to adapt to shiftwork more easily than morning-types; larks are more physically fit during the morning shift, and owls are more fit during the evening shift; and the sleep of morning-types is more disturbed when working the nightshift than it is for evening-types.[4,112] Of concern with respect to safety, Moore-Ede's group[101] has found that extreme morning-types are more likely to doze on the nightshift. Finally with respect to morning- and evening-types, a disproportionately large number of shiftwork "dropouts" are morning-types.[4]

The magnitude of the amplitude of the circadian temperature rhythm has been related to shiftwork tolerance. Wever[167,168,170] points out that (1) the larger the amplitude of the rectal temperature rhythm, the more persistent the rhythm is and the longer the time requirement for re-entrainment after a zeitgeber shift, and (2) for persons with an early phase of the temperature rhythm—i.e., morning-types—a shift in zeitgebers causes more interference with performance and more subjective symptoms of ill-being. Reinberg et al.[118] studied differences between male workers with good tolerance to shiftwork and those with poor tolerance (defined as a history of persisting fatigue or sleep disturbance, changes in mood

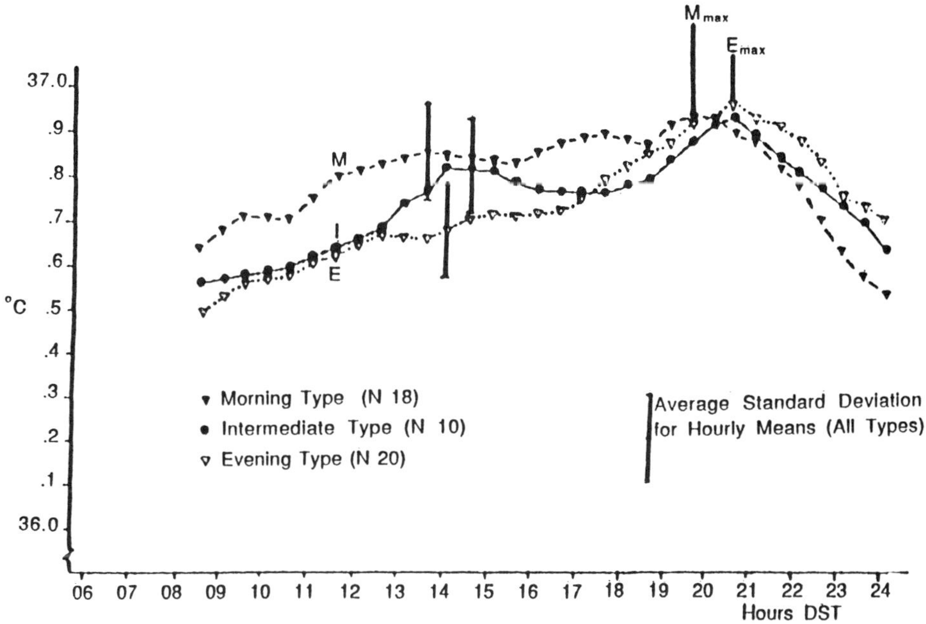

FIGURE 6. Mean oral temperature curves of morning and evening types (types determined by questionnaire). Used with permission from Horne JA, Ostberg O: A self-assessment questionnaire to determine morningness-eveningness in human circadian rhythms. Int J Chronobiol 4:97–110, 1976.

and behavior, and digestive problems). Thirty-one out of 38 men with good tolerance were found to have circadian temperature rhythms of 24 hours on their normal wake/sleep routine. Only 5 out of 27 men with poor tolerance had a 24-hour period. It thus appeared that the temperature rhythm was free-running in the shiftworkers with poor tolerance, who demonstrated periods either less than or longer than 24 hours. A subject with poor tolerance who was found to have a period of 26.6 hours was also studied after his transfer to a day schedule and was then found to have a period of 24 hours. Thus, it was observed that the majority of subjects with poor tolerance to shiftwork (after several months or years) had a desynchronization of the activity/rest period from the temperature rhythm. Results of this study did not appear to be influenced by age, experience on shiftwork, type of shift rotation, or type of industry.

Reinberg and colleagues[124,125] have also found a negative correlation between the amplitude of the temperature and PEFR rhythms and the magnitude of the rhythm shift in workers after the first nightshift. A small amplitude for these rhythms may be an index of relatively easy adjustment to changes in the activity/rest schedule and, thus, of good short-term tolerance. Ease in adjustment to a shift in the synchronizer schedule does not, however, imply good *long-term* tolerance to shiftwork. The opposite appears to be true—a large circadian amplitude for certain rhythms gives resistance to zeitgeber changes and has been associated with good long-term tolerance to shiftwork.[120,123] Resistance allows the circadian system to remain relatively unchanged with respect to daytime activity while on the nightshift. On the other hand, shiftworkers with symptoms of poor tolerance after several years of shiftwork have been found to have small amplitudes in the circadian body temperature rhythm.[7,8] Interindividual differences have also been observed with respect to the sensitivity of some circadian rhythms to exogenous influence.[93]

Age is another consideration with respect to tolerance of shiftwork. Shiftworkers may become intolerant of their work schedules when they reach their forties or fifties though they have done shiftwork successfully for many years.[3,123] Foret et al.[46] surveyed more than 700 oil refinery workers and found that age was an important factor for sleep quality and vigilance. Forty years of age seemed to be the point at which increased frequency of poor sleep became pronounced. A decreased amplitude in the heart rate rhythm (which has been associated with increased risk of coronary heart disease) may occur with increasing age.[24] Lastly, a 2-year study of international aircrew sleep found older flight crew members (especially those past 50) slept less and had a poorer quality of sleep than younger crewmen.[58]

Sleep habits may also affect tolerance of shiftwork. Some people require a strict sleep schedule, even when on a dayshift, in order to sleep well and try to keep that schedule on weekends and holidays. Such sleep rigidity may predispose these people to especially difficult problems in adjusting to shiftwork with respect to insomnia and its related symptoms.[101] Persons who complain of poor sleep and fatigue should be expected to find their problem aggravated by shiftwork. It is suggested from laboratory sleep studies that although these people may actually sleep what is believed to be an adequate amount for an adult, they *need* more sleep than normal.[2]

Differences between men and women with respect to toleration of shiftwork are not clear.[25] With respect to sleep loss, women with children are more apt to be unable to get adequate sleep owing to family responsibilities. In order to keep up with home chores and child care, sleep is apt to be sacrificed.[52] Smith et al.[137] found a significant association between sex and the number of sick days taken; 76% of female shiftworkers took an absence as compared to 56% of males. This difference was not evaluated, however, for the effect of domestic responsibilities on the women studied. Colligan et al.[26] in their NIOSH study of several hundred food preparers, also found a sex difference; more male than female shiftworkers used increased amounts of stomach and digestion medication.

Finally, both male and female workers differ in their social and family responsibilities as well as their housing situations. For instance, economic pressures may lead a worker to moonlight and thus to increase his risk of sleep deprivation and fatigue. For workers whose schedules involve a compressed work week with shifts of 10–12 hours, fatigue toward the end of the shift may pose a safety hazard both on the job and on the commute home.[18,27,91,140] Long commuting distances to and from work effectively lengthen the work day. For workers driving long distances home after work, the possibility of falling asleep at the wheel is a legitimate concern.

With respect to pre-employment screening, based on the preceding discussion of the effect of shiftwork on health, and keeping interindividual differences in tolerance to shiftwork in mind, the following should generally be considered contraindications for shiftwork.

Relative contraindications (most appropriately used for counseling prospective employees and for establishing adequate medical surveillance for those who decide to undertake such a schedule) include:

extreme "morningness"
sleep rigidity
insomnia
mild asthma
non-insulin-dependent diabetes mellitus
age over forty
cardiac risk factors such as cigarette smoking, family history of coronary artery disease, elevated cholesterol, or hypertension
history of depression
use of a medication known to have a circadian variation in effectiveness
history of seizures, but not currently requiring medication and no episodes for at least a year
frequent indigestion
mild irritable bowel syndrome
Crohn's disease
family instability
excessive family responsibilities
and a long commute to work.

Applicants with any of the preceding should be counseled with respect to the potential for shiftwork to aggravate their condition(s), and their personal physicians should be consulted with respect to the stability and severity of any medical disorders. Those disorders listed because of their potential to be aggravated by chronic sleep deprivation (e.g., epilepsy) may not be of concern if the shift is a permanent afternoon shift (permanent afternoon shiftworkers actually tend to get more sleep than dayworkers), and sleep deprivation may actually be of more concern if a very early starting time is required for the morning (day) shift, e.g., 0600, or if the worker is required to get up before 0500 owing to a long travel time to work.

Definite contraindications, which should lead the physician to consider recommending a medical restriction from shiftwork, include:

epilepsy requiring medication with the last year
coronary artery disease, especially if there is unstable angina or history of myocardial infarction
asthma requiring regular medication, especially if the patient is steroid dependent
insulin-dependent diabetes mellitus (IDDM) (IDDM workers may be able to tolerate a permanent nightshift if regularity in meals, activity, and medication can be maintained during work days *and* days off)
hypertension requiring multiple drugs
polypharmacy in general if there are circadian variations in the effectiveness of any medication—especially if a rotating schedule is being considered
recurrent peptic ulcer disease
irritable bowel syndrome if symptoms are severe
chronic depression or other psychiatric disorder requiring medication
a history of shift maladaptation syndrome

Screening the prospective shiftworker does not necessarily require a physical examination. A well-designed questionnaire that elicits information adequate to determine if any of the above contraindications exist can be used initially. People whose responses indicate possible contraindications can be further questioned and examined as appropriate for their condition(s).

Once a person has embarked on shiftwork, he or she should receive medical surveillance appropriate for the type of work being done and should be assessed periodically for signs and symptoms of medical, psychiatric, or social or family problems that may be associated with shiftwork.

The frequency of medical surveillance to monitor the effects of shiftwork depends on whether the worker is at increased risk for problems, as revealed by the pre-employment evaluation. If a physical examination is not required for any other work stressor, a questionnaire may be sufficient. For most workers, yearly surveillance is probably adequate. Evidence of medical disorders mentioned earlier should be looked for, and the worker should be questioned concerning symptoms of sleep deprivation, such as irritability and chronic fatigue. Family or other social conflicts that may have developed should also be explored. Weight loss should be monitored, as well as general nutritional status. Questions related to the use of caffeinated beverages, alcohol, sleeping pills, and cigarettes should be included.[137]

It is important to remember that ill-effects from shiftwork may not show up for several years. Angersbach et al.[9] did not see a difference between dayworkers and shiftworkers in the incidence of GI disease until after 5 years on their respective schedules. Costa et al.[33] found the interval between beginning shiftwork and the appearance of symptoms of disease to be 3.6 years for neurotic disorders, 4.7 years for gastroduodenitis, and 5 years for peptic ulcers. As pointed out earlier, a shiftworker may tolerate symptoms of poor health for economic gain until a physician advises a change of work schedule. Decreasing tolerance to shiftwork with increasing age has already been discussed. Toleration of shiftwork for 20 years does not mean the worker will not develop problems upon reaching middle age.

For workers requiring periodic testing of pulmonary function, the time of day of the testing must be noted. Guberan et al.[59] found, in a study controlled for respiratory exposures, that the forced expiratory volume of normal men increased 4.1% between the beginning and end of the morning shift, decreased 1.5% between the beginning and end of the afternoon shift, and had no significant change between the beginning and end of the nightshift.

In closing, it is still appropriate for physicians to heed the advice that Murphey[106] gave in 1979: "The most valid criteria for a counterindication to shiftwork remains the individual's own assessment of his ability to adapt to his particular shift system–living circumstances combination, *based on his experience on the job* and aided by counsel from his physician" (p. 322).

Finally, a few words concerning the practical application of the above recommendations. Competing interests of management, individual workers, and unions in hiring and job placement may make it difficult to implement medical decisions made during screening and surveillance of shiftworkers. "Failing" a preplacement medical examination may cause an applicant to be put in a "handicapped" status. Unions may resist the removal of a worker from nightwork if the dayshift has been designated for workers with the most seniority. Management may accuse a worker diagnosed with SMS of malingering. A worker may exaggerate problems associated with shiftwork in order to be placed on a more sociably desirable shift, or may deny symptoms in order to remain on the more economically rewarding nightshift. Nevertheless, the occupational physician should be consulted in decisions concerning the work schedule of employees. Workers should be cleared medically before they attempt shiftwork, and medical surveillance should be provided for shiftworkers. Clearly, the medical staff must educate all parties concerning the stress that shiftwork places on the human circadian system and what can be done both on the job and at home to minimize it.

REFERENCES

1. Aanonsen A: Medical problems of shift-work. Ind Med Surg 28:422–427, 1959.
2. Adam K, Tomeny M, Oswald I: Do poor sleepers have less restorative sleep than good sleepers? In Koella WP, Ruther E, Shulz H (eds): Sleep '84. New York, Gustav Fischer, 1985, pp 48–49.
3. Akerstedt T, Froberg J: Interindividual differences in circadian patterns of catecholamine excretion, body temperature, performance, and subjective arousal. Biol Psychol 4:277–292, 1976.
4. Akerstedt T, Froberg JE: Shift work and health—Interdisciplinary aspects. In Rentos PG, Shepard RD (eds): Shift Work and Health. Department of Health, Education, and Welfare publication no. (NIOSH) 75-203, 1976, pp 179–197.
5. Akerstedt T, Gillberg M, Wetterberg L: The circadian covariation of fatigue and urinary melatonin. Biol Psychiat 17(5):547–554, 1982.
6. Alfredsson L, Karasek R, Theorell T: Myocardial infarction risk and psychosocial work environment: An analysis of male Swedish working force. Soc Sci Med 16:463–467, 1982.
7. Andlauer P, Fourre L: Le travail en equipes alternantes. Etude de la naisance comparée à deux modalités d'alternance. Rev Fr Travail 19:35–51, 1965.
8. Andlauer P, Reinberg A: Amplitude of the oral temperature circadian rhythm and tolerance to shift work. Chronobiologia 6(Suppl 1):67–73, 1979.
9. Angersbach D, Knauth P, Loskant H, et al: A retrospective cohort study comparing complaints and diseases in day and shift workers. Arch Occup Envir Health 45:127–140, 1980.
10. Armstrong BG, Nolin AD, McDonald AD: Work in pregnancy and birthweight for gestational age. Br J Ind Med 46:196–199, 1988.
11. Aschoff J: Circadian rhythms in man. Science 148:1427–1432, 1965.
12. Aschoff J: Circadian timing and perception. NY Acad Sci 423:422–467, 1984.
13. Aschoff J, Fatranska M, Giedbe H: Human circadian rhythms in continuous darkness: Entrainment by social cues. Science 171:213–215, 1971.
14. Aschoff J, Hoffman K, Pohl H, Wever R: Re-entrainment of circadian rhythms after phase shifts of zeitgeber. Chronobiologia 2:23–78, 1975.
15. Aschoff J, Wever R: Spontanperiodik des menschen dei ausschulub aller zeitgeber. Naturwissenschaften 49:337–342, 1962.
16. Axelsson G, Rylander R, Molin I: Outcome of pregnancy in relation to irregular and inconvenient work schedules. Br J Ind Med 46:393–398, 1989.
17. Bergonzi P, Chuunvilla C, Tempesta E: Selective deprivation of sleep stages in epileptics. In Koella WP, Levin P (eds): Sleep: Physiology, Biochemistry, Psychology, Pharmacology, Clinical Implications. 1st Eur Congr Sleep Res. Basil, Kayer, 1973.
18. Brief RS, Scala RA: Occupational health aspects of unusual work schedules: A review of Exxon's experience. Am Ind Hyg Assoc J 47(4):199–202, 1986.
19. Brown D: Shiftwork: A survey of the sociological implications of studies of male shiftworkers. J Occup Psychol 48:231–240, 1975.
20. Brunel S, de Montigny C: Diurnal rhythms in the responsiveness of hippocampal pyramidal neurons to serotonin, norepinephrine, gamma-aminobutryric acid and acetylcholine. Brain Res Bull 18:205–212, 1987.
21. Carandente F, Halberg F: Chronobiologic view of shift work and ulcers. Shift Work and Health. Department of Health, Education, and Welfare publication no (NIOSH) 76-203, 1976, pp 273–283.
22. Carpentier J, Cazamian P: Night Work: Its Effects on the Health and Welfare of the Worker. Geneva, ILO, 1977.
23. Centers for Disease Control: Leading work-related diseases and injuries. MMWR 35(39):613–614, 619–621, 1986.
24. Cinelli P, Scalzi M, Fabiano F, et al: Risk factors in chronoelectrocardiology: Age. Med Sci 11:361–362, 1983.
25. Colligan MJ: Methodological and practical issues related to shiftwork research. J Occup Med 22(3):163–166, 1980.
26. Colligan MJ, Frock IJ, Tasto D: Shift work—The incidence of medication use and physical complaints as a function of shift. In Department of Health, Education, and Welfare Occupational and Health Symposia—1978. (NIOSH) publication no 80-105, 1980, pp 47–57.

27. Colligan MS, Tepas DL: The stress of hours of work. Am Ind Hyg Assoc J 47:686–695, 1986.
28. Colquhoun WP: Circadian variations in mental efficiency. In Colquhoun WP: Biological Rhythms and Human Performance. London, Academic Press, 1971, pp 39–107.
29. Colquhoun WP, Rutenfranz J (eds): Studies of Shiftwork. London, Taylor & Francis, 1980.
30. Conroy RTWL, Elliot AL, Mills JN: Circadian rhythms in plasma concentration of 11-hydroxycorticosteroids in men working on night shift and in permanent night workers. Br J Ind Med 27:170–174, 1970.
31. Conroy RTWL, Elliot AL, Mills JN: Circadian excretory rhythms in night workers. Br J Ind Med 27:356–363, 1970.
32. Cooper C, Marshall J: White Collar and Professional Stress. New York, John Wiley, 1980, pp 25–147.
33. Costa G, Apostali P, d'Andrea F, Gaffuri E: Gastrointestinal and neurotic disorders in textile shift workers. In Reinberg A, Vieux N, Andlauer P (eds): Night and Shift Work: Biological and Social Aspects. Oxford, Pergamon Press, 1981, pp 187–196.
34. Czeisler CA, Moore-Ede MC, Coleman RM: Resetting circadian clocks: Applications to sleep disorders, medicine, and occupational health. In Guilleminault C, Lugaresi E (eds): Sleep/Wake Disorders: Natural History, Epidemiology, and Long-Term Evolution. New York, Raven Press, 1983, pp 243–260.
35. Czeisler CA, Richardson GS, Coleman RM, et al: Chronotherapy: Resetting the circadian clocks of patients with delayed sleep phase insomnia. Sleep 4(1):1–21, 1981.
36. Czeisler CA, Richardson GS, Zimmerman JC, et al: Entrainment of human circadian rhythms by light-dark cycles: A reassessment. Photochem Photobiol 34:329–247, 1981.
37. Czeisler CA, Weitzman ED, Moore-Ede MC, Zimmerman CJ: Human sleep: Its duration and organization depend on its circadian phase. Science 210:1254–1267, 1980.
38. Daan S, Lewy AJ: Scheduled exposure to daylight: A potential strategy to reduce 'jet lag following transmeridian flight. Psychopharmacol Bull 20(3):566–568, 1984.
39. Darlington AC: Shift maladaptation syndrome. Paper presented at Occup Med Assoc, Postgraduate sem #12, April 27, 1987.
40. DeBacker G, Kornitzer M, Peters H, Dramaix M: Relation between work rhythm and coronary risk factors. Eur Heart J 5(suppl 1):307, 1984.
41. DeGraff W, Poelstra PAM, Visser P: The diagnostic value of sleep quality for the general practitioner. In Koella WP, Ruther E, Schulz H (eds): Sleep '84. New York, Gustave Fischer, 1985, pp 474–475.
42. DelPonte A, Capani F, Domani A, Sensi S: Diurnal variation of hypoglycemic action of insulin in diabetics—Preliminary results. In Reinberg A, Halberg F (eds): Chronopharmacology. Proc 7th Int Cong Pharmacol, Paris. New York, Pergamon Press, 1979, pp 311–314.
43. DelPonte A, Capani F, Sensi S: Circadian variation of digoxin effects in healthy subjects. In Reinberg A, Halberg F (eds): Chronopharmacology. Proc 7th Int Cong Pharmacol, Paris. New York, Pergamon Press, 1979, p 135.
44. Englund CE: Human chronopsychology: An introduction and report of an autorhythmometric study of circadian periodicity in learning, mood, and task performance. Paper presented at 1981 APA Annual Meeting. San Diego, Naval Health Research Center, 1981.
45. Faravelli C, la-Malfa G, Romano S: Circadian rhythm in primary affective disorders. Comp Psychiat 26(4):364–369, 1985.
46. Foret J, Bensimon G, Benoit O, Vieux N: Quality of sleep as a function of age and shiftwork. In Reinberg A, Vieux N, Andlauer P (eds): Night and Shift Work: Biological and Social Aspects. Oxford: Pergamon Press, 1981, pp 149–154.
47. Fort A, Ferguson DB, Kitcher KMPE, Botchway CA: The use of saliva in monitoring adjustment to experimental phase shifts (abstract). Ergonomics 21(10):865, 1978.
48. Freedman RC, Bigger JT, Kornfeld DS: The intern and sleep loss. N Engl J Med 285(4):201–203, 1971.
49. Freese M, Okenek K: Reasons to leave shiftwork and psychological and psychosomatic complaints of former shiftworkers. J Appl Psychol 69(3):509–514, 1984.
50. Froberg JE: Twenty-four hour patterns in human performance: Subjective and psychological variables and differences between morning and evening active subjects. Biol Psychol 5:119–134, 1977.
51. Froberg JE, Karlson CG, Levi L, Lidberg L: Circadian rhythms of catecholamine excretion, shooting range performance and self-ratings of fatigue during sleep deprivation. Biol Psychol 2:175–188, 1975.

52. Gadbois C: Women on night shift: Interdependence of sleep and off-the-job activities. In Reinberg A, Vieux N, Andlauer P (eds): Night and Shift Work: Biological and Social Aspects. Oxford, Pergamon Press, 1981, pp 187–196, 223–227.
53. Gander PH, Kronauer RE, Czeisler CA, Moore-Ede MC: Simulating the action of zeitgebers on a coupled two-oscillator model of the human circadian system. Am J Physiol 247(16):R418–R426, 1984.
54. Ghata J, Reinberg A: Circadian rhythm studies of blood glucose and urinary potassium in normal adult males and in similarly aged insulin dependent diabetic subjects. In Reinberg A, Halberg F (eds): Chronopharmacology. Proc 7th Int Congr Pharmacol, Paris. New York, Pergamon Press, 1979, pp 315–321.
55. Ghata J, Reinberg A, et al: Adjustment of the circadian rhythm of urinary 17-OHCS, 5-HIAA, catecholamines, and electrolytes in oil refinery operators to a rapidly rotating shift system. Ergonomics 21(10):861–874, 1978.
56. Gillberg M, Akerstedt T: Body temperature and sleep at different times of day. Sleep 5(4):378–388, 1982.
57. Gordon NP, Cleary PD, Parker CE, Czeisler CA: The prevalence and health impact of shiftwork. Am J Public Health 76(10):1225–1228, 1986.
58. Graeber RC, Lauber JK, Connel LJ, Gander PH: International aircrew sleep and wakefulness after multiple time-zone flights: A cooperative study. Aviation Space Environ Med 57(12):B3–B9, 1986.
59. Guberan E, Williams MK, Walford J, Smith MM: Circadian variation of F.E.V. in shift workers. Br J Ind Med 26:121–125, 1969.
60. Hadjelova J, Daliva M: Daily variations of the urinary excretion of some corticosteroids and catecholamines in workers under different working conditions (abstract). Ergonomics 21(10):866, 1978.
61. Halberg F: Some physiological aspects of 24-hour periodicity. Lancet 73:20, 1953.
62. Halberg F, Halberg E, Barnum CP, Bitterer J: Circadian rhythm—Coined. In Withrow RB (ed): Photoperiodism and Related Phenomenon in Plants and Animals. Washington D.C., AAAS, 1959, pp 803–878.
63. Halberg F, Reinhardt J, Bartter FC, et al: Agreement in endpoints from circadian rhythmometry on healthy human beings living on different continents. Experientia 25:107–112, 1969.
64. Healy ES, Kales A, Monroe LJ, et al: Onset of insomnia: Role of life-stress events. Psychosom Med 43:439–451, 1981.
65. Horne JA, Ostberg O: A self-assessment questionnaire to determine morningness-eveningness in human circadian rhythms. Int J Chronobiol 4:97–110, 1976.
66. Ilmarian J, Ilmarien R, Korhonen O, Nurminen M: Circadian variation of physiologic functions and their relation to oral temperature. In Reinberg A, Vieux N, Andlauer P (eds): Night and Shift Work: Biological and Social Aspects. Oxford, Pergamon Press, 1981, pp 91–98.
67. Jenkins CD: Recent evidence supporting psychologic and social risk factors for coronary disease. N Engl J Med 294:987–995, 1976.
68. Johnson LC, Spin-Weber CL: Quality of sleep and performance in the navy: A longitudinal study of good and poor sleepers. In Guilleminault C, Lugaresi E (eds): Sleep/Wake Disorders: Natural History, Epidemiology, and Long-Term Evaluation. New York, Raven Press, 1983, pp 13–28.
69. Johnston WB, Packer AE: Workforce 2000 (Work and Workers for the Twenty-First Century). Indianapolis, Hudson Institute, 1987, pp xiii–xxiii.
70. Kerkoff G: Individual differences in circadian rhythms. In Folkard S, Monk T (eds): Hours of Work: Temporal Factors in Work-Scheduling. New York, John Wiley, 1985, pp 29–35.
71. Klein KE, Wegman HM, Hunt BI: Desynchronization as a function of body temperature and performance circadian rhythm as a result of outgoing and homecoming transmeridian flights. Aerospace Med 43:119–132, 1972.
72. Kleitman N: Sleep and Wakefulness, rev ed. Chicago, University of Chicago Press, 1963.
73. Knauth P, Rutenfranz J: Experimental shift work studies of permanent night and rapidly rotating shift systems: 1. Circadian rhythm of body temperature and reentrainment at shift change. Int Arch Occup Environ Health 37:125–137, 1976.
74. Knutsson A, Akerstedt T, Jonsson BG, Orth-Gomer K: Increased risk of ischemic heart disease in shift workers. Lancet 12:89–92, July, 1986.
75. Kogi K, Ong CN, Cabantog C: Some social aspects of shift work in Asian developing countries. Int J Ind Ergon 4:151–159, 1989.
76. Koller M, Kundi M, Cervinka R: Field studies of shift work at an Austrian oil refinery. I. Health and psychosocial well-being of workers who drop out of shiftwork. Ergonomics 21(10):835–847, 1978.

77. Kripke DF, Simons RN, Garfinkel L, Hammond EC: Short and long sleep and sleeping pills. Arch Gen Psychiat 36:103–116, 1979.
78. Lewy AJ, Sack RL, Miller S, Hoban TM: Antidepressant and circadian phase-shifting effects of light. Science 135:352–354, 1987.
79. Little MA, Rummel JA: Circadian variations in thermal and metabolic responses to heat exposure. J Appl Physiol 31:556–561, 1971.
80. Lobban MC, Folkard S, Monk TH: Circadian rhythms of renal excretion in nurses on night duty (abstract). Ergonomics 21(10):865, 1978.
81. Lynch HJ, Wurtman RJ, Moskawitz MA, et al: Daily rhythm in human urinary melatonin. Science 187:169–171, 1975.
82. Mamalle N, Laumon B, Lazar P: Prematurity and occupational activity during pregnancy. Am J Epidemiol 119:309–322, 1984.
83. Margolis BL: Stress is a work hazard, too. Ind Med Surg 42(Oct):20–21, 1973.
84. Matsumoto K, Yusuke M: Effects of night time nap and age on sleep patterns of shift workers. Sleep 10:580–589, 1987.
85. McDonald AD, Armstrong B, Cherry N, et al: Spontaneous abortion and occupation. J Occup Med 28:1232–1238, 1986.
86. McDonald AD, McDonald JC, Armstrong B, et al: Prematurity and work in pregnancy. Br J Ind Med 45:56–62, 1988.
87. McDonald AD, McDonald JC, Armstrong B, et al: Fetal death and work in pregnancy. Br J Ind Med 45:148–157, 1988.
88. McGurwin L: Scientists adjust the hands of time to ease shift-change stress on workers. N Engl Bus 9(2):39, 1987.
89. Meers A, Maasen A, Verhaegan P: Subjective health after six months and after four years of shift work. Ergonomics 21:857–859, 1978.
90. Michel-Briand C, Chopard JL, Guiot A, et al: The pathological consequences of shiftwork in retired workers. In Reinberg A, Vieux N, Andlauer P (eds): Night and Shift Work: Biological and Social Aspects. Oxford: Pergamon Press, 1981, pp 399–407.
91. Mills DQ: Does organized labor want the 4-day week? In Poor R, Samuelson PA (eds): 4 Days, 40 Hours. Cambridge, MA, Bursk & Poor, 1970, pp 61–69.
92. Mills JN, Minors DS, Waterhouse JM: The circadian rhythms of human subjects without time pieces or indication of the alternation of day and night. J Physiol 240:567–594, 1974.
93. Mills JN, Minors DS, Waterhouse JM: The physiological rhythms of subjects living on a day of abnormal length. J Physiol 268:803–826, 1977.
94. Minors DS, Mills JN, Waterhouse JM: The circadian variations of the rates of excretion of urinary electrolytes and of deep body temperature. Int J Chronobiol 4:1–28, 1976.
95. Minors DS, Scott AR, Waterhouse JM: Circadian arrhythmia: Shiftwork, travel, and health. J Soc Occup Med 36(2):39–44, 1986.
96. Minors DS, Waterhouse JM: Circadian Rhythms and the Human. Boston, Wright, PSG, 1981, pp 211–243.
97. Mirouze J, Monnier L, Othoniel MF, et al: Effects of diurnal changes in food intake on diabetic control and plasma glucose circadian rhythms in insulin-dependent diabetics. In Reinberg A, Halberg F: Chronopharmacology. Proc 7th Int Congr Pharmacol, Paris. New York, Pergamon Press, 1979, pp 325–330.
98. Monk TH, Folkard S: Concealed inefficiency of late-night study. Nature 273:296–297, 1978.
99. Monk TH, Tepas DI: Shift work. In Cooper CL, Smith MJ (eds): Job Stress and Blue Collar Work. London, John Wiley, 1985, pp 65–84.
100. Moore JC, Englert E: Circadian rhythms of gastric acid secretion in man. Nature 226:1261–1262, 1970.
101. Moore-Ede MC: Screening shiftwork candidates. Moore-Ede Associates Letter on Human Performance in Round-the-Clock Operations 11(2):3–5, 1984.
102. Moore-Ede MC, Czeisler CA, Richardson GS: Circadian timekeeping in health and disease. N Engl J Med 309:469–476, 530–536, 1983.
103. Moore-Ede MC, Krieger GR, Darlington AC: Shiftwork maladaptation syndrome: Etiology, diagnosis, and management. Notes, Occup Med Assoc Postgraduate Sem #12, April 27, 1987.
104. Moore-Ede MC, Richardson GS: Medical implications of shift work. Ann Rev Med 36:607–617, 1985.
105. Mott PE, Mann FC, McLaughlin Q, Warwick DP: Shiftwork: The Social, Psychological, and Physical Consequences. Ann Arbor, University of Michigan Press, 1965.
106. Murphey TJ: Fixed vs. rapid rotation shift work. J Occup Med 21:319–322, 1979.

107. Murphy JF, Dauncey M, Newcombe R: Employment in pregnancy: Prevalence, maternal characteristics, perinatal outcome. Lancet 1:1163–1166, 1984.
108. Newton RW, Hunt LP: Psychosocial stress in pregnancy and its relation to low birth weight. Br Med J 288:1191–1194, 1984.
109. Nilsson C: Social consequences of the scheduling of working hours. In Reinberg A, Vieux N, Andlauer P (eds): Night and Shift Work: Biological and Social Aspects. Oxford, Pergamon Press, 1981, pp 187–196.
110. Orth-Gomer K: Intervention on coronary risk factors by changing working conditions of Swedish policemen. In Harvath M, Frankth E (eds): Psychophysiologic Risk Factors of Cardiovascular Diseases. Prague, Avicenum-Czechoslavak, 1982.
111. Orth-Gomer K: Intervention on coronary risk factors by adapting a shiftwork schedule to biologic rhythmicity. Psychosom Med 45:407–415, 1983.
112. Ostberg O: Interindividual differences in circadian fatigue patterns in shift workers. Br J Ind Med 30:341–351, 1973.
113. Pratt KL, Mattson RH, Wubers NJ, Williams R: EEG activation of epileptics following sleep deprivation: A prospective study of 114 cases. Electroencephalogr Clin Neurophysiol 24:11–15, 1968.
114. Preston FS, Bateman SC, Short RV, Wilkinson RT: The effects of flying and of time changes on menstrual cycle length and on performance in airline stewardesses. In Ferin M, Halberg F, Richard RM, Van der Wiele RL (eds): Biorhythms and Human Reproduction. New York, John Wiley, 1974, pp 501–512.
115. Reinberg A: Advances in human chronopharmacology. Chronobiologia 3:151–165, 1976.
116. Reinberg A: Clinical chronopharmacology. In Reinberg A, Smolensky MH (eds): Biological Rhythms and Medicine: Cellular, Metabolic, Physiopathologic, and Pharmacologic Aspects. New York, Springer-Verlag, 1983, pp 211–257.
117. Reinberg A: Strategy for chronotherapy of insulin dependent diabetes mellitus. Paper presented at Clin Appl Chronobiol Sem, NIH, June 20, 1989.
118. Reinberg A, Andlauer P, DePrins J, et al: Desynchronization of the oral temperature circadian rhythm and intolerance to shiftwork. Nature 308:272–274, 1984.
119. Reinberg A, Andlauer P, DePrins J, Smolensky M: Tolerance to shift work: A chronobiological approach. Adv Biol Psychiat 11:35–47, 1983.
120. Reinberg A, Andlauer P, Guillet P, et al: Oral temperature, circadian rhythm amplitude, aging, and tolerance to shift-work. Ergonomics 23(1):55–64, 1980.
121. Reinberg A, Guillet P, Gervais P, et al: One-month chronocorticotherapy (Dutimilan, 8–15). Control of the asthmatic condition without adrenal suppression and circadian rhythm alteration. Chronobiologia 4:295–312, 1977.
122. Reinberg A, Vieux N, Andlauer P, et al: Concluding remarks on shiftwork tolerance: Perspectives based on findings derived from chronobiologic field studies on oil refinery workers. Chronobiologia 6(suppl 1):105–110, 1979.
123. Reinberg A, Vieux N, Andlauer P, et al: Tolerance of shift work, amplitude of circadian rhythms and aging. In Reinberg A, Vieux N, Andlauer P: Night and Shift Work: Biological and Social Aspects. Oxford, Pergamon Press, 1981, pp 341–354.
124. Reinberg A, Vieux N, Ghata J, et al: Circadian rhythm amplitude and individual ability to adjust to shift work. Ergonomics 21(10):763–766, 1978.
125. Reinberg A, Vieux N, Ghata J, et al: Consideration of the circadian amplitude in relation to the ability to phase shift circadian rhythms of shift workers. Chronobiologia 6(suppl 1):57–63, 1979.
126. Reynolds CF III, Coble PA, Kupfer DJ, Shaw DH: Depressive patients and the sleep laboratory. In Guilleminault C (ed): Sleeping and Waking Disorders: Indications and Techniques. Menlo Park, CA, Addison-Wesley, 1982, pp 245–263.
127. Reynolds CF III, Saloff PH, Kupfer DJ, et al: Depression in borderline patients: A prospective EEG sleep study. Psychiat Res 14:1–15, 1985.
128. Rockwell DA, Hodgson MG, Beljan JR: Psychologic and psychophysiologic responses to 105 days of social isolation. Aviat Space Environ Med 47:1087–1093, 1976.
129. Rockwell DA, Winget CM, Rosenblatt ZS, et al: Biological aspects of suicide. J Nerv Ment Dis 166:851–859, 1978.
130. Rutenfranz J, Kanuth P, Angersbach D: Shiftwork research issues. In Johnson LC, Tepas DI, Colquhoun WP, Colligan MJ (eds): The Twenty-Four Hour Workday. Proc Symp Variations in Work-Sleep Schedules. Department of Health and Human Services publication no. (NIOSH) 81-127, 1981.
131. Sack DA, Nurnberger J, Rosenthal NE, et al: Potentiation of antidepressant medications by phase advance of the sleep-wake cycle. Am J Psychiat 142:606–608, 1985.

132. Saurel MJ, Kaminski M: Pregnant women at work. Lancet 1:475, 1983.
133. Saurel-Cubizolles MJ, Kaminsky M: Pregnant women's working conditions and their changes during pregnancy: A national study in France. Br J Ind Med 44:236–243, 1987.
134. Scheving LE, Kanabrocki EL, Brewer RL, et al: Chronobiology and how it might apply to the problems of shift work: Discussion I. In Shift Work and Health. Department of Health, Education, and Welfare publication no. (NIOSH) 76-203, 1976, pp 118-139.
135. Sensi S, Capani F, Bertini M, et al: Circadian variation in insulin response to tolbutamide and related hormonal levels in fasting healthy subjects. Int J Chronobiol 3:141–153, 1976.
136. Smith MJ, Colligan MJ, Hurrell JJ Jr: A review of the psychological stress research carried out by NIOSH, 1971–1976. In New Developments in Occupational Stress. Cincinnati, Department of Health and Human Services, 1980, pp 1–9.
137. Smith MJ, Colligan MJ, Tasto DL: Health and safety consequences of shift work in the food processing industry. Ergonomics 25(2):133–144, 1982.
138. Smolensky MH: Aspects of human chronopathology. In Reinberg A, Smolensky MH (eds): Biological Rhythms and Medicine: Cellular, Metabolic, Physiopathologic, and Pharmacologic Aspects. New York, Springer-Verlag, 1983, pp 131–209.
139. Smolensky MH: The chronobiology and chronotherapy of asthma. Paper presented at Clin Appl Chronobiol, NIH, June 20, 1989.
140. Steele JL, Poor R: Work and leisure: The reactions of people at 4-day firms. In Poor R (ed): 4 Days, 40 Hours. Cambridge, MA, Bursk & Poor Publishing, 1970, pp 105–122.
141. Stewart AJ, Wahlquist ML: Effect of shiftwork on canteen food purchase. J Occup Med 27(8):552–554, 1985.
142. Stogatz SH, Kronauer RE, Czeisler CA: Circadian regulation dominates homeostatic control of sleep length and prior wake length in humans. Sleep 9(2):353–364, 1986.
143. Tammeling GJ, Kruyt EW, Olievier CN, Sluiter HJ: Circadian pattern of the ventilatory function of healthy subjects and patients with obstructive lung disease. Int J Chronobiol 3:155–169, 1975.
144. Tasto DL, Colligan MJ, Polly SJ: The health consequences of shift work. In Occupational Stress. Department of Health, Education, and Welfare publication no (NIOSH) 78-154, 1978, pp 37–41.
145. Taub JM: Behavioral and psychophysiological correlates of irregularity in chronic sleep routines. Biol Psychol 7:37–53, 1978.
146. Taylor PJ, Pocock SJ, Sergean R: Absenteeism of shift and day workers. Br J Ind Med 29:208–213, 1972.
147. Tepas DI: Shiftwork eating and drinking behavior: Myth, theory, and reality. Presentation at 1st Ann Conf Shiftwork Management, Chicago, August 3, 1989.
148. Tepas DI, Mahan RP: The many meanings of sleep. Work Stress 3(1):93–102, 1989.
149. Tharp B: Epilepsy and sleep. In Guilleminault C (ed): Sleeping and Waking Disorders: Indications and Techniques. Menlo Park, CA, Addison-Wesley, 1982, pp 373–381.
150. Thiis-Evensen E: Shiftwork and health. Ind Med Surg 27:493–497, 1958.
151. Tilley AJ, Wilkinson RT, Drug M: Night and day shifts compared in terms of the quality and quantity of sleep recorded in the home and performance measured at work: A pilot study. In Reinberg A, Vieux N, Andlauer P (eds): Night and Shift Work: Biological and Social Aspects. Oxford, Pergamon Press, 1981, pp 187–196.
152. Tsaneva N, Daleva M: Field study of the diurnal changes of the adrenal system (abstract). Int J Chronobiol 3:1–17, 1975.
153. Verhaegen P, Maasen A, Meers A: Health problems in shiftworkers. In Johnson LC, Tepas DI, Colquhoun WP, Colligan MJ (eds): Advances in Sleep Research. Vol 7. Biological Rhythms, Sleep, and Shift Work. New York, Spectrum, 1981, pp 271–287.
154. Vittek J, Rappaport SC, Gordon GG, Southren AL: Circadian rhythms in the concentration of salivary steroid hormones in post menopausal females. IRCS Med Sci 11:768–769, 1983.
155. Walker J: Social problems of shiftwork. In Folkard S, Monk TH (eds): Hours of Work—Temporal Factors in Work Scheduling. Chichester, John Wiley, 1985, pp 211–225.
156. Webb WB, Agnew HW: Regularity in the control of the free-running sleep-wakefulness rhythm. Aerospace Med 45:710–714, 1974.
157. Webber WRS, Jones DP, Wright P: Measurements of tear turnover in normal healthy persons by fluorophotometry suggests a circadian rhythm. IRCS Med Sci 12:683–684, 1984.
158. Wedderbrun AAI: How important are the social effects of shiftwork? In Johnson LC, Tepas DI, Colquhoun WP, Colligan MJ (eds): Advances in Sleep Research. Vol 7. Biological Rhythms, Sleep, and Shift Work. New York, Spectrum, 1981, pp 257–269.

159. Wehr TA, Goodwin FK: Biological rhythms and psychiatry. In Arieti S, Brodie K (eds): American Handbook of Psychiatry. Vol 7, 2nd ed. New York, Basic Books, 1981, pp 46–107.
160. Wehr TA, Goodwin FK: Introduction. In Wehr TA, Goodwin FK (eds): Circadian Rhythms in Psychiatry. Los Angeles, Boxwood Press, 1983, pp 1–39.
161. Weitzman ED: Circadian rhythms: Discussion. In Shift Work and Health. Department of Health, Education, and Welfare publication no. (NIOSH) 76-203, 1976, pp 51–69.
162. Weitzman E, Czeisler C, Moore-Ede MC: Sleep-wake, endocrine and temperature rhythms in man during temporal isolation. In Johnson LC, Tepas DI, Colquhoun WP, Colligan MJ (eds): Biological Rhythms, Sleep and Shift Work. Advances in Sleep Research, Vol 7. New York, Spectrum, 1981, pp 75–91.
163. Weitzman E, Czeisler CA, Zimmerman JC, et al: Chronobiological disorders: Analytical and therapeutic techniques. In Guilleminault C: Disorders of Sleep and Waking: Indications and Techniques. Menlo Park, CA, Addison Wesley, 1982, pp 297–329.
164. Weitzman ED, Godmacher D, Kripke D, et al: Reversal of sleep-waking cycle: Effect on sleep stage pattern and certain neuro-endocrine rhythms. Trans Am Neurol Assoc 93:153–157, 1968.
165. Wever R: The circadian multi-oscillator of man. Int J Chronobiol 3:19–55, 1975.
166. Wever R: The Circadian System of Man: Results of Experiments under Temporal Isolation. New York, Springer-Verlag, 1979.
167. Wever R: Phase shifts of human circadian rhythms due to shifts of artificial zeitgebers. Chronobiologia 7:303–327, 1980.
168. Wever R: On varying work-sleep schedules: The biological rhythm perspective. In Johnson LC, Tepas DI, Colquhoun WP, Colligan MJ (eds): Biological Rhythms, Sleep and Shift Work. Advances in Sleep Research, Vol 7. New York, Spectrum, 1981, pp 36–60.
169. Wever R: Organization of the human circadian system: Internal interactions. In Wehr TA, Goodwin FK (eds): Circadian Rhythms in Psychiatry. Los Angeles, Boxwood Press, 1983, pp 17–32.
170. Wever R: Sex differences in human circadian rhythms: Intrinsic periods and sleep fractions. Experientia 40:1226–1234, 1984.
171. Wever R: Man in temporal isolation: Basic principles of the circadian system. In Folkard S, Monk TH: Hours of Work—Temporal Factors in Work Scheduling. Chichester, John Wiley, 1985, pp 15–28.
172. Wever R, Polasek J, Wildgruber N: Bright light affects human circadian rhythms. Pflugers Arch 396:85–87, 1983.
173. Wirz-Justice A: Antidepressant drugs: Effects on the circadian system. In Wehr TA, Goodwin FK: Circadian Rhythms in Psychiatry. Los Angeles, Boxwood Press, 1983, pp 235–243.
174. Wyatt S, Marriott R: Night work and shift changes. Br J Ind Med 10:164–172, 1953.

ROGER J. COLE, PhD
RICHARD T. LOVING, RN, MN
DANIEL F. KRIPKE, MD

PSYCHIATRIC ASPECTS OF SHIFTWORK

From the Department of Psychiatry
University of California, San Diego and San Diego Veterans Affairs Medical Center
San Diego, California

Reprint requests to:
Roger J. Cole, PhD
Department of Psychiatry, 116-A
Veterans Affairs Medical Center
3350 La Jolla Village Drive
San Diego, CA 92161

Supported by MH18398, MH00117 US Naval Health Research Center, San Diego, and the Department of Veterans Affairs.

Not to be abed after midnight is to be up betimes.
Shakespeare, *Twelfth Night*

In the opening scene of *Hamlet*, two guards meet in darkness at midnight on a castle wall. Oddly, it is the approaching guard, come to start his shift, who issues the challenge, "Who's there?" This seems irregular. Has the on-duty guard been sleeping, or is the relief guard acting inappropriately owing to sleep deprivation or disturbed circadian rhythms?

Are mental dysfunctions caused by shiftwork?

Shiftwork produces serious disruption of the circadian system,[5,17,43,71] as well as social isolation and various other stressors.[40,41,53,66] Both circadian disturbances[68] and psychosocial stress are thought to contribute to psychiatric illness. Does working shifts therefore increase a person's risk of developing psychiatric disturbances?

What follows is a critical review of the relationship of shiftwork to psychiatric morbidity, the possible mechanisms by which shiftwork might contribute to psychiatric disturbances, and a note on the potential of artificial bright light to reduce psychiatric shiftwork problems.

METHODOLOGICAL COMMENT

A major methodological difficulty in studying effects of shiftwork on psychiatric (or medical) morbidity is that shiftworkers are a self-selected group. For example, Meers et al.[37] found that of 104 new shiftworkers who entered employment at a wire mill, 40 (38%) dropped out within four years. Many shiftworkers transfer to daywork for health reasons or because of psychological difficulties.[8,18,19] Thus, cross-sectional or retrospective studies of shiftworkers could be misleading. If shiftwork causes psychiatric problems and some people drop out because of them, a study that focuses only on "survivors" who continue to work shifts might overlook the people who are most adversely affected. On the other hand, if we study shiftwork dropouts and find an increased incidence of psychiatric morbidity, how can we distinguish whether this morbidity was caused by working shifts or whether the psychiatric problems developed independently?

Other factors complicate the picture still further. Some shiftwork settings involve reduced social demands that might attract psychiatrically compromised workers. Some supervisors might find it easier to assign workers with psychiatric difficulties to nightshifts than to deal with them on dayshifts. Clearly, either longitudinal studies of new shiftworkers or randomizing studies to separate cause and effect are needed in this area. Unfortunately, to our knowledge, no sufficiently well-controlled studies exist to determine if shiftwork *causes* psychiatric difficulties. Available data are at best a basis for speculation.

SHIFTWORK AND PSYCHIATRIC MORBIDITIES

Psychiatric Hospitalization

Koller et al.[28] interviewed all patients admitted to an Austrian psychiatric hospital over four months. The proportion of psychiatric patients who were working shifts or irregular hours prior to admission was higher than would be expected in the general population. However, this difference reached statistical significance only for occasional nightworkers, not for permanent ones. This study suggested that shiftworkers might be at increased risk for psychiatric hospitalization, but it did not show whether work schedules cause psychiatric problems.

One mechanism by which shiftwork could theoretically induce psychiatric disturbances is by disrupting circadian rhythms. Jet travel across time zones causes circadian disruption similar to that caused by shiftwork.[20] Jauhar and Weller[26] retrospectively studied all admissions to a psychiatric hospital near London's Heathrow Airport over a 2-year period. Compared to the hospital's entire catchment area, the airport accounted for a disproportionate number of admissions for schizophrenia. Because a large proportion of airport patients had just flown across time zones, this finding is consistent with a hypothesis that rhythm disruption might precipitate psychiatric episodes serious enough to require hospitalization; however, alternative explanations are possible.

Substance Use Disorders

Shiftworkers have higher rates of pharmacologic substance use when compared to dayworkers. Based on interviews with 573 male textile workers, Costa et al.[7] reported, "the percentage of those habitually taking drugs was higher among rotating three-shift workers (48%) and permanent nightworkers (28%) than among two-shift (day and evening) workers (12%) and dayworkers (15%): the drugs consumed were mainly hypnotic and sedative (72%)—for sleep and neurotic troubles—and digestive (15%) and analgesic (9%)." In a telephone survey of 3,025 U.S. adults, Gordon et al.[23] found that the rate of self-reported use of sleep medications among female shiftworkers was more than double that of female nonshiftworkers. Tranquilizer use was also elevated among female shiftworkers. No such relationships were found among males; however, heavy alcohol use was elevated in both male and female shiftworkers. A survey study by Tasto et al.[59] of 1,219 nurses and 1,298 food-processing workers indicated significantly higher rates of consumption of both alcohol and sleep-enhancing medications among rotating shiftworkers than nonrotating day, evening, and nightworkers. Shiftworkers complain of difficulty sleeping during the day,[3] which probably accounts for their increased use of sleeping medications. Their increased use of alcohol and tranquilizers could be due to sleep problems, psychological difficulties, or both.

Tasto et al.[59] also found increased stimulant use in rotating shiftworkers. Because shiftworkers complain that they can't stay awake at night,[5] this is not unexpected. Thelle et al.[64] reported increased cigarette smoking among shiftworkers, but Gordon et al. did not find increased consumption of cigarettes or coffee.[23]

We are aware of no studies assessing the prevalence with which shiftworkers meet DSM III-R criteria for substance use disorder.[9] A caveat applies in this area: "Since denial is a basic defense in drug and alcohol abusers, historical data cannot be assumed to be correct."[46] It would be of interest to determine whether the proportion of shiftworkers among people in treatment for substance use disorders is higher than in the general population.

In advising shiftworkers, it must be emphasized that use of drugs is generally counterproductive. Alcohol can act as a depressant and make it seem easier to fall asleep, but chronic use[22,27] or use to promote daytime sleep[52] produces fragmented sleep with frequent awakenings. For most shiftworkers, sleep disruption is a chronic condition.[3] There is no evidence that prescription hypnotics are effective for long-term use and, in particular, no evidence that they enhance long-term performance.[58]

Neuroticism

Many studies have described associations between neuroticism and shiftwork. Tasto et al.[59] explored dozens of possible predictors of shiftwork difficulties by administering questionnaires and examining medical records of 1,219 nurses and 1,298 workers in the U.S. food-processing industry. A high neuroticism score on the Eysenck Personality Inventory predicted poor adaptation to shiftwork more strongly than any other variable. Harma et al.[24] assessed factors affecting the shiftwork tolerance of Finnish women. In 128 nurses and nursing aides, they found that neuroticism, measured on the Eysenck scale, was the most powerful predictor of gastrointestinal problems and other symptoms of intolerance to the work schedule. Nachreiner[41] administered the MPI (a German personality inventory) and other survey instruments to 1,005 workers in the chemical industry. Compared to nonneurotics, neurotics reported more dissatisfaction with shiftwork and a greater desire to change to daywork. Based on the responses of former shiftworkers, it appeared that neurotics dropped out of shiftwork sooner than nonneurotics. All of these effects were especially pronounced in introverted subjects.

Costa et al.[7] defined criteria for neurotic disorder as "symptoms of anxiety or depression that required treatment with psychotropic drugs for more than three months or hospitalization." They studied 573 Italian male textile workers, and found a 5-fold higher incidence in three-shift workers than in dayworkers, and a 15-fold higher incidence in permanent nightworkers. Aanonsen[1] studied "nervous disorders" among 731 Norwegian shiftworkers and former shiftworkers and 345 dayworkers. "Nervous disorders" were assessed by direct interview and included "slight to serious neuroses," "various degrees of depression," and lasting symptoms for which "no organic cause could be demonstrated." Although no statistical tests were reported, the rate of these disorders was higher among shiftworkers and former shiftworkers (18.6%) than among dayworkers (13.3%).

Two studies found no relationship between neuroticism and shiftwork tolerance. Taylor et al.[61] reviewed institutional records of 965 matched pairs of British shift- and dayworkers in 29 companies. They found no difference in the absence rate of shiftworkers compared to dayworkers when the main cause of absence was classed as "mental and psychoneurotic." However, the validity of retrospective classifications of "psychoneurotic" problems from diverse company records is questionable. Furthermore, the relationship between absence rates and overall shiftwork tolerance is not clear. Mott et al.[40] administered the Cattell 16PF inventory to 1,045 workers in five U.S. plants. The level of neuroticism was unrelated to the level of difficulty workers experienced with their shift schedules. They found, however, that the more the shift schedule conflicted with other life roles, the more problems the worker had. They speculated that it is the situational demands of shiftwork, not underlying neuroticism, that produces difficulties.

All of the data presented so far on shiftwork and neuroticism have been cross-sectional or retrospective and therefore subject to various systematic biases. Meers et al.[37] provided prospective evidence that neurotics adapt poorly to shiftwork. They followed 104 newly enrolled shiftworkers over four years. Individuals who had higher scores on a scale of "psychoneurotic complaints" (as opposed to somatic neurotic complaints) at the time of enrollment were more likely to drop out of shiftwork than those with lower scores for the same complaints.

Lund[35] found a possible physiological basis for the greater difficulty neurotics have with shiftwork. They studied 34 subjects in a temporal isolation unit during "free run." In free run, circadian rhythms are allowed to cycle at their own pace in the absence of external time cues (zeitgebers). Seven subjects experienced internal desynchronization of the core body temperature rhythm from the sleep/wake rhythm. Compared to subjects who did not become internally desynchronized, these seven people had significantly higher scores on a German test of neuroticism, which was administered before the subjects entered the isolation unit. The authors concluded that neurotic people have less stable circadian rhythms than nonneurotics. If this is so, then neurotics might be expected to suffer more pronounced disruption of circadian rhythms than normals when placed in a shiftwork situation.

Lund[36] has also suggested that shiftwork can cause neuroticism. He reported that "in (laboratory) experiments where 'forced internal desynchronization' was achieved by exposing subjects to 30 days of (light-dark) schedules ranging (in period) from 20 to 32 hours, posttrial neuroticism scores were significantly increased." Of course, living in temporal isolation could theoretically increase neuroticism for reasons unrelated to circadian desynchronization. Lund's report did not give enough details of the investigation to determine whether this may have been the case.

In summary, studies from several countries, employing diverse methodologies, converge (with few exceptions) in concluding that neurotics adapt more poorly to shiftwork than nonneurotics and are more likely to drop out. Preliminary evidence suggests that neurotics may have less stable circadian rhythms than nonneurotics. This might explain their poor adaptation to shiftwork. One study suggested that circadian disturbances such as those produced by shiftwork might induce neuroticism; this possibility deserves further investigation.

In the modern DSM III-R nosology,[9] the general concept of neurotic disorders has been reclassified as mood disorders, anxiety disorders, various personality disorders, and so forth. It is important to reexamine which specific DSM III-R disorders are elevated with shiftwork. Possibly, many of the neurotic complaints described would currently be regarded as symptoms of depression.

Depression

Prevalence

Few studies have formally assessed depression among shiftworkers. Tasto et al.[59] found elevated depression scores on the Profile of Mood States (POMS) among 309 nurses working rotating shifts, compared to 910 nonrotating day or night nurses. However, they found no elevation of depression among 634 night or rotating food-processing workers. As mentioned above, Costa et al.[7] included depression in their definition of "neurotic disorders" and found a 5- to 15-fold higher rate in shiftworkers than in dayworkers. Similarly, Aanonsen[1] included "various degrees of depression" in his definition of "nervous disorders," and reported a high rate among shiftworkers. Akerstedt and Theorell[4] performed a factor analysis on a self-rating questionnaire administered repeatedly to 17 male railway repair workers. They found that depression was part of a cluster of "sleep/mood" complaints that also included sleep/wake disturbances, apathy, anxiety, fatigue, and restlessness. Sleep/mood complaints increased significantly when the workers were shifted from day to night schedules, then dropped toward baseline upon return to daywork.

Many other studies have found increased psychological and somatic complaints among shiftworkers, including "severe emotional problems," "extreme job stress,"[23] fatigue, apathy, palpitations, nervousness, gastric complaints,[37] "irritation/strain,"[19] muscle pain,[65] reduced subjective well-being,[16] and other symptoms.[2] Some of these complaints could be interpreted as signs of depression. However, since standard psychological inventories were not used, we have no basis for distinguishing symptoms caused by affective disorders from symptoms caused by other psychological problems or by physical ailments related to shiftwork.

Three retrospective studies on shiftwork and depression produced conflicting results. Michel-Briand et al.[38] performed psychiatric interviews on 99 retired shiftworkers and 93 retired dayworkers. Twenty-nine percent of the former shiftworkers were depressed, as compared to 17% of the former dayworkers. Although the two groups were well matched on age and certain other variables, socioeconomic differences between them may have contributed to the results. Koller et al.,[28] studying 188 Austrian patients hospitalized for strictly defined depressive syndromes, found that the proportion who had been employed in shiftwork was no higher than the proportion of shiftworkers in the general population. It should be noted, however, that depressed patients suffering from additional psychiatric disorders or alcoholism were systematically excluded from this study. This could have reduced the number of shiftworkers in the sample.

Taylor and Pocock[60] found no excess mortality due to suicide among shiftworkers or former shiftworkers, compared to dayworkers, in a twelve-year prospective study of 8,603 male manual laborers. Classification as a shiftworker in this study required at least ten years' employment on a shift schedule without any interruption exceeding six months. Thus, the shiftwork group represented "survivors" who tolerated their schedules well enough not to change them over many years. The possibility cannot be ruled out that shiftwork may have induced serious depression in some people who transferred to daywork (or committed suicide) before they were on the job long enough to be included in the shiftwork group.

The evidence regarding shiftwork and depression is incomplete and conflictual. Some of the contradictions might be better understood through considering hypothesized mechanisms by which shiftwork might be related to depression.

Circadian Mechanisms

Patients with a major depressive disorder experience early onset of REM sleep and early morning awakening, indicating a possible phase advance of one or more circadian oscillators.[29,67] This and other findings have led to the hypothesis that depression may occur when circadian oscillators are phase-advanced relative to environmental zeitgebers.[29] Some shiftwork schedules can place the worker's rest/activity rhythm in a phase-advanced position relative to the environment, and this could theoretically induce depression. A related hypothesis holds that depression might result not from a global phase advance of all oscillators, but rather from the advance of one oscillator relative to another, resulting in an abnormal phase angle between them.[29] If this is correct, then perhaps depression might occur when oscillators are forced out of their normal phase position with respect to one another (e.g., by the introduction of conflicting zeitgebers, as occurs during a nightshift).

Depression is also associated with circadian disturbances other than phase advance and phase angle changes. Major depressives who are free-running may exhibit an abnormally short period of the sleep/wake rhythm.[44] Disturbances of the circadian rhythm of body temperature[67] and cortisol[54] in major depressives have also been reported. A 48-hour sleep/wake rhythm has been reported in some cases of bipolar disorder.[67] Patients with another form of depression, seasonal affective disorder (SAD), appear to have a delayed circadian rhythm of melatonin secretion and tend to sleep late, suggesting delayed circadian phase.[32,33]

The fact that depressed people have disturbed circadian rhythms raises the question of whether disruption of rhythms by external causes, such as shiftwork, can induce or exacerbate depression. Most of the evidence relevant to this question is indirect.

Sleep disturbances similar to those seen in major depression can be induced by forcing normal subjects to adopt an abnormal sleep/wake schedule. For example, Weitzman et al.[70,72] simulated shiftwork in the laboratory by shifting the sleep/wake schedule of normal subjects by 12 hours. This procedure produced short REM latencies, an increase in the amount of REM sleep early in the sleep period, early awakening, and general disruption of sleep. All of these disturbances resemble those seen in depressives during night sleep. Many of them persisted through three weeks on the reversed schedule.[71] Studies of the sleep of actual shiftworkers have shown similar effects.[3,6,30,59]

Thus, disruption of circadian rhythms can produce some symptoms similar to those seen in depression. It is not clear, however, whether rhythm disruption can produce the disturbances of affect typical of depression.

Free-running in temporal isolation for a sufficient period of time can produce internal desynchronization of rhythms, yet most subjects report no major disturbances of affect when this occurs.[73] On the other hand, some people have been anecdotally reported to experience severe depression, undetected by the investigators, during internal desynchronization in free-run experiments.[56,57] In free-run, different rhythms may assume different periods, so that the phase angle between them constantly changes. According to a phase disturbance hypothesis of depression, free-run might therefore be expected to produce negative affect at some times but not at others.

Shiftworkers differ from free-running subjects in that they experience an abrupt phase shift of the rest/activity cycle relative to most environmental zeitgebers. There is some evidence that phase shifting of zeitgebers can produce disturbances of affect. Rockwell et al.[48] reported a case in which a subject committed suicide two weeks after completing a 27-day laboratory circadian phase-shift protocol. This person showed abnormal phase relationships between various rhythms at baseline and, compared to 14 other subjects, experienced excessive internal desynchronization and very poor rephasing of many rhythms in response to a 12-hour shift of the light/dark cycle. Although this tragic case is open to several interpretations, one possibility is that the subject was predisposed to depression, and that the disruption of his rhythms induced by the extreme phase shift of the zeitgeber during the experiment triggered a major depressive episode, which led to his suicide. In an earlier study, Rockwell et al.[47] found that six subjects living in groups of three in a laboratory isolation unit experienced increased depression (as measured by the POMS, the Zung depression scale, and other scales) following an eight-hour phase shift of the light/dark cycle.

Subjects phase-shifted in other laboratory isolation studies have reported subjective symptoms and behavioral impairments resembling jet lag, but depression was not measured.[74,75] Jauhar and Weller,[26] in their Heathrow Airport study, found that patients admitted to a psychiatric hospital for depression were significantly more likely to have arrived on an east-to-west flight. Because east-to-west flight places a person's circadian rhythms in an advanced phase relative to local time, these results are consistent with the phase-advance hypothesis of depression. It is interesting to speculate from these data that mania might be exacerbated by forcing a person into a delayed phase. Likewise, one might speculate that seasonal affective disorder, in which patients apparently suffer a delayed circadian phase of at least some pacemakers,[32,33] could be exacerbated by west-to-east flight.

We noted earlier that studies of depression among shiftworkers have yielded contradictory results. These contradictions may be due in part to differences in methodology between studies; however, according to the theories we have discussed, it is also possible that shiftwork itself might have conflicting effects on depression. Wehr et al.[69] reported a case in which a six-hour phase advance of the sleep/wake cycle temporarily alleviated depression. Depending on the work schedule and the way the worker adapts to it, shiftwork might induce either a delay, an advance, or no change in the sleep/wake phase. Thus, according to Wehr's results and the phase-advance hypothesis, shiftwork could theoretically cause depression, alleviate it, or have no effect at all. Similarly various shiftwork schedules and adaptation strategies could advance or delay circadian rhythms other than sleep/wake or change the phase angle between different circadian oscillators. Thus, according to phase-angle hypotheses, and depending on the individual's baseline phase angles, shift schedule, and personal predispositions, shiftwork could either exacerbate or ameliorate depression. In addition, several studies have shown that partial or total sleep deprivation can reduce depression.[14,15,21,25] Shiftwork frequently involves sleep deprivation[3] and thus might be prophylactic or therapeutic for some people who are predisposed to depression. Incidentally, in-flight sleep deprivation might also account for some of the jet-lag results discussed above.

Photic Mechanisms

Seasonal affective disorder deserves special mention with regard to shiftwork. This syndrome is characterized by recurrent depressions that occur annually, especially in the winter.[51] Preliminary studies suggest that up to 25% of the population may suffer from SAD,[62] and that the prevalence in northern latitudes may be higher.[45] About 53% of SAD patients experience clinically significant relief of symptoms (often total remission) in response to morning bright-light treatments (usually of 1–3 hours' duration).[63] In order to be effective, phototherapy must be much brighter than ordinary indoor illumination (e.g., 2500 lux or more, as compared to 500 lux for a brightly lit office). It is also of interest to note that a significant number of patients suffering nonseasonal depressions respond favorably to bright light therapy.[50]

The high prevalence of SAD in extreme latitudes during the fall and winter and its response to light therapy suggest that SAD may be triggered by reduced light exposure. It is therefore interesting to speculate how shiftwork might affect people who are susceptible to SAD. At first, one might imagine that a person who works all night and sleeps during the day might be particularly "light deprived" compared to a dayworker. On the other hand, dayworkers employed indoors frequently are exposed to bright outdoor illumination at only two times each day—while traveling to work and while traveling home.[55] In winter, when the sun rises late and sets early, dayworkers may therefore experience no outdoor light at all. Nightshift workers, on the other hand, may be more likely to be out and about during the day, because this is free time for them, day sleep is often difficult, and some types of business can be conducted only during the day. Thus, night and rotating shiftworkers, if they go out in the daylight, may actually be at an advantage over dayworkers when it comes to avoiding SAD.

On the other hand, it has been proposed that SAD might be induced by mistimed light exposure rather than by insufficient light exposure. Some SAD patients derive therapeutic benefit only from bright light exposure in the morning, others respond only to evening light, and some respond to both.[63] Circadian studies suggest that light exposure in the middle of the day may have relatively little biological effect.[8] The timing of outdoor light exposure may therefore be critical in the induction or avoidance of depression. However, "the timing of light exposure" refers not simply to clock time but to the individual's internal circadian time. Thus, the effects of a shift schedule on SAD (or nonseasonal depression) may depend on a complex interplay between individual predispositions, initial circadian phase, lighting conditions on the job, and the timing of daylight exposures during nonwork hours.

The possible association between shiftwork and premenstrual depression also deserves special mention here. In a study of 1,199 female nurses, Tasto et al.[59]

found that "rotating shift nurses suffered more tension, nervousness, weakness, and sickness at menstruation than did all other shifts, as well as significantly longer menstrual periods than all other shifts." Rotating nurses also made more clinical visits for menstrual problems in this study. Thus, it is possible that shiftwork may disrupt not only circadian cycles but monthly cycles as well. Parry et al.[42] have recently demonstrated in a controlled trial that (nonshift-working) women who suffer from premenstrual depression experience significant relief of symptoms in response to evening treatment with bright light during the late luteal phase. This suggests that inadequate (or perhaps mistimed) bright light exposures could be a source of premenstrual symptoms among shiftworkers.

Thus we see that shiftwork holds the potential, at least theoretically, for either exacerbating or alleviating various types of depression. We know that many people quit nightwork because it makes them feel worse. Perhaps others actually seek it because it makes them feel better. To date, the empirical evidence in this area is too sparse to identify reliable effects of shiftwork on depression.

BRIGHT LIGHT TREATMENT, SHIFT WORK, AND PSYCHIATRIC DISTURBANCE

If disruption of circadian rhythms contributes to psychiatric problems, or if people with certain psychiatric problems are especially adversely affected by shiftwork because they have unstable circadian rhythms, then it would be desirable to find a method of restoring circadian synchronization among those on shift schedules. Properly timed exposure to bright light holds great promise as a means of achieving this.

It has long been known that light is a powerful circadian zeitgeber in virtually all plant and animal species.[39,49] Early experiments suggested that light was not a very effective zeitgeber in humans. However, Lewy et al.[34] demonstrated that the pineal hormone melatonin, considered a marker for circadian rhythms, could be suppressed by light in humans if the light was of sufficient intensity. This opened the way for a flood of studies showing that very bright light is indeed a powerful zeitgeber for humans and that it has effects qualitatively similar to those already well recognized in other species.[8,11,75]

One way in which the effects of light on circadian rhythms can be described is by the phase-response curve. This is a graph showing the direction and magnitude of the phase shift in a particular rhythm that occurs in response to bright light pulses occurring at various times of the day and night. Although the phase-response curve to bright light in humans has yet to be filled out in detail, preliminary results indicate that bright light pulses administered early in the morning cause phase advances in various rhythms, while pulses administered late in the night cause phase delays.[8,10,11,75] Repeated bright light exposures at appropriate times can cause dramatic phase shifts in circadian rhythms, resynchronizing people to new 24-hour schedules in a matter of days.[8]

Thus, the potential relevance of bright light treatment to the wide variety of shiftwork problems discussed in this volume is clear. Used correctly, bright light (and judicious avoidance of mistimed bright light) could theoretically help people rapidly adapt to shift schedules, overcoming problems with sleep, performance, psychological well-being, and perhaps medical well-being. We will focus here on the implications of bright light for alleviating psychiatric problems in shiftwork.

As discussed above, neurotic people seem to have the hardest time adjusting to shiftwork; they also seem to have circadian rhythms that are easily dissociated from one another. There is good reason to believe that bright light treatment could strengthen the synchronization of these people to their shift schedules. Perhaps this would alleviate the subjective distress their schedules cause and thereby decrease the likelihood that they will leave their jobs.

We have mentioned that both seasonal and nonseasonal depressions respond favorably to bright light treatment. Perhaps the shiftworker suffering from these disorders could kill two birds with one stone by using the same light treatment as therapy for depression and as a tool for achieving adaptation to the shift schedule. A caveat is in order here. We must emphasize that the role, if any, of circadian phase maladjustment in depression is not clear. It is therefore possible that light treatments timed to optimize shift scheduling might not have the desired antidepressant effects. Furthermore, if circadian phase problems do cause depression, it is conceivable that the same light-induced phase shift that helps a worker adopt a new schedule might somehow worsen depression. Moreover, in susceptible people, bright light can evidently trigger mania.[31] Many more laboratory, clinical, and field studies will be necessary to determine the effects of various lighting schedules on shift adaptation and depression.

Eastman[12,13] used bright light treatment to help subjects adapt to simulated shiftwork in their home environment. She developed a special schedule in which the subjects tried to live 26-hour days to help them rotate between shifts. The schedule was based on the fact that in the absence of outside time cues, people tend to free-run with circadian rhythms longer than 24 hours. She used timed bright light exposures late in the subject's "night," plus avoidance of bright light early in the "day," in an effort to help them phase-delay their circadian rhythms in keeping with the new schedule. Bright light appeared to help three of the first four subjects' core temperature rhythms entrain to the new schedule; however, similar trials on an additional eight subjects produced only partial phase shifts of the temperature rhythm to the new schedule. It is possible that competing 24-hour zeitgebers interfered with the 26-hour schedule. Perhaps more important is the fact that, based on recent quantitative analyses of human circadian responses to bright light exposure,[8] the timing of Eastman's light treatments (two hours before bedtime) and their magnitude (2000 lux) may have been insufficient to produce the intended phase shifts. Brighter light treatments later at night might have produced more dramatic results. Despite the fact that subjects in this study experienced large changes in the phase angle between their circadian temperature rhythm and their sleep/wake rhythm, no significant impairments of mood (as measured by the POMS) were reported.

Eastman's work demonstrates that although light may have promise for shiftworkers, the optimal patterns of administration cannot readily be predicted. Extensive empirical trials are needed *for each pattern of shiftwork* to test phototherapy designs. Because millions of workers are impaired by work shifts yearly, a major program of experimental research is appropriate.

Another strategy for use of light would be to attempt nonspecific increases in illumination of nocturnal workplaces, especially in the areas where workers take meals and breaks. Such increases in illumination seem likely to accelerate circadian phase adjustments.

A final strategy would be to empirically examine what patterns of timing and intensity of spontaneous, uncontrolled illumination among actual shiftworkers minimize symptoms. A recently developed methodology of continuous illumination monitoring[50] would make it possible to record large numbers of shiftworkers to find which light exposure patterns are associated with minimal symptoms for various shiftwork schedules.

SUMMARY

There is little rigorous evidence that shiftwork produces specific psychiatric disturbances. Substantial evidence suggests that shiftworkers are prone to increased drug and alcohol consumption, but the frequency with which this leads to actual drug abuse disorders has never been adequately defined. A preponderance of studies suggests that symptoms of a "neurotic" character are overrepresented among nightshift workers. The nature of these symptoms needs to be clarified with modern psychiatric nomenclature. It seems likely, based on certain experimental work, that nightshift work may at times exacerbate mood disorders, leading to an impression of "neurotic" disturbance. At the same time, some conditions of shiftwork might actually palliate mood disorders. Therefore, a reexamination of these issues is needed with improved research designs and more careful characterization of the nature of workers' complaints, their psychiatric histories (i.e., personal and family histories of mood disorders and other psychopathology), and possible specific effects of particular shiftwork rotation schedules. Use of bright light to alleviate mood disturbances associated with shiftwork needs extensive empirical testing.

REFERENCES

1. Aanonsen A: Shift work and health. Universitetsforlaget, 1964, pp 13–81.
2. Agervold M: Shiftwork: A critical review. Scand J Psychol 17:181–188, 1976.
3. Akerstedt T, Gillberg M: Displacement of the sleep period and sleep deprivation. Hum Neurobiol 1:163–717, 1982.
4. Akerstedt T, Theorell T: Exposure to night work: Serum gastrin reactions, psychosomatic complaints and personality variables. J Psychosom Res 20:479–484, 1976.
5. Akerstedt T, Torsvall L, Gillberg M: Sleepiness in shiftwork: A review with emphasis on continuous monitoring of EEG and EOG. Chronobiol Int 4:129–140, 1987.
6. Bryden G, Holdstock TL: Effects of night duty on sleep patterns of nurses. Psychophysiology 10:36–42, 1973.
7. Costa G, Apostoli P, d'Andrea G, Gaffuri E: Gastrointestinal and neurotic disorders in textile shift workers. In Reinberg A, Vieux N, Andlauer P (eds): Night and Shift Work: Biological and Social Aspects. Oxford, Pergamon Press, 1981, pp 215–221.
8. Czeisler CA, Kronauer RE, Allan JS, et al: Bright light induction of strong (type O) resetting of the human circadian pacemaker. Science 244:1328–1332, 1989.
9. Diagnostic and Statistical Manual of Mental Disorders, 3rd rev ed. Washington, DC, American Psychiatric Association, 1987.
10. Dijk DJ, Beersma DG, Daan S, Jaffe RB: Bright morning light advances the human circadian system without affecting NREM sleep homeostasis. Am J Physiol 256(1 PT 2):R106–R1011, 1989.
11. Drennan M, Kripke DF, Gillin JC: Bright light can delay the human temperature rhythm independent of sleep. Am J Physiol 257:R136–R141, 1989.
12. Eastman CI: Bright light in work-sleep schedules for shift workers: Application of circadian rhythm principles. In Rensing L, van der Heiden U, Mackey MC (eds): Temporal Disorder in Human Oscillatory Systems. New York, Springer Verlag, 1987, pp 176–185.
13. Eastman CI: Circadian rhythms during gradually advancing and delaying bright light and sleep schedules. Sleep Res 18:418, 1989.
14. Elsenga S, van den Hoofdakker RH: Clinical effects of sleep deprivation and clomipramine in endogneous depression. J Psychiatr Res 17:361–374, 1982.
15. Elsenga S, van den Hoofdakker RH: Clinical effects of several sleep/wake manipulations on endogenous depression. Sleep Res 12:326, 1983.
16. Folkard S, Lobban M, Nessling R, Haines SM: A field study of thermal comfort, performance efficiency and feelings of well-being in shift working nurses. Paper presented to the XVII International Conference on Occupational Health, Brighton, England, 14–19 September, 1975.

17. Folkard S, Minors DS, Waterhouse JM: Chronobiology and shift work: Current issues and trends. Chronobiologia 12:31–54, 1985.
18. Frese M, Okonek K: Reasons to leave shiftwork and psychological and psychosomatic complaints of former shiftworkers. J Appl Psychol 69:509–514, 1984.
19. Frese M, Semmer N: Shiftwork, stress, and psychosomatic complaints: A comparison between workers in different shiftwork schedules, non-shiftworkers, and former shiftworkers. Ergonomics 29:99–114, 1986.
20. Fuller CA, Sulzman FM, Moore-Ede MC: Shift work and the jet lag syndrome: Conflicts between environmental and body time. In Johnson LC, Tepas DI, Colquhoun WP, Colligan MJ (eds): The Twenty-four Hour Workday: Proceedings of a Symposium on Variations in Work-Sleep Schedules. DHHS (NIOSH) publication no 81-127, 1981, pp 305–320.
21. Gillin JC: The sleep therapies of depression. Prog Neuropsychopharmacol Biol Psychiatry 7:351–364, 1983.
22. Gillin JC, Kripke DF, Butters N, et al: A longitudinal study of sleep in primary alcoholism. Sleep Res 15:92, 1986.
23. Gordon NP, Cleary PD, Parker CE, Czeisler CA: The prevalence and health impact of shiftwork. Am J Public Health 76:1225–1228, 1986.
24. Harma M, Ilmarinen J, Knauth P: Physical fitness and other individual factors relating to the shiftwork tolerance of women. Chronobiol Int 5:417–424, 1988.
25. Holsboer-Trachsler E, Ernst K: Sustained antidepressive effect of repeated partial sleep deprivation. Psychopathology 19(Suppl 2):172–176, 1986.
26. Jauhar P, Weller MPI: Psychiatric morbidity and time zone changes: A study of patients from Heathrow Airport. Br J Psychiatry 140:231–235, 1982.
27. Johnson LC, Burdick JA, Smith J: Sleep during alcohol intake and withdrawal in the chronic alcoholic. Arch Gen Psychiatry 22:406–418, 1970.
28. Koller M, Haider M, Kundi M, et al: Possible relations of irregular working hours to psychiatric psychosomatic disorders. In Reinberg A, Vieux N, Andlauer P (eds): Night and Shift Work: Biological and Social Aspects. Oxford, Pergamon Press, 1981, pp 465–472.
29. Kripke DF: Phase advance theories for affective illnesses. In Wehr T, Goodwin F (eds): Circadian Rhythms in Psychiatry: Basic and Clinical Studies. Pacific Grove, CA, Boxwood Press, 1983, pp 41–69.
30. Kripke DF, Cook B, Lewis OF: Sleep of night workers: EEG recordings. Psychophysiology 7:377–384, 1971.
31. Kripke DF, Gillin JC, Mullaney DJ, et al: Treatment of major depressive disorders by bright white light for 5 days. In Halaris A (ed): Chronobiology and Psychiatric Disorders. New York, Elsevier, 1987, pp 207–218.
32. Lewy AJ, Sack RL, Miller LS, Hoban TM: Antidepressant and circadian phase-shifting effects of light. Science 235:352–354, 1987.
33. Lewy AJ, Sack RL, Singer CM: Winter depressives may have phase delayed phase response curves. Soc Biol Psychiatry 43:309–310, 1988.
34. Lewy AJ, Wehr TA, Goodwin FK, et al: Light suppresses melatonin secretion in humans. Science 210:1267–1269, 1980.
35. Lund R: Personality factors and desynchronization of circadian rhythms. Psychosom Med 36:224–228, 1974.
36. Lund R: Instability of circadian rhythms and personality factors. Ergonomics 21:863, 1978.
37. Meers A, Maasen A, Verhaegen P: Subjective health after six months and after four years of shift work. Ergonomics 21:857–859, 1978.
38. Michel-Briand C, Chopard JL, Guiot A, et al: The pathological consequences of shift work in retired workers. In Reinberg A, Vieux N, Andlauer P (eds): Oxford, Pergamon Press, 1980, pp 399–407.
39. Moore-Ede MC, Sulzman FM, Fuller CA: The Clocks That Time Us: Physiology of the Circadian Timing System. Cambridge, MA, Harvard University Press, 1982.
40. Mott PE, Mann FC, McLoughlin Q, Warwick DP: Shift Work: The Social, Psychological, and Physical Consequences. Ann Arbor, University of Michigan Press, 1965.
41. Nachreiner F: Role perceptions, job satisfaction, and attitude towards shiftwork of workers in different shift systems as related to situational and personal factors. In Colquhoun WP, Rutenfranz J (eds): Studies of Shiftwork. London, Taylor and Francis, Ltd., 1980, pp 150–161.
42. Parry BL, Berga SL, Mostofi N, et al: Morning versus evening bright light treatment of late luteal phase dysphoric disorder. Am J Psychiatry 146:1215–1217, 1989.

43. Plett R, Colquhoun WP, Condon R, et al: Work at sea: A study of sleep, and of circadian rhythms in physiological and psychological functions, in watchkeepers on merchant vessels. III. Rhythms in physiological functions. Int Arch Occup Environ Health 60:395–403, 1988.
44. Pollak CP, Alexopoulos GS, Moline ML, Wagner DR: Circadian period and phase of body temperature and plasma cortisol rhythms of depressives living in isolation from all temporal cues. Sleep Res 18:438, 1989.
45. Potkin SG, Zetin M, Stamenkovic V, et al: Seasonal affective disorder: Prevalence varies with latitude and climate. Clin Neuropharmacol 9:181–183, 1986.
46. Robbins DB: Psychiatric conditions in worker fitness and risk evaluation. In Himmelstein JS, Pransky GS (eds): Occupational Medicine: Worker Fitness and Risk Evaluations. Philadelphia, Hanley & Belfus, Inc., 1988, pp 309–321.
47. Rockwell DA, Hodgson MG, Beljan JR, Winget CM: Psychologic and psychophysiologic response to 105 days of social isolation. Aviat Space Environ Med 47:1087–1093, 1976.
48. Rockwell DA, Winget CM, Rosenblatt LS, et al: Biological aspects of suicide: Circadian disorganization. J Nerv Ment Dis 166:851–858, 1978.
49. Roelfsema F: The influence of light on circadian rhythms. Experientia 43:7–13, 1987.
50. Rosenthal NE, Blehar NC: Seasonal Affective Disorders and Phototherapy. New York, Guilford Press, 1989.
51. Rosenthal NE, Sack DA, Gillin JC, et al: Seasonal affective disorder: A description of the syndrome and preliminary findings with light therapy. Arch Gen Psychiatry 41:72–80, 1984.
52. Rouhani S, Tran G, LePlaideur F, et al: EEG effects of a single low dose of ethanol on afternoon sleep in the nonalcohol-dependent adult. Alcohol 6:87–90, 1989.
53. Rutenfranz J, Colquhoun WP, Knauth P, Ghata JN: Biomedical and psychosocial aspects of shift work. Scand J Work Environ Health 3:165–182, 1977.
54. Sachar EJ, Roffwarg HP, Gruen PH, et al: Neuroendocrine studies of depressive illness. Pharmakopsychiat Neuro-Psychopharmakol 9:11–17, 1976.
55. Savides TJ, Messin S, Senger C, Kripke DF: Natural light exposure of young adults. Physiol Behav 38:571–574, 1986.
56. Siffre M: Six months alone in a cave. National Geographic 147:426, 1975.
57. Sobel D: In the sleep lab: Losing touch. New York Times, July 1, 8, 15, 22, 1980, Sect c, pp 1ff.
58. Solomon F, White CC, Parron DL, Mendelson WB: Sleeping pills, insomnia and medical practice. N Engl J Med 300:803–808, 1979.
59. Tasto DL, Colligan MJ, Skjei EW, Polly SJ: Health Consequences of Shift Work. Cincinnati, US Department of Health, Education , and Welfare, 1978.
60. Taylor PJ, Pocock SJ: Mortality of shift and day workers 1965–68. Br J Ind Med 29:201–207, 1972.
61. Taylor PJ, Pocock SJ, Sergean R: Absenteeism of shift and day workers: A study of six types of shift system in 29 organizations. Br J Ind Med 29:208–213, 1972.
62. Terman M: On the question of mechanism in phototherapy for seasonal affective disorder: Considerations of clinical efficacy and epidemiology. J Biol Rhythms 3:155–172, 1988.
63. Terman M, Terman JS, Quitkin FM, et al: Light therapy for seasonal affective disorder: A review of efficacy. Neuropsychopharmacol 2:1–22, 1989.
64. Thelle DS, Forde OH, Try K, Lehmann EH: The Tromsø heart study: Methods and main results of the cross-sectional study. Acta Med Scand 200:107–118, 1976.
65. Ursin H, Endresen M, Ursin G: Psychological factors and self-reports of muscle pain. Eur J Appl Physiol 57:282–290, 1988.
66. Walker J: Social problems of shiftwork. In Folkard S, Monk TH (eds): Temporal Factors in Work-scheduling. Chichester, John Wiley, 1985, pp 211–225.
67. Wehr TA, Goodwin FK: Biological rhythms in manic-depressive illness. In Wehr TA, Goodwin FK (eds): Circadian Rhythms in Psychiatry. Pacific Grove, CA, Boxwood, 1983, pp 129–184.
68. Wehr TA, Goodwin FK: Circadian Rhythms in Psychiatry. Pacific Grove, CA, Boxwood, 1983.
69. Wehr TA, Wirz-Justice A, Goodwin FK, et al: Phase advance of the circadian sleep-wake cycle as an antidepressant. Science 206:710–713, 1979.
70. Weitzman ED, Goldmacher D, Kripke DF, et al: Reversal of sleep-waking cycle: Effect on sleep stage pattern and neuroendocrine rhythms. Trans Am Neurol Assoc 93:153–157, 1968.
71. Weitzman ED, Kripke DF: Experimental 12-hour shift of the sleep-wake cycle in man: Effects on sleep and physiologic rhythms. In Johnson LC, Tepas DI, Colquhoun WP, Colligan MD (eds): Advances in Sleep Research: Biological Rhythms, Sleep and Shift Work. New York, Spectrum, 1981, pp 93–110.

72. Weitzman ED, Kripke DF, Goldmacher D, et al: Acute reversal of sleep-waking cycle in man: Effect on sleep stage patterns. Arch Neurol 22:483–489, 1970.
73. Wever RA: The circadian system of man: Results of experiments under temporal isolation. New York, Springer-Verlag, 1979.
74. Wever RA: Use of light to treat jet lag: Differential effects of normal and bright artificial light on human circadian rhythms. In Wurtman RJ, Baum JM, Potts JT Jr (eds): The Medical and Biological Effects of Light. New York, The New York Academy of Sciences, 1985, pp 282–304.
75. Wever RA: Light effects on human circadian rhythms: A review of recent Andechs experiments. J Biol Rhythms 4:161–185, 1989.

MICHAEL J. COLLIGAN, PHD
ROGER R. ROSA, PHD

SHIFTWORK EFFECTS ON SOCIAL AND FAMILY LIFE

From the National Institute for Occupational Safety and Health
Cincinnati, Ohio

Reprint requests to:
Michael J. Colligan, PhD
National Institute for Occupational Safety and Health
Division of Training and Manpower Development
Cincinnati, OH 45226

A critical review of the literature concerned with the impact of shiftwork on physical, psychological, and social adjustment reveals a complicated and apparently contradictory picture. Although a number of studies provide convincing evidence that shiftwork adversely affects functioning and well-being,[6,22,24] others report that it does not.[8,20] In large part, this confusion may represent a necessary and productive step in the learning process. It is becoming apparent that earlier research methodologies and conceptual approaches to the study of shiftwork were too broad and insensitive to permit a clear picture of what is in reality a complicated problem. Even the term *shiftwork* is somewhat misleading because it implies a unified, single schedule or system of work. Conventionally, shiftwork has been defined as any work schedule in which half of the scheduled hours fall between 1600 and 2400 (evening shift) or between 2400 and 0800 (nightshift).[9] A worker's scheduled hours may be the same every working day (fixed or permanent shift schedule), or they may vary on a daily, weekly, or monthly basis (rotating shift schedule). Within these parameters there are numerous different possibilities for working hours. The International Association of Fire Fighters, for example, reported that their membership uses more than 150 different work schedules.[4] These shift rotas or routines differ in starting and ending times, ratio of days on- to days off-duty, number of consecutive days on a particular shift, direction of shift rotation (day–evening–night or day–night–evening), and whether the operation is continuous (7 day) or discontinuous (weekends off). Each schedule may produce a different set of effects on worker adjustment and life-style. A particular work schedule may be disadvantageous to a worker in certain respects (e.g., resulting in reduced sleep or disrupted physiological circadian rhythms) and advantageous in other respects (e.g., permitting more time for hobbies or church activities, or for being with the children). Thus, it is quite difficult to make simple generalizations about the "goodness" of a particular schedule or shift rota because large populations of workers have heterogeneous needs and backgrounds.

Previous research into the effects of shiftwork on family and social relations has relied almost exclusively on univariate, cross-sectional, self-report surveys of male shiftworkers. These study designs are subject to response bias and rarely permit conclusions about the direction of causality. For example, from such an approach, we cannot determine whether rotating shiftwork causes marital dissatisfaction, or whether unhappily married people choose rotating shifts to escape domestic strife. Other variables that may affect adjustment (such as age, education, number and ages of children) have not been adequately examined or controlled. Response biases, differential attrition across shifts, sampling deficiencies, measurement errors, and other methodological problems of earlier shiftwork research have been noted elsewhere.[4] These deficiencies limit our ability to describe the effects of "shiftwork" on family and social life. Therefore, this review must be considered a heuristic exercise rather than a definitive statement. We have accepted the modest goal of providing a general impression or overview of the ways in which shiftwork may affect individual, social, and family life-styles. In reviewing the literature, we will divide shiftwork into fixed and rotating schedules.

FIXED DAYS

One of the most comprehensive studies of the effects of shiftwork on worker family and social adjustment was done by Mott and his associates at the University of Michigan.[15] They surveyed 661 male shiftworkers (fixed afternoon, fixed night, and rotators) and their wives about the perceived impact of work schedules on a variety of spouse and parent role activities. The responses were compared to those of 252 male workers on fixed dayshifts. (Practical considerations precluded surveying the wives of dayworkers.) The results, as expected, were better for the permanent dayshift in almost every indicator of personal and social adjustment. Permanent dayworkers showed the highest overall level of shift satisfaction; only 6% expressed a desire for a different work schedule. They also indicated the highest marital satisfaction, family integration and coordination, and avoidance of domestic friction. They had the highest rate of membership in formal organizations (e.g., churches, fraternal societies, athletic clubs), and they were more likely to hold offices in these organizations than workers on other shifts.

Subsequent studies confirmed and extended these findings. Frost and Jamal[6] reported that dayworkers scored higher on a Maslow-derived measure of work need fulfillment (indicating greater job satisfaction) and evidenced better overall mental health than nondayworkers. Dayworkers also spent more hours participating in social organizations, and they anticipated staying longer with their employer.

Khaleque and Rahman[13] studied fixed and rotating shiftworkers employed in either a jute mill or a cigarette factory in India. They reported that 75% of the permanent dayworkers were positively disposed toward their work schedule as compared to 30% on the afternoon shift, 45% on the nightshift, and 38% on a rotating schedule. The day schedule was also reported least disruptive in relation to a variety of nonwork activities such as family life, leisure pursuits, and regular meal times.

Daywork is not superior to other shifts in all respects, however. Mott et al.[15] found that dayworkers reported having less time to help with housework than workers on other shifts. Workers on dayshift spent about the same amount of time as other shiftworkers visiting family. And workers on fixed afternoon, night, and rotating schedules actually felt that their shifts made it easier to engage in solitary activities such as gardening, fishing and hunting, or building and fixing things around the home.

FIXED AFTERNOONS

The afternoon shift (typically extending from 1500 or 1600 to 2300 or 2400) might be expected to produce ambiguous effects. On the one hand, it is not physiologically disruptive because it is highly compatible with the normal diurnal activity cycle. This shift requires people to work during usual waking hours and allows them to sleep during the nighttime hours. Consequently, problems with physical health and fatigue attributable to disruption of physiological circadian rhythms should not occur. Related biological activities such as sleeping and eating should also be unaffected. On the other hand, the afternoon shift is disruptive because many recreational and family interactions take place in the early evening. Family suppers, interactions with spouse and children, visiting with friends and relatives, and similar activities are likely to be altered or impaired by the evening work schedule. Therefore, one might expect this shift to be benign from a physiological perspective but to pose some problems in terms of social adjustment and role fulfillment. These expectations are confirmed in the literature.

Mott et al.[15] found that male workers on fixed afternoon shifts reported more sleep and fewer health complaints than fixed night or rotating shiftworkers. These results have subsequently been reported by a number of other investigators.[17,19,21] With respect to family responsibilities, however, afternoon workers reported the most dissatisfaction with the amount of time available for companionship with their wives and for relaxation and diversions from household responsibilities. They also expressed concern about being unavailable to provide protection and security to their wives during the later hours of their shift. Wedderburn[23] in a survey of 815 steelworkers in the United Kingdom similarly found that 79% of the workers on an afternoon schedule felt that their shift restricted their social and family life, compared to 17% of workers on a dayshift.

The responses of the wives of afternoon workers in the survey by Mott et al. were similar to those of their husbands. They felt that their husbands' work schedules interfered more than day schedules would with their own abilities to provide companionship to their husbands. The wives also expressed concern about their husbands' inability to provide security and protection for the family when working an afternoon or evening shift. These findings suggest that evening hours are perceived as an important time by both husbands and wives to "catch up" on the day's activities, share personal problems and concerns, and enjoy each other's company.

The most dissatisfaction associated with the fixed afternoon schedule, however, appears to be related to its impact on the parenting role. Workers on a fixed afternoon, Monday–Friday schedule who have school-age children routinely spend 5 days of every week without seeing their children. The children are at school in the morning and early afternoon, when the worker is at home, and they are home in the late afternoon and early evening, when the worker is at his job. Thus Mott et al.[15] reported that workers on fixed afternoon shifts expressed more difficulty communicating with their children than workers on any other shift. Tasto et al.[19] reported similar results from a survey of approximately 1200 nurses and food processors on fixed and rotating shift schedules. Afternoon shiftworkers were more dissatisfied with the amount of time spent with their children and reported less involvement in rearing and disciplining their children than did workers on dayshifts. They were also most unhappy with the amount of time available for participating in sports, social gatherings, and personal activities.

The same type of complaint was reported from an analysis of the 1977 Quality of Life Survey by Staines and Pleck.[18] Afternoon shiftworkers reported having more time available for housework than dayworkers had, but they also reported more conflict between their work schedule and the requirements of family life. The specific effects of lost parenting time on the children of workers on fixed afternoon shifts have not been studied.

FIXED NIGHTS

The nightshift is consistently regarded as the most disruptive of all shifts in terms of physiological adjustment and well-being. Workers on this shift have poorer sleep (in quantity and quality), more frequent health complaints, and more difficulties with meal taking than either day or afternoon shiftworkers.[12,17] Concern about these and other possible health effects from long-term circadian asynchrony is quite high in the European community. As a result, many of these countries have outlawed fixed night schedules except in critical occupations.[17] From the perspective of family and social adjustment, however, the fixed night shift may actually be preferred to the afternoon shift because it allows the worker to be awake and at home with the family during the morning and early evening hours. Thus, Mott et al.[15] reported that nightshift workers had fewer problems providing their wives with companionship, and they reported being more available to help with the housework, than afternoon and rotating shiftworkers. In a related finding, nightworkers reported spending more time in organizational activities, despite holding fewer memberships in social clubs and fraternal orders, than dayworkers. Nightshift workers also found more time for solitary activities such as gardening, hunting and fishing, and home maintenance than did workers on fixed dayshifts.

Tasto et al.[19] replicated these results in a study of nurses and food processors. Workers on fixed night schedules were more satisfied than afternoon or rotating shiftworkers (but not dayworkers) with the amount of time they had for (1) being with their children, (2) child-rearing and disciplining activities, (3) personal activities and running errands, and (4) sports and other social activities.

Khaleque and Rahman[13] reported results consistent with these. In their study of shiftworkers in India, 85% of the fixed afternoon workers and 61% of the rotating shiftworkers felt that their schedules interfered with their social life, but only 33% of the nightshift workers expressed this view.

The above results suggest that, relative to the afternoon and rotating shifts, the fixed night schedule affords more usable time for family and social interaction. Little is known, however, about the impact of nightwork on the nature and quality of family life, or on the costs involved in maintaining "normal" relationships. Some preliminary evidence suggests that the fixed nightshift may exact a toll. For example, it appears that the fulfillment of family obligations may be accomplished at the physiological cost of lost sleep. In a study of 898 female nurses in 61 French hospitals, Gadbois[7] reported that 85% of the nurses requested nightshift because it allowed time at home with their young children. The amount of sleep obtained by nurses with two or more children, however, averaged 1.33 hours less than that obtained by nurses without children. This sleep debt was attributed to the delay of sleep until parenting responsibilities were completed in the morning. Further evidence of the impact of nightwork on the quality of social life was provided by Adams et al.[1] In their study of nurses on fixed nightshifts, those most able to adjust physically to nightwork scored high on introversion and had few social responsibilities or commitments.

Another complaint of workers on fixed nightshift is sexual dissatisfaction.[15,19] The demands of work, of child-rearing, domestic, and social obligations, and of sleep schedules make it difficult for couples to coordinate time for privacy with a sexual partner.

Finally, there is evidence that the nightshift produces greater strain on family members who must accommodate their life-styles to this schedule. For example, the wives of workers on fixed nightshift (surveyed by Mott et al.[15]) were even less satisfied than their husbands with the amount of time for companionship allowed by the work schedule. This discordance may reflect different perceptions within the marriage about the quality of interactions among nightshift couples. It may indicate that maintenance of the relationship involved higher costs for the wife than for the husband. The husband's satisfaction with the companionship he was receiving may have resulted from the wife's working harder to support his shift adjustment. Some evidence for this point is presented by Lee et al.,[14] who found that wives of shiftworkers expressed a stronger desire than their husbands for a "nonshift" schedule, even if it meant lower wages. These wives indicated that the activities of the family had to be severely restricted to ensure a good sleeping environment for the husbands on shiftwork. Thus, it appears that fixed nightwork may allow more "clock time" for family interactions than does an afternoon schedule. The cost of this extra time, however, may be health problems for the worker and life-style disruptions for family members.

ROTATING SHIFT SCHEDULES

Workers on rotating shifts experience some of the best advantages and worst disadvantages of each of the fixed shifts. On dayshift, the workers sleep and eat according to a diurnal schedule. They are free to socialize during evening hours but are occupied during daylight hours. Thus, daywork prohibits daytime leisure activities such as hunting, golfing, and shopping. The afternoon shift also follows the normal diurnal physiological pattern and allows for a lengthened sleep period. The disadvantage of afternoon shift is the forfeiture of those family and social activities that take place in the evening. On the nightshift, the worker experiences reduced sleep and physiological asynchrony but has time for daytime and early evening activities.

Perhaps the major advantage of rotating shiftwork is that it diffuses the deleterious physiological effects of working nights across the entire work force. If all workers rotate shifts, then each worker only periodically experiences the asynchrony associated with nightwork. Most European countries have replaced permanent nightwork with rotating schedules in order to avoid physiological asynchrony. Lately, even rotating shift schedules in Europe are designed to keep the number of consecutive nightshifts to a minimum.

In terms of social and family adjustment, rotating schedules produce some unique problems. Not surprisingly, Mott et al.[15] reported that the wives of rotating shiftworkers complained of problems scheduling events because of their husbands' variable schedules. Both workers and wives listed fewer friends than fixed dayshift workers and reported more family friction and interference between work schedule and family activities. Men on rotating shifts also reported problems with sexual relations, finding time for companionship with their wives, and communicating with the children.

Another survey[10] of 82 rotating shiftworkers at a Swedish plant indicated that the activities most hindered by work schedules were sleep, meal taking, seeing family and friends, and watching television. Housework, shopping, house maintenance, and gardening were reported to be easier on a rotating schedule compared to dayshift. It was concluded that time-inflexible activities (i.e., those requiring the presence and availability of others or having a fixed time period) were impaired by a rotating schedule, whereas time-flexible activities (e.g., some shopping, solitary hobbies) were facilitated.

Jamal and Jamal[11] compared fixed and rotating schedules in 383 manufacturing workers and 440 nurses. Manufacturing workers on rotating shifts reported spending less time with friends (but not family) than their fixed shift counterparts. Nurses on fixed shifts spent more time with family than nurses on rotating shifts.

Tasto et al.[19] reported that both nurses and food processors in their sample indicated more dissatisfaction with a rotating schedule than with a fixed schedule for social activities, hours spent with spouse, and hours spent with children. (Not all employees questioned were working the same rotating schedules. Rapid, slow, and weekly rotations were in use. Possible differences with respect to type of rotating schedule were not assessed.)

The underlying theme from these studies is that rotating schedules allow free time at different points in the 24-hour day as workers move from shift to shift. Their days are free to golf or shop when working nights, their evenings are free to spend with their spouses and children when working days, and their mornings are free for sleep or work around the house when working afternoons. The effective use of this time, however, may be severely curtailed by carryover effects and strain associated with a variable schedule. Support for this position comes from evidence that rotating shiftworkers get less overall sleep than workers on fixed shifts[21] and that they experience a higher incidence of depression, confusion, tension/anxiety, and fatigue.[11,19] Thus, while rotating shiftworkers may have flexible time for certain activities relative to workers on fixed shifts, feelings of general malaise and lethargy may reduce their ability to use this time effectively.

It should also be noted that rotating shifts are a problem for parents of young children. It is difficult to find child care providers who will work the same rotating shifts as these workers. Gadbois[7] noted that the most frequently cited reason why nurses agree to work fixed nightshifts rather than rotating schedules was concern about child care. This problem intensified in households where only one parent is present or both parents work. Presser[16] has observed that if one parent is working a rotating schedule, the second parent can be severely limited in employment opportunities because of the need to be available for child care.

A final consideration for rotating shiftwork is the frequent use of such schedules by continuous (i.e., 7-day) operations. Workers in the situations often work on Saturdays and Sundays—the most desirable times for recreational and social activities. A number of studies have indicated that weekend work, more than the actual hours of work, is the most dissatisfying aspect of shiftwork. Chadwick-Jones[3] reported that weekend work was the major work schedule complaint in a survey of Welsh steelworkers. Similar results were reported by Banks,[2] who interviewed wives of British steelworkers. Working Saturday or Sunday was extremely unpopular because of its perceived effects on family and social activities. Staines and Pleck[18] reported that working nonstandard schedules (weekends and irregular patterns of days) was associated with poorer quality of family life and an average of 3.8 fewer hours per week with one's children. These findings suggest that workers and their spouses may be more willing to tolerate the inconveniences of shiftwork throughout the week if they are provided some weekends off.

CONCLUSION

As this brief review indicates, each shift produces a set of advantages and disadvantages in terms of social satisfaction and adjustment for the worker and his or her family. Our understanding of the impact of shiftwork on all aspects of social and family adjustment is still quite sketchy, however. Studies to date have focused too often on male shiftworkers in single-earner families and have used univariate, cross-sectional survey designs. Future research should consider more objective indicators of social and family adjustment among shiftworkers. Such indices as divorce rate, frequency of participation in marital counseling and individual psychotherapy, and the children's academic performance, delinquency and truancy rates, frequency of participation in extracurricular activities, and number of friends could be compared between shiftworkers and conventional dayworkers in multivariate designs. More surveys of nonshiftworking spouses, direct surveys of the children of shiftworkers, and longitudinal studies of changes in social and family adjustment are also needed. These techniques could be employed to identify and characterize families showing successful adjustment to shiftwork.

Rapid changes in the complexion of the workforce and composition of the American family must also be considered in future research. By recent estimates,[16] 56% of all married women now work and one of every four couples employed full-time has at least one spouse who works a nonday schedule. A larger number of multiple-shiftworker families and single-parent households increases the potential for conflict between working hours and family and social life. These changes call for resources to be directed toward the identification and development of coping techniques that will enhance social satisfaction and adjustment for shiftworkers and their families.

REFERENCES

1. Adams J, Folkard S, Young M: Coping strategies used by nurses on night duty. Ergonomics 29:185–196, 1986.
2. Banks O: Continuous shiftwork: The attitude of wives. Occup Pyschol 30:68–69, 1956.
3. Chadwick-Jones JK: Automation and Behaviour: A Social Psychological Study. London, John Wiley, 1969.
4. Colligan MJ: Methodological and practical issues related to shiftwork research. J Occup Med 22:163–166, 1980.

5. Dirkin JM: Industrial shiftwork: Decrease in well-being and specific effects. Ergonomics 9:115–124, 1966.
6. Frost PJ, Jamal M: Shiftwork, attitudes, and reported behavior: Some association between individual characteristics and hours of work and leisure. J Appl Psychol 64:77–81, 1979.
7. Gadbois C: Women on night shift: Interdependence of sleep and off-the-job activities. In Reinberg A, Vieux N, Andlauer P (eds): Night and Shiftwork: Biological and Social Aspects. Oxford, Pergamon, 1981, pp 223–228.
8. Harrington JM: Shiftwork and health: A critical review of the literature. London, Her Majesty's Stationary Office, 1978.
9. Hedges JN, Sekscenski ES: Workers on late shifts in a changing economy. Monthly Labor Rev 14–22, Sept 1977.
10. Herbert A: The influence of shiftwork on leisure activities: A study with repeated measures. Ergonomics 26:565–574, 1983.
11. Jamal M, Jamal SM: Work and nonwork experiences of fixed and rotating shifts: An empirical assessment. J Vocat Behav 20:282–293, 1982.
12. Johnson LC, Tepas DI, Colquhoun WP, Colligan MJ: The Twenty-four-Hour Workday: Proceedings of a Symposium on Variations in Work-Sleep Schedules. DHHS (NIOSH) publication no. 81-127, 1981.
13. Khaleque A, Rahman A: Shiftworkers' attitudes towards shiftwork and perception of quality of life. Int Arch Occup Environ Health 53:291–297, 1984.
14. Lee TJ, Moon WK, Cho KS: Sociological observation of effects of shiftwork on the functions of the family. J Hum Ergol (Tokyo) 11(suppl):519–526, 1982.
15. Mott PE, Mann FC, McLoughlin Q, Warwick DP: Shiftwork: The Social, Psychological and Physical Consequences. Ann Arbor, University of Michigan Press, 1965.
16. Presser AB: Shiftwork among American couples: The relevance of job and family factors. In Haider M, Keller M, Cervinka R (eds): Night and Shiftwork: Long-term Effects and Their Prevention. Frankfurt, Peter Lang, 1986, pp 149–156.
17. Rutenfranz J, Colquhoun WP, Knauth P, Ghata JN: Biomedical and psychosocial aspects of shiftwork. Scand J Work Environ Health 3:165–182, 1977.
18. Staines GL, Pleck JH: Nonstandard work schedules and family life. J Appl Psychol 69:515–523, 1984.
19. Tasto DL, Colligan MJ, Skjei EW, Polly SJ: The Health Consequences of Shiftwork. DHEW (NIOSH) publication no. 78-154, 1978.
20. Taylor PJ, Pocock SJ: Mortality of shift and day workers 1956–1968. Br J Ind Med 29:201–207, 1972.
21. Tepas DI, Walsh J, Armstrong D: Comprehensive study of the sleep of shiftworkers. In Johnson LC, Tepas DI, Colquhoun WP, Colligan MJ (eds): The Twenty-four-Hour Workday: Proceedings of a Symposium on Variations in Work-Sleep Schedules. DHHS (NIOSH) publication no. 81-127, 1981, pp 419–434.
22. Thiis-Evensen E: Shiftwork and health. Ind Med Surg 27:493–497, 1958.
23. Wedderburn AAI: Some suggestions for increasing the usefulness of psychological and sociological studies of shiftwork. Ergonomics 21:827–833, 1978.
24. Wyatt S, Marriott R: Night work and shift changes. Br J Ind Med 10:164–172, 1953.

CARLOS A. COMPERATORE, PHD
GERALD P. KRUEGER, PHD

CIRCADIAN RHYTHM DESYNCHRONOSIS, JET LAG, SHIFT LAG, AND COPING STRATEGIES

From the U.S. Army Aeromedical Research Laboratory
Fort Rucker, Alabama

The views presented in this paper are those of the authors and do not reflect the official policy or position of the Department of the Army, the Department of Defense, or the U.S. Government.

Reprint requests to:
Carlos A. Comperatore, PhD
U.S. Army Aeromedical Research Laboratory
Fort Rucker, AL 36362-5292

BACKGROUND

The human body uses predictable environmental events such as sunrise and sunset to maintain a consistent internal organization of physiological functions. Peak levels of physiological rhythms are specifically timed to occur at the appropriate phase of the daily light/dark (LD) cycle. This internal synchronization of physiological rhythmicity results in the availability of metabolic energy, neurotransmitter synthesis, enzyme activity, and hormone production at critical times of the day. The mechanism that mediates the interdependence of human physiology with environmental cycles of light and dark has been referred to as the circadian timing system (CTS).[55] It is generally accepted that the CTS synchronizes physiological and behavioral rhythms to a circadian period (*circa*, about; *dies*, a day) and that the phase of these rhythms can be reset by the influence of the environmental LD cycle. Other environmental rhythmic cues (e.g., social interaction, meal timing) also serve to synchronize the CTS, but the LD cycle is of overriding importance.

The Human Circadian Timing System (CTS). The CTS is composed of structures such as the suprachiasmatic nuclei (SCN) and the pineal gland, which together contribute to the synchronization of physiological and behavioral rhythms. These structures are usually referred to as oscillators or biological clocks because of their periodic contribution to the generation of circadian rhythmicity. Research on the mechanism of CTS function suggests that this system is composed of coupled multiple oscillators, many of them yet unknown. Cyclic environmental events with periods of approximately 24 hours, such as the earth's LD cycle, entrain (or synchronize) the rhythmic output of the CTS. In the absence of the entraining influence of sunrise and sunset or social cues, the CTS endogenously maintains physiological and behavioral rhythmicity (e.g., sleep/wake cycle and rhythms of REM sleep, body core temperature, plasma cortisol, adrenalin, noradrenalin, and melatonin) with a period of approximately 24 hours.

In humans, under normal LD cycles, physiological and behavioral rhythms exhibit consistent peaks (acrophases) and troughs in either the day or the night (light or dark phase of the LD cycle). Table 1 is an extensive, but not exhaustive, list of physiological and behavioral rhythms. Several of these rhythms (e.g., activity/rest, body core temperature, adrenalin and noradrenalin production, vigilance, decision making, problem solving) exhibit peaks in the light phase of the LD cycle (diurnal). Others, such as the hormone melatonin, exhibit peak levels during the night phase (nocturnal) of the LD cycle.[55,86]

Internal and External Synchronization. Under a consistent environmental LD cycle, physiological and behavioral rhythms maintain a relative synchronization with each other (internal synchronization) and with the daily rhythm of sunrise and sunset (external synchronization). That is, in steady state conditions, they exhibit their peaks and troughs at approximately the same time of day or night, depending on their natural expression. If meal times are regular and sleep periods are consistent, other physiological rhythms such as premeal duodenal disaccharidase activity and motility also contribute to the establishment of internal synchronization.[19,70] In steady state, it is possible to maximize the ability to maintain normal energy levels and the best possible state of health.

DESYNCHRONOSIS: JET LAG AND SHIFT LAG

Workers often forfeit the comfort of internal and external rhythm synchronization in situations that require an alteration of the activity/rest cycle (day: activity; night: rest). Two categories of work-related circadian rhythm disruption are common: (1) transcontinental or international travel necessitating rapid changes in the phase of the light/dark cycle (e.g., transmeridian flights) and (2) transition in a shiftwork rotation schedule that changes the activity/rest cycle (e.g., altering workshifts from days to evenings or nights).

Individuals who engage in rapid transmeridian travel (e.g., international business-people, airline crews, and military personnel) undergo alterations in the timing of the CTS. These changes manifest in the desynchronization of physiological and behavioral rhythms. Upon arrival, travelers encounter a new rhythm of sunrise and sunset and a time-altered activity and social schedule. The impact of these changes on body physiology results in several days of fatigue, sleepiness, lethargy, insomnia, gastrointestinal track disorders, and poorer mental agility and performance. The syndrome is commonly known as **jet lag.**[88] Essentially, the body takes a while to synchronize its rhythms to the new time zone.

Similarly, shiftworkers (e.g., factory workers, police officers, hospital attendees, communication technicians) who alter their work schedule to include duty during the evening or night, also disrupt the synchronization of the CTS, with results resembling jet lag. Shiftwork changes usually disrupt the timing of sleep and activity and have noticeable effects on alertness, fatigue, and work

TABLE 1. Physiological and Behavioral Rhythms Exhibiting 24-Hour Periodicities

Rhythm	Acrophase
Sleep/Activity	
Sleep	Night
REM sleep	Night
Exercise capacity	Day
Activity	Day
Endocrine Metabolism/Homeostasis	
Core temperature	Day
Urine production	Day
Catecholamine excretion	Day
17-Hydroxicorticosteroid excretion in plasma and urine	Day
Electrolyte and corticosteroid excretion in urine	Day
Melatonin synthesis	Night
Adrenalin and noradrenalin production	Day
Cognitive performance	
Addition of numbers	Day
Auditory vigilance	Day
Decision making	Day
Reasoning	Day

effectiveness. Kogi[47] refers to the detrimental effects of shiftwork changes as "shift lag" because of the similarity with the jet lag syndrome both in generation and symptomology.[47,89]

The adverse effects of jet lag and shift lag result from the desynchronization of physiological and behavioral rhythms, a condition referred to as internal dissociation or, by some authors, circadian rhythm **desynchronosis.** Although jet lag and shift lag are both forms of desynchronosis, they are somewhat different from one another. The transmeridian traveler experiences a rapid change in the timing of sunrise and sunset (LD cycle) and has to adjust, often only briefly, to the destination's schedule of life events. On the other hand, the shiftworker has to adjust to (1) a change in work schedule (e.g., day to evening or night, night to day or evening), (2) a change in sleeping schedule (often from nighttime to daytime), and (3) family and societal schedules that are mostly diurnal. Shiftworkers exacerbate the body's adjustment by changing schedules again on off-duty days (e.g., weekends) in an attempt to maintain a normal social life.

Desynchronosis adversely affects worker performance and health. Today, with the volume of work-related international travel, jet lag directly impacts on the effectiveness of many business interactions. At the least, jet lag has become a commonplace nuisance in international business. At worst, for international airline pilots and crews who travel back and forth across time zones, jet lag, when combined with shift lag, may affect the safety of airline travel.[30,31] (Pilot scheduling and airline safety are discussed in depth in Chapter 10).

Shift lag, too, is an increasing problem in occupational medicine. Research on the performance implications of human circadian rhythms, and on the medical and social difficulties experienced by shiftworkers, clearly suggests that it is important for occupational medicine specialists to understand shift lag and possible preventive measures.[79–81]

The long-term health risks associated with continued use of shiftwork schedules are becoming better known.[45,47,48,52,67–69,89] The physiological impact of rotating shifts particularly affects nightworkers, whose rhythms of body temperature and sleep do not completely reverse to match their duty schedules.[43,44,84]

Among nightshift workers, the immunological functions of lymphocytes in peripheral blood show a circadian variation and are lowered at night.[56] Gastrointestinal diseases such as gastric or duodenal ulcers occur more frequently among these workers.[1,6] Shiftworkers, in general, complain more frequently of respiratory and motor organ disorders, shortages of quality sleep, increased fatigue levels, and lapses in performance (for review see Chapter 6 and Kogi[47]).

International travelers, employers of shiftworkers, and many employees themselves may underestimate the impact of desynchronosis associated with jet lag and shift lag. This chapter reviews the mechanism of generation of both jet lag and shift lag and highlights the complexity of coping with desynchronosis.

Transmeridian Flights and Desynchronosis (Jet Lag). Because the earth rotates on its axis every 24 hours, the globe has been divided into 24 one-hour time zones, each with 15 meridians. Daylight travels from one meridian to another in 4 minutes. Therefore, individuals who travel rapidly across several time zones can expect not only a change in their activity/rest rhythm to accommodate to the new time zone, but a change in the environmental LD cycle as well. On the day of travel eastward travelers experience a reduction of day length while their bodies respond as if they were still in the departure time zone (they lag behind).

To adjust the body's rhythms to an eastward destination the CTS needs to be ***advanced*** as many hours as time zones crossed. In contrast, westbound travelers experience an extension of the day of travel. In this case, adjustment of the CTS to the destination time zone requires a ***delay*** of as many hours as time zones traversed.[88]

The greater the number of time zones traversed in a single day, the greater the time adjustment required for the resynchronization of internal rhythms with the new LD cycle and activity/rest cycle. The human CTS can adapt to advance or delay shifts of no more than 60 to 90 minutes per day.[10,11] Beyond this range, the CTS begins to lag behind the LD cycle and internal desynchronization ensues.[40,42] The inability of the human CTS to rapidly readjust beyond its limits of entrainment results in a transitional period of desynchronosis, commonly referred to as jet lag. This syndrome usually lasts a few days, but depending on the number of time zones crossed and individual differences, it may last up to 18 days.[12,39]

Since activity/rest rhythms exhibit an endogenous period greater than 24 hours (approximately 25 hours per day), it is easier to adjust to westbound travel, which results in a longer travel day. Eastward travelers experience a shortening day and longer resynchronization periods.[41] The severity of jet-lag desynchronosis symptoms depends on the amount of time shift and on individual chronotypic characteristics (see Table 2). For example, after flying eastward across six time zones from New York to Europe, on the day of arrival at 0900 the body's CTS still functions as it would at 0300 in New York (it lags behind), and the traveler undoubtedly is very sleepy. Conversely, if local time is 2400 and the body's biological time is 1800, the traveler will likely have trouble falling asleep.

Travelers who fly over the top of the Arctic Circle cross more time zones faster and sometimes experience even more dramatic symptoms, including disorientation, decreased concentration, and muscle aches.[15] For example, crossing 11 time zones on a 10-hour flight from Europe to Alaska would produce the full range of jet-lag symptoms and require at least one week to adjust; yet passengers flying from North to South America, staying within one or two time zones, may experience fewer and less acute jet-lag symptoms.

TABLE 2. Factors Influencing Rate of Adjustment to Time Zone or Shift Change

Direction of change (time advance or delay)[40,86,87]
Rhythm stability (stable or labile)[78]
Rhythm amplitude (low or high)[5,86,87]
Personality traits (extraversion or introversion, neuroticism)[16,34]
Rhythm chronotype (morning person or evening person)[16]
Age (young or old)[33]
Motivation (high or low)[30]
Sleep habits (rigid or flexible)[27,28]
Performance task (high or low cognitive load)[27,30]

Effects of Jet Lag on Performance. Rapidly crossing time zones affects both physiological and performance rhythms. The latter are of major operational significance when people are required to carry out complex psychomotor or intellectual tasks soon after arrival. In general, psychomotor performance after a 6-hour transmeridian flight suffers a reduction of 8–10% of preflight levels during the first day after arrival. This is disquieting because such impairment is comparable to that observed when the blood alcohol concentration is 0.05%.[41] In general, several performance rhythms (see Table 3) have been shown to be adversely affected after both westward and eastward transmeridian flights, but

TABLE 3. Performance Degradation Effects of Time and Schedule Changes

Subjects and Alterations	Degradation Effects
Pilots and students 6 time zones eastward	Flight simulator skills 24 h, means 3–4% from preflight Reaction time Complex sensory motor skills (to operate simulator) Digit summation Digit cancelation
6 time zones westward	Psychomotor performance in simulator reduced Digit summation Digit cancelation
6–9 time zones eastward	Efficiency in simulator performance reduced Psychomotor performance 1.8–3.5% from preflight Hand-eye coordination, 8% from preflight
Military personnel 6 time zones eastward	50% of personnel experienced fatigue and sleep difficulties; 40% reported subjective weakness Dynamic arm strength reduced by 6.1–10.8% Elbow flexor strength reduced 8.4–12% Lift and carry tasks reduced 9.5% Logical reasoning reduced 15%
Student volunteers 2–4 h phase change of sleep/wake period	Significant decrement in vigilance, calculation proficiency, mood
Female volunteers 8 h advance of sleep/wake period	Short-term memory reduced Visual search performance reduced
Student pilots 2.5 h advance of sleep/wake period	Sleep impairment 35% increased errors in flight performance 1–15% decrease in letter cancelation
Nurses Reversal of sleep/wake period; shift from day to night duty	Short-term memory reduced

eastward travel has more pronounced effects. Upon arrival, westward time-zone crossings usually affect performance during the afternoon and early evening hours, whereas eastward crossings affect performance during the morning and early afternoon hours.[41] In general, these effects have been shown to persist up to 5 days postflight, but differences between pre- and postflight performance are not significant 3 days after arrival.

Partial adjustment of these rhythms can be observed on the first day after arrival. However, after eastward flights inducing a 6-hour phase advance, readjustment is slower than after a 6-hour westward flight (phase delay).

COPING WITH JET LAG

Monk[54] distinguishes several jet-lag stress effects stemming from the particular physical and psychological aspects of international travel (e.g., making connections at airports, luggage hassles, and customs checks) and the flight itself (e.g., dehydration, changes in altitude effects) from those that are a product of the need to reset the biological clock upon arrival (i.e., CTS desynchronosis). Since circadian rhythm desynchronosis involves the loss of internal and external synchronization, coping strategies must ameliorate both physiological and cognitive effects associated with the jet-lag syndrome. The following strategies help alleviate jet lag.

Adjusting to the New Time Zone. Transmeridian travelers who expect to remain in the new time zone for weeks should quickly change the timing of behavior patterns to match local events; that is, sleep and wake-up times, meal times, and social events should match local schedules as soon as possible. To speed up the rate of readjustment, it is necessary to (1) immerse oneself in local society, maintaining normal social activity patterns, (2) engage in physical exercise, and (3) maintain regular exposure to daylight.[38,86] Outdoor activities are recommended because daylight assists in the adjustment of melatonin rhythms (see "Pharmacological Alternatives," below), which significantly contributes to the resynchronization of the CTS.[49,73] Late wake-up and sleep times and social isolation impede adjustment and are therefore discouraged.[40] Lastly, following local meal schedules significantly aids in the process of resynchronization.[29]

Because it takes several days to adjust to jet lag, it is recommended that travelers arrive a few days early to allow time for the CTS to resynchronize before they conduct important meetings, negotiations, or other business that may require decision making.

Remaining on Home Base Time. In certain circumstances, travelers can attempt to maintain the time schedule of their departure location by not resetting their watches and by scheduling events, meals, and sleep times to match their home base clocks. This technique avoids most of the CTS disruption of travel except for the change in LD cycle. For compatibility with societal expectations, it is often difficult to arrange things in the new environment to the traveler's own time preference. However, a California businessman can arrange late afternoon meetings on the East Coast on the day of travel, and a New York worker can conduct business at midday on the West Coast.

Sleep Timing. Because getting uninterrupted restful sleep upon arrival is often difficult, the traveler should be fully rested at departure so that there is no "sleep debt."[54] A wristwatch can be set to the destination time zone and activities pursued according to the new clock time. Bedtime should be shifted progressively earlier each night (phase advance) for a few days before an eastward flight and progressively later (phase delay) in anticipation of a westward flight. The time of awakening must also be adjusted.

On long flights, naps should be short to avoid interfering with sleep planned for the first night after arrival. Upon arriving, it is recommended to remain awake until normal bedtime for the destination time zone.

Meal Timing and the Use of Diets. Diet has been proposed to be useful in the amelioration of jet-lag symptoms,[23] particularly because certain foods (carbohydrates) induce sleep by facilitating serotonin synthesis and others (proteins) promote alertness by stimulating the synthesis of catecholamines. Within this context, choice of diet before and during the trip may help in the adjustment to the destination's timing of life events such as sleep and meal schedules.

Diet has not, however, been shown to aid in actual resynchronization of the CTS. Recent research in circadian rhythms of the gastrointestinal (GI) track of rats indicates the existence of a motility rhythm that can be entrained by the consistent timing of meals.[19] Irregular contractions (IC), possibly similar to hunger contractions in humans, recorded from the antrum and duodenum, were shown to occur throughout 3, and sometimes 5, hours before a scheduled meal. The involvement of a biological clock in the timing of these contractions was shown during phase shifts of meal timing and fasting. Transient changes in the phase of the IC rhythm lasting 4 to 6 days were observed after delays in meal timing of 6 and 8 hours; such delays were similar, for humans, to eating dinner later after a westward flight. In addition, the IC rhythm exhibited a circadian variation during food deprivation. Similar experiments with rhythms of duodenal dissacharidases also indicate the influence of a biological clock on physiological rhythms of the GI track.[17] Consequently, resynchronization of the GI track after changes in meal timing must be treated in a similar form as resynchronization of rhythms driven by the suprachiasmatic nuclei (SCN). In both cases the timing of the exogenous environmental cycles, light/dark for the SCN and feeding/fasting for the GI track, is critical for the reestablishment of steady state synchronization. Although choice of meals may possibly aid in inducing sleep or alertness, it is the consistent timing of meals and fasting periods that will serve as phase information for the oscillator influencing the GI track and that will ultimately play a significant role in facilitating CTS resynchronization.

Bright Light Therapy and Jet Lag. In 1980, Lewy and co-workers[49] demonstrated that high irradiances (1000 lux) of broad-spectrum white light influence human endocrine function, specifically secretion of the hormone melatonin (see "Pharmacological Alternatives," below). This finding implied that bright artificial light influenced the SCN and its control of pineal activity. The SCN receives light/dark cycle phase information by way of the retinohypothalamic tract and regulates pineal function via a multisynaptic pathway and the paraventricular nucleus of the hypothalamus, the superior cervical ganglia, and sympathetic fibers ending in the nervi coronarii innervating the gland. Consequently, because the SCN has been associated with synchronization of endogenous physiological rhythms to the exogenous influence of sunrise and sunset, bright artificial lights may be used to mimic the destination LD cycle before the transmeridian flight. In this manner, travelers may reduce the desynchronosis experienced upon arrival. Conceivably, aircraft passenger cabins specially configured with bright lights could speed up CTS entrainment on overseas flights; such cabins may have special military applications.

SHIFTWORK SCHEDULES, LIGHT/DARK CYCLES, AND DESYNCHRONOSIS

Shiftwork and Shift Lag. Historically (circa 1890s), two alternating teams of employees, each working 12 hours per day, (0600–1800 and 1800–0600) 7 days per week, kept industries such as steel mills operating continuously.[4] After World War I, operations were divided into three 8-hour shifts per day, with employees working 7 days or 56 hours per week. Since World War II, shifts work a conventional 40-hour work week combining any five 8-hour workdays of the 7-day week. Three different teams work 8 hours per shift with a 1-hour or shorter rest and meal break midshift: 0730–1630 (dayshift), 1530–2430 hours (evenings) and 2300–0800 (nights). To provide continuous operations (CONOPS), many different schemes are used to rotate employees from one shift to another[83] and to determine which 5 of the 7 days in the week they work. The schemes ensure that workers work each schedule equally.

Traditional shiftwork schedules fail to account for many circadian rhythm variables, especially the limitations of sleep/wake cycles. In particular, shifting between day- and nightwork results in sleep disruption, decreases alertness on the job, and interferes with established family and social activity schedules.[83]

In a common shiftwork weekly schedule change, each employee works 7 consecutive nights, followed by 2 days off; then 7 evening shifts, followed by a day off; then 7 consecutive day shifts, followed by 4 days off (7N–2 Off–7E–1 Off–7D–4 Off).[15] If a worker begins this schedule on a Wednesday, a 4-day weekend—Saturday, Sunday, Monday, Tuesday—serves as the only weekend respite in four weeks. The schedule includes a stretch in which employees work 14 or 15 days with an average work week of 42 hours. Workers rotate shifts every week, but they experience shift lag upon each weekly change. Coleman and Czeisler call this the "weekly phase advance" schedule because it forces employees to advance their work schedule eight hours earlier in the ***counterclockwise*** (backward) direction (nights to evenings to days) each week.[15] In effect, at shift change, the body must adjust to a shorter day, necessitating going to bed earlier than normal.

Regularly changing shiftwork schedules (e.g., from day- to nightshift) bring about sudden substantial rescheduling of the activity/rest rhythm and meal times. Depending upon the circumstances, the most immediate consequence is redistribution and especially loss of sleep due to changes in sleep and wake-up times. In addition, synchronization of body core temperature with the activity/rest rhythm is disrupted because temperature rhythms adapt very slowly to new schedules,[17,18,84,89] whereas activity/rest rhythms are immediately altered by changing sleep and wake-up times.

After transmeridian travel, the synchronicity of the new LD cycle and social cues with the local sleep/wake cycle promotes readjustment of travelers' CTS to diurnal activity. In contrast to transmeridian travel, after a shiftwork change from day- to nightshift, the temporal relationship between sunrise and sunset and the new sleep/wake schedule is in conflict. Internal synchronization is lost, and external synchronization to the LD cycle is also severely disrupted. Cognitive performance usually deteriorates with changes in shiftwork schedules because its 24-hour distribution becomes desynchronized relative to the new activity/rest rhythm.[24-26] Thus, after changes in work schedules, the shift-lag syndrome persists until the CTS resynchronizes to the new duty/rest schedule. This process is made more difficult during shift lag than during jet lag because daily exposure to sunlight tends to entrain the SCN to diurnal activity.

Aviation Crews, Jet Lag, and Shift Lag. Commercial and military air crews must be able to perform safely and effectively at various times of the day and night that are often in conflict with their circadian rhythms. Pilots frequently fly "long-haul" routes through the night, across multiple time zones, and experience jet lag upon arrival. Graeber[31] points out that many pilots begin 3- to 4-day trips with a slight sleep debt, and they accumulate a substantial amount of sleep loss during a trip. On short layovers, rest time often is inadequate, and its timing in conflict with the preflight sleep/wake cycle. That is, it is difficult to sleep when the body temperature is rising. Lodging accommodations are not always conducive to restful sleep, and amounts and quality of sleep often are inadequate.

Soon, after short layovers, pilots resume flying, sometimes in the same direction, but more often on a return trip in the reverse direction across the same time zones just traversed. Resulting circadian rhythm desynchronization can have a variety of effects on individual crew members, including disturbances in manual flying skills.[31] Klein et al.[37] showed clear directional differences in disruption of performance in postflight simulator tests and in the rate of recovery in the new time zone. Flight simulator performance was more degraded after an eastward return flight than after a westward outbound flight.

Some pilots and crew members not only work unusual flight schedules imposed by their employers but add to their CTS desynchronization by becoming long-haul commuters. Some of them fly as passengers from their residence across time zones to report to work at their employer's home base airfield. There, they "begin" their several days of scheduled flying. When these same pilots get rescheduled for flights departing at substantially different times of the day, they subject themselves to complicated interactions between jet lag and shift lag, become fatigued, and are likely to put themselves and their passengers at risk.

COPING WITH SHIFT LAG

Various countermeasures can prevent shift-lag desynchronosis or, when it is inevitable, can facilitate coping with or adjusting to it. We include practical and optimal coping strategies without limiting the scope to procedures that are most economical to the industrial community.

Fixed Shift Schedules. One countermeasure to prevent shift-lag desynchronosis is for employees *not to change shift times at all.* People may choose from many available jobs that do not involve rotating shiftwork schedules. A select few CONOPS industries lock into a fixed shift system whereby some employees work exclusively nights or evenings for extended periods, months, even years at a time.

With a steady work schedule the presumption is that desynchronosis should not be a problem. Research indicates, however, that the circadian distribution of physiological rhythms does not completely reverse even after several months on nightshift. The body's core temperature rhythm does not exhibit a complete reversal with a nocturnal redistribution of its acrophase. In most cases, acrophase tends to occur at the beginning of the nocturnal work period but drops abruptly thereafter.[84] Even in cases of consistent long-term schedules, body temperature is not fully inverted; instead, a nocturnal tendency of the acrophase is followed by a flattening of the rhythm.[2,43,66,84] It is not clear how much of the temperature pattern is self-induced by nightworkers, who, on their off-duty days, revert to a day schedule, altering their meal and sleep times to accommodate other societal expectations.[82]

Decreased Rate of Rotation. Most CONOPS organizations rotate employee shifts weekly. Changing schedules every 3 to 4 weeks would allow more time for CTS adjustment between less frequent shift changes. Workers who are able to maintain similar sleep and wake-up times during off-duty days are more likely to exhibit consistent physiological adaptation than those who change meal and sleep times to a diurnal schedule on their off-duty days. Staying on schedule allows rhythms of body temperature and of rest and activity to maintain a constant relative syncrhonization after initial adaptation. Performance is then more consistent from one workday to another.

Clockwise or Forward Rotation of Shifts. For many years industrial plants used a "phase advance" (counterclockwise: days to nights to evenings), backward shift rotation system.[85] Circadian rhythm principles suggest that workers should instead rotate toward later shifts in a *clockwise,* forward (days to evenings to nights) "phase delay" fashion. That is, because the body naturally adjusts its free-running rhythms toward a longer day (25 hours), it is easier to delay the time one goes to bed for about 3–4 hours (for clockwise shift changes) than it is to move bedtimes counterclockwise to earlier hours. Thus working days, then evenings, and then nights permits an easier circadian rhythm adjustment to a new schedule.

Slow Drift Rotation. To avoid weekly abrupt 8-hour shift transitions, Coleman and Czeisler recommend that workers make a gradual transition to the new shift by starting work 2½ hours later than on the previous day the last three days before the actual change to a new schedule. Coleman,[15] however, suggests that this kind of schedule is hard to get used to; it makes it difficult for workers and their families to anticipate when the employee is to be working and when off duty.

Rapid Rotation. In quick succession, employees are expected to work 1 or 2 dayshifts, then 1 or 2 evenings, followed by 1 or 2 nights. This rapid clockwise rotation purports to allow circadian rhythms to remain synchronized with the dayshift.[15,83] Employees do not spend enough time on the evening or night schedules for their internal rhythms to adjust to nightwork. That is, the diurnal acrophase of the body temperature rhythm is not noticeably altered, internal synchronization is not lost, and disruption of sleep/wake cycles is only slight.[26] Workers tough out the nightshift and rotate quickly through it, but during the night they experience lowest daily body temperatures, increased fatigue, and a considerable decrement in performance.

For more detailed review of the problems of shift lag and coping strategies, see Chapter 12.

RESYNCHRONIZATION RATE FOR ADJUSTING TO JET LAG AND SHIFT LAG

The rate of adjustment to changing light/dark cycles or shift schedules depends on a number of physiological and individual factors (see Table 2).[88]

Phase Delay Versus Phase Advance. In general, the human CTS exhibits a preference for quicker reestablishment of internal syncrhonization after a ***delay*** in the activity/rest rhythm or the LD cycle. Consequently, the human CTS readjusts more rapidly when crossing time zones traveling west. Similarly, changing from morning to evening to night schedules (phase delay) is more desirable than the reversed pattern of change (phase advance).

Individual Differences. People who are more apt to rapidly adjust to changing LD cycles and rotating work schedules are distinguished by rhythm amplitude and stability and by their wake-up time preference. Some researchers suggest that low-amplitude body temperature rhythms may identify people with a tendency to adjust rapidly to changes in the activity/rest schedules.[9,65,86,88]

In contrast, some workers tolerate long-term shiftwork without experiencing sleep disturbances even after 25 years. Unlike people who can rapidly reentrain to changing work schedules, these workers exhibit large-amplitude body temperature rhythms and adjust slowly to new schedules. They suffer short-term desynchronosis but experience fewer sleep and work-performance alterations after resynchronization owing to the stability of their circadian rhythms.[5,63]

Russian researchers developed a method to measure rhythm stability.[77,78] People can be classified into three categories—"inert," "intermediate," and "labile"—depending on the stability of their rhythms. Inert people have more rigid circadian rhythms; they experience more difficulty during rapid changes of work schedules or crossing of time zones than their labile counterparts.[76–78] Intermediate individuals fall somewhere between the two extremes.

Morning people ("larks"), with strong preference for early morning wake-up times, exhibit early morning peaks and large amplitudes in their temperature rhythms. These characteristics make the circadian system rigid and result in greater resistance to resynchronization. In contrast, evening people ("owls") appear to have a more labile circadian system exhibiting smaller amplitudes in temperature rhythm than "larks"; their peaks occur later in the day.[35]

In general, young extroverted people exhibiting labile rhythms and an affinity for late morning awakening ("owls") and having flexible sleeping habits and high motivation are more apt to readjust rapidly to sudden changes in light/dark cycles or work schedules. On the other hand, the choice between rapidly changing and long-term shiftwork schedules becomes an operational question affected by the type of work (whether lowly or highly cognitive tasks), the duration of individual shifts, the total duration of shiftwork (whether it is chronic or temporary), and the individual characteristics (rhythm chronotypes) of shiftworkers employed.

PHARMACOLOGICAL ALTERNATIVES

The Problem of Rapid Resynchronization of the CTS. The central problem in ameliorating the desynchronization syndrome is rapid and complete reestablishment of internal synchronization. Both internal and external synchronization can be recovered by inducing significant changes in the timing of the CTS. This concept applies for rapid crossing of time zones during transmeridian flights and for dramatic changes in shiftwork schedules (going from day- to nightshifts).

The most immediate problem of the transmeridian traveler (eastward and westward) is to rapidly adjust the sleep period to coincide with the destination night and to obtain sufficient restful sleep on that new schedule. Nightshift workers must sleep during late morning and afternoon hours, and evening shiftworkers must sleep in the early and late morning hours. In these cases, the change in timing results in desynchronization of the temperature and activity/rest rhythms, as well as of the many rhythmic physiological functions controlled by the circadian timing system (Table 1). Consequently, any drug used against desynchronization must quicken the resynchronization rates of various rhythms that are dependent on the CTS, and in particular that of the body's temperature rhythm.

Hypnotics induce sleep but do not necessarily resynchronize the CTS. Complete resynchronization of the CTS not only induces sleep, but also reestablishes the normal architecture of the sleep period, total sleep time, sleep continuity, normal sleep inertia, and normal relationship of the acrophase of the body core temperature rhythm with the activity phase of the sleep/wake cycle. Consequently, a drug that artificially induces sleep does not alter the physiological and cognitive consequences of desynchronosis if it does not influence the timing of the CTS. Sleep induced by hypnotics masks the status of the CTS, which may remain desynchronized with the new schedule. The restorative value of such a sleep period may also be questioned because endogenous physiological rhythms are still in the process of resynchronization. In fact, the use of a synthetic substance that may influence the activity and effect of endogenous neurotransmitters (e.g., benzodiazepines affect GABA receptors) may retard the process of resynchronization (not often studied in human volunteers). In brief, the evaluation of potentially chronobiotic drugs (those that affect the CTS) depends upon their effects on the process of CTS resynchronization, and not simply on their effects on individual symptoms associated with desynchronosis (e.g., sleep loss and fatigue).

One variable that reflects CTS phase status with relation to a new work schedule or LD cycle is body core temperature. Consequently, following changes in the phase relationship of the temperature rhythm with a newly implemented schedule after the administration of a drug is likely to reflect the influence of the drug on the status of the CTS. Proper phase relationships between the temperature rhythm and the activity/rest rhythm imply that normal sleep patterns may have been reestablished. The effects on cognitive performance must also be considered since cognitive degradation is one of the most detrimental consequences of desynchronosis in terms of individual and industrial productivity. Unfortunately, very few studies with human subjects provide this information.

Current Pharmacological Alternatives. Although, there is not enough clinical evidence that any chronobiotic drug rapidly resets the CTS, or all of the rhythms under its control, a number of substances appear to be potentially helpful in combatting desynchronosis.[64]

Benzodiazepines are currently used to combat desynchronization. Temazepam has been effective to induce sleep in humans without severe side effects.[51] Two desirable characteristics of temazepam are its short half-life (5–8 hours) and the fact that its metabolism does not result in active metabolites.[13] Psychomotor performance after single doses of temazepam (5, 15, and 30 mg) was somewhat impaired after the 30-mg dose up to 2 hours postadministration.[50] In a visuomotor task, Nicholson and Stone[58] showed that single administrations (10, 20, and 30 mg) of temazepam had no significant effect after 10–16 hours. On the other hand, when subjects were tested sooner after administration impairment was more striking. In the same study, subjects who ingested temazepam in morning hours experienced significant impairment of visuomotor coordination up to approximately 6.5 hours postadministration. Similar studies also report impairment of visuomotor coordination 2 hours postingestion of 30 mg of temazepam.[14,57] Although temazepam is considered safe by some authors,[51] its detrimental effects on visuomotor coordination may extend up to 12 hours postadministration. Consequently the U.S. Army discourages the use of temazepam as a sleep aid in situations requiring completion of certain complex tasks (e.g., helicopter flight) within 12 hours of administration.[3]

As is the case with other tranquilizer and hypnotic drugs (diazepam, oxazepam, triazolam, and botizolam), there is no evidence that temazepam reentrains physiological and behavioral rhythms, such as those of body core temperature and performance, to new work schedules or LD cycles. Its value, in terms of combatting desynchronosis symptomology, resides in the induction of sleep and the consequent reduction of fatigue in the subsequent day.

Another benzodiazepine, triazolam, has been shown to entrain activity rhythms of the hamster,[36,85] a photoperiodic animal that hibernates and shows gonadal regression during the short days of winter. Most of the reported effects of triazolam on hamster activity rhythms, particularly those involving changes in the length of the period of the rhythm, were induced in constant lighting conditions (either darkness or light) or with blind subjects. These experimental results must be interpreted with caution and very carefully generalized for clinical applications.

To date there is no evidence that triazolam actually resynchronizes human circadian rhythms by directly influencing the timing of the CTS. Although, triazolam has been recently recommended for study and use in combatting desynchronosis,[64] the drug has been shown to impair cognitive function 1 hour (0.125-mg dose)[21] and 8 hours after administration (0.5-mg dose).[60] Its role in the improvement of sleep is also not clear; a 0.5-mg dose of triazolam administered in the laboratory improved the duration and continuity of sleep,[59] but during a less controlled eastward transmeridian troop transport flight, it failed to improve the continuity or to increase the duration of sleep of human subjects.[60]

Xanthene drugs are also potentially useful during transmeridian flights because they are readily available (in coffee, tea, and cola drinks) and have been shown to phase-advance and -delay temperature rhythms in animals, depending on the time of administration (advance: at fall of cycle; delay: at rise of cycle). Rats given an intraperitoneal injection of 1,3-dimethylxanthene (aminophylline; 7.5 mg/100 g) showed a phase advance of the body core temperature rhythm of 5–7 hours and, in other cases, a phase delay up to approximately 12 hours.[23] In addition, these animals exhibited a dramatic reduction of body temperature after receiving injections of trimethylxanthene. This effect is pharmacologically induced; it does not physiologically influence CTS phase status.

The use of caffeine to delay sleep onset is a common practice. However, in order to mimic the effects obtained by Ehret and co-workers[23] in humans, subjects must receive comparably large doses of caffeine. A cup of coffee contains approximately 100 mg of trimethylxanthene (i.e., caffeine), tea contains a bit less, and a cola has approximately 50 mg. Ehret's dose corresponds to approximately 5¼ g for a 70-kg person. Consequently, a cup of coffee before bedtime may delay sleep onset but may not affect the phase of the CTS and dependent rhythms unless the right amount of caffeine is ingested. Over-the-counter, high-caffeine drugs designed to fight sleepiness may be useful when sleep onset must be delayed in order to adopt a new sleep/wake schedule.

Other Alternatives. **Nomifensine,** an antidepressant drug, has been shown to increase the rate of reentrainment of the body core temperature rhythm of rats with bilateral SCN lesions.[32] Thus in the absence of the SCN, and therefore of the LD cycle timing system, nomifensine may influence the oscillator system associated with the timing of the body core temperature rhythm. In the cases of jet lag and shift lag, the possibility of rapidly readjusting the temperature rhythm implies reestablishment of normal sleep, less fatigue during resynchronization, and improved performance during the first days after time zones are crossed or workshift is changed. Research in the use of nomifensine to readjust body temperature rhythms is inconclusive but deserves further attention.

Quiadon (3-alkylpyrazolyl piperazine), a tranquilizer that depletes serotonin availability, has also been tested as a possible chronobiotic.[74,75] Subjects exposed to a simulated 8-hour phase shift of the LD cycle were given approximately a 10-mg dose of Quiadon or placebo just before the new sleep period. During the sleep period, these subjects exhibited fewer awakenings than control subjects given a placebo. Although the two groups did not differ upon awakening in terms of subjective rating of restfulness, subjects given placebos were more tired on retiring. Quiadon may be a potentially useful sleep-inducing drug, and its use may reduce fatigue in the context of jet lag or shift lag. Little is known of the effects of this drug on cognitive performance and timing of body core temperature rhythms. Consequently, its possibility as an effective chronobiotic is still unclear.

Research on tranquilizing drugs of similar biochemical structure may provide viable alternatives to the use of benzodiazepines.

Future Alternatives. An alternative to the use of benzodiazepines, antidepressants, or tranquilizers entails the hormone **melatonin.** In humans, as well as in other species (rodents, lizards, and nonhuman primates), melatonin is synthesized in the pineal gland in the dark phase of the light/dark cycle (during sleep in humans). Exogenously administered melatonin has been shown to induce a slowing of the EEG, sleep, vivid dreams, and a reduction of tremors in patients with Parkinson's disease.[7,8,20]

In 1983 Redman and co-workers[62] showed that exogenously administered melatonin influenced entrainment of activity rhythms in albino rats. Preliminary data in studies of single human subjects suggest that melatonin may increase the rate of readjustment of the CTS after a rapid change in the phase of the LD cycle without undesirable physiological effects.[73] Short and Armstrong[73] reported that 5 mg of melatonin administered 20 minutes before bedtime and upon awakening in the middle of the sleep period induced sleep and rapid reentrainment of body core temperature rhythms after transmeridian flights. In the day after the flight, subjects reported feeling rested and capable of performing academic functions. Petrie and co-workers[61] recently showed that administration of 5 mg of melatonin once a day 3 days before an eastward transmeridian flight, both during the flight and for 3 days after arrival, significantly reduced feelings of fatigue and inertia and facilitated reestablishment of normal sleep patterns.

Short[72] reported evidence in a single-subject experiment that melatonin facilitates rapid adjustment of the acrophase of body core temperature to the dark phase of the LD cycle, thus promoting the daytime synchronization of the sleep period. However, further research efforts must confirm this hypothesis because, unlike jet lag, nightworker shift lag involves the additional problem of sleeping during daytime hours and thus requires a permanent reversal of temperature and activity/rest rhythms with relation to the environmental rhythm of day and night. At present, the use of this hormone in the facilitation of rapid adaptation to shifts from day- to nightwork schedules requires more extensive investigation. Although melatonin currently remains in experimental status in the United States, its future use to combat desynchronosis is probable, particularly because there are indications that, unlike benzodiazepines, melatonin appears to directly affect the status of the CTS.

SUMMARY

Jet lag and shift lag affect many employees in our fast-paced working world. Understanding circadian rhythm desynchronosis is important for successful implementation of coping strategies. The complex interaction between endogenous physiological rhythms and exogenous entraining rhythms (e.g., the light/dark cycle and the timing of eating and fasting) must be acknowledged in evaluating the prevention of jet lag, shift lag, or a combination of the two. Jet lag and shift lag have similar physiological consequences; both result in fatigue, loss of sleep, gastrointestinal disorders, and reduced performance. Jet lag is short lived (it generally lasts fewer than 3 days but can last as long as 18 days); it varies with the number of time zones crossed, individual differences in rhythm chronotype, and the number of days of layover before the return flight. In contrast, shift lag constitutes a more complex problem, particularly in cases where the LD cycle must remain in the opposite phase position from the duty/rest schedule. The severity and persistence of this syndrome also depends on the direction of the shift change (e.g., dayshift to nightshift or daylight to evening work), individual differences, and the number of days scheduled on a given shift (e.g., fixed shifts, slow rotations, fast rotations). The most severe desynchronosis may be experienced by airline personnel involved in transmeridian flights. The jet-lag syndrome can be exacerbated by shift lag depending on the schedule of return flights and on the contiguity of subsequent assignments.

Eastward travelers, in particular, can expect difficulty in readjusting to the destination schedule because the light/dark cycle and life events occur earlier relative to preflight clock times. The general coping strategy is to quickly adopt the destination schedules for sleep and meal times, as well as for social activities. Hypnotic drugs such as benzodiazepines (e.g., temazepam) may serve to induce sleep, but they do not resynchronize the CTS. Use of sleep aids must be carefully monitored because side effects may impact complex cognitive or visuomotor task performance upon awakening and also because repeated use carries some risk of addiction. A less risky sleep induction aid is the timely consumption of carbohydrate-rich meals.

On the other hand, the westward traveler has only to phase-delay sleep and meal times to the destination schedule. This is relatively easier than a phase advance and can be facilitated with readily available substances such as tea, coffee, or over-the-counter caffeine tablets. Meals rich in proteins rather than carbohydrates may also prolong wakefulness until the desired sleep time.

Shift lag poses a more difficult problem than jet lag, although the general strategy for coping with it is similar. The first step is to ensure that during the transition to a new workshift, a new sleep schedule is quickly established. In this case, the direction of the shift (e.g., phase delay: days to evenings, or phase advance: days to nights) determines the degree of difficulty associated with the implementation of the new sleep/wake schedule. In any case, pharmacological aids should be used with particular caution because adjustment to long-term shift rotation may lead workers to abuse benzodiazepines inadvertently. The best strategy for shift lag may be the application of circadian principles by employers to the development of shift schedules. Using rhythm chronotype screening, implementing phase delay rotations, and using fixed, fast, and slow rotating shifts as determined by personnel characteristics and mission significantly ameliorate the impact of shift lag on the individual and ultimately on the organization.

Current research efforts to elucidate the mechanism of action of the circadian timing system and to identify various contributing biological clocks promise future solutions for coping with desynchronosis. For example, research on melatonin to facilitate resynchronization of the body temperature rhythm suggests that interventions in the biosynthesis of this hormone or exogenous administrations of it may be useful in combatting symptoms related to desynchronosis.

Until these and other questions are answered, however, desynchronosis can be best managed by educating workers, employers, labor and management representatives, and occupational specialists about the issues associated with the symptomology and mechanism of generation of the jet-lag and shift-lag syndromes.

Acknowledgment. We wish to thank Ms. Gloria Kennedy for assistance in the preparation of our manuscript.

REFERENCES

1. Aanonsen A: Shift Work and Health. Oslo, Universitetsforlaget, 1964.
2. Akerstedt T: Adjustment of physiological circadian rhythms and the sleep-wake cycle to shiftwork. In Folkard S, Monk TH (eds): Hours of Work. New York, John Wiley, 1985, pp 185–197.
3. Alfonso C: Halcion (triazolam). Soc U S Army Flight Surgeons Newsletter 3(4):2, 1989.
4. Alluisi EA, Morgan BB: Temporal factors in human performance and productivity. In Alluisi EA, Fleishman EA (eds): Human Performance and Productivity. Vol 3. Stress and Performance Effectiveness. Hillsdale, NJ: Lawrence Erlbaum, 1982, pp 165–247.
5. Andlauer P, Reinberg A: Amplitude of the oral temperature circadian rhythm and tolerance of shiftwork. Chronobiologia 6:67–73, 1979.
6. Angersbach D, Knauth P, Loskant H: A retrospective cohort study comparing complaints and diseases in day and shift workers. Int Arch Occup Environ Health 45:127–140, 1980.
7. Anton-Tay F: On the effect of melatonin upon the human brain: Its possible therapeutic implications. Life Sci 10:841–850, 1971.
8. Anton-Tay F: Melatonin: Effects on brain function. Adv Biochem Psychopharmacol 11:315–424, 1974.
9. Aschoff J: Internal dissociation and desynchronization of circadian systems. Twenty-first International Congress of Aviation and Space Medicine, preprint 255, 1973.
10. Aschoff J: Problems of re-entrainment of circadian rhythms: Asymmetry effect, dissociation and partition. In Assenmacher J, Farner DS (eds): Environmental Endocrinology. New York, Springer Verlag, 1978, pp 185–195.
11. Aschoff J: Circadian rhythms within and outside their ranges of entrainment. In Assenmacher J, Farner DS (eds): Environmental Endocrinology. New York, Springer Verlag, 1978, pp 172–181.
12. Beljan JR, Rosenblatt LS, Hetherington NW, et al: Human performance in the aviation environment. Final report (five parts). NASA Contract NAS2-6657, 1972.
13. Breimer DD: Pharmacokinetics and metabolism of various benzodiazepines used as hypnotics. Br J Clin Pharmacol 8:7–13, 1979.
14. Clark CH, Nicholson AN: Immediate and residual effects in man of the metabolites of diazepam. Br J Clin Pharmacol 6:325–332, 1978.
15. Coleman RM: Wide Awake at 3:00 A.M.: By Choice or by Chance? New York, W.H. Freeman, 1986.
16. Colquhoun WP: Phase shift in temperature rhythm after transmeridian flight, as related to pre-flight phase angle. Int Arch Occup Environ Health 42:149–157, 1979.
17. Colquhoun WP, Blake MJF, Edwards RS: Experimental studies of shift work. I. A comparison of "rotating" and "stabilizing" 4-hour systems. Ergonomics 11:437–453, 1968a.
18. Colquhoun WP, Blake MJF, Edwards RS: Experimental studies of shift work. III. Stabilized 12-hour shift system. Ergonomics 12:865–882, 1968b.
19. Comperatore CA, Stephan FK: Entrainment of duodenal activity periodic feeding. Biol Rhythms 2(3):227–242, 1987.
20. Cramer H: Melatonin and sleep. In Popoviciu L, Asgian G (eds): Sleep. Basel, Karger, 1980, pp 204–210.

21. Duncan RL, Simon LM, O'Donnell VM, et al: The effect of triazolam on cognitive performance. Abstracts of the 1989 American Psychological Association Annual Convention, New Orleans, 11–15 August 1989.
22. Ehret CF, Groh KR, Meinert JC: Consideration of diet in alleviating jet lag. In Scheving LE, Halberg F (eds): Principles and Applications to Shift in Schedules. Rockville, MD, Sijthoff and Noordhoff, 1980, pp 393–402.
23. Ehret CF, Potter VR, Dobia KW: Chronobiological action of theophylline and of pentobarbital as circadian zeitgebers in the rat. Science 188:1212–1214, 1975.
24. Folkard S: Shiftwork and its effects on performance. In Scheving LE, Halberg F (eds). Chronobiology: Principles and Applications to Shifts in Schedules. Rockville, MD, Sijthoff and Noordhoff, 1980, pp 293–306.
25. Folkard S: Shiftwork and performance. In Johnson LC, Tepas DI, Colquhoun WP, Colligan MJ (eds): Biological Rhythms, Sleep and Shift Work. New York, Spectrum, 1981, pp 283–305.
26. Folkard S, Knauth P, Monk TH, Rutenfranz J: The effect of memory load on the circadian variation in performance efficiency under a rapidly rotating shift system. Ergonomics 19:479–488, 1976.
27. Folkard S, Monk TH: Shiftwork and performance. Hum Factors 21:483–492, 1979.
28. Folkard S, Monk TH: Individual differences in the circadian response to a weekly rotating shift system. In Reinberg A, Vieux N, Andlauer P (eds): Night and Shiftwork: Biological and Social Aspects. Oxford, Pergamon, 1981, pp 367–374.
29. Goetz F, Bishop J, Halberg F, et al: Timing of single daily meal influences relations among human circadian rhythms and urinary cyclic AMP and hemic glucagon, insulin and iron. Experentia 15:1081–1084, 1976.
30. Graeber RC: Alterations in performance following rapid transmeridian flight. In Brown FM, Graeber RC (eds): Rhythmic Aspects of Behavior. London, Lawrence Erlbaum, 1982, pp 173–212.
31. Graeber RC: Aircrew fatigue and circadian rhythmicity. In Weiner EL, Nagel DC (eds): Human Factors in Aviation. New York, Academic Press, 1988, pp 305–344.
32. Halberg F, Lubanovic WA, Brockway B, et al: Nomifensine chronopharmacology, schedule-shifts and circadian temperature rhythms in di-suprachiasmatically lesioned rats: Modeling emotional chronopathology and chronotherapy. Chronobiologia 6:405–424, 1979.
33. Hauty GT, Adams T: Phase shifts of the human circadian system and performance deficit during the periods of transition. III. North-South flight. Aerospace Med 73:1257–1262, 1966.
34. Hildebrandt G, Stratmann I: Circadian system response to night work in relation to the individual circadian phase position. Int Arch Occup Environ Health 43:73–83, 1979.
35. Horne JA, Ostberg O: Individual differences in human circadian rhythms. Biol Psychol 5:179–190, 1977.
36. Joy JE, Losee-Olson S, Turek FW: Single injections of triazolam, a short-acting benzodiazepine, lengthen the period of the circadian activity rhythm in golden hamsters. Experientia 45:152–154, 1989.
37. Klein KE, Bruner H, Holtmann H, et al: Circadian rhythm of pilots' efficiency and effects of multiple time zone travel. Aerospace Med 41:125–132, 1970.
38. Klein KE, Wegmann HM: The resynchronization of human circadian rhythms after transmeridian flights as a result of flight direction and mode of activity. In Scheving LE, Halberg F, Pauly JE (eds): Chronobiology. Toyko, Igaku, 1974, pp 564–570.
39. Klein KE, Wegmann HM: Circadian rhythms in air operations. In Nicholson AN (ed): Sleep, Wakefulness, and Circadian Rhythms. Neuilly sur Seine, France, NATO Advisory Group for Aerospace Research and Development 10.1–10.25, 1979.
40. Klein KE, Wegmann HM: Significance of circadian rhythms in aerospace operations. AGARD dograph no. 247, Advisory Group for Aerospace Research and Development, NATO. London, Technical Editing and Reproduction, 1980.
41. Klein KE, Wegmann HM, Athenassenas G, et al: Air operations and circadian performance rhythms. Aviat Space Environ Med 47:221–230, 1976.
42. Klein KE, Wegmann HM, Hunt BI: Desynchronization of body temperature and performance circadian rhythm as a result of outgoing and homecoming transmeridian flights. Aerospace Med 43:119–132, 1972.
43. Knauth P, Emde E, Rutenfranz J, et al: Reentrainment of body temperature in field studies of shift work. Int Arch Occup Environ Health 49:137–149, 1981.
44. Knauth P, Rutenfranz J: Duration of sleep related to the type of shift work. In Reinberg A, Vieux N, Andlauer P (eds): Night and Shift Work: Biological and Social Aspects. Oxford, Pergamon, 1981.

45. Kogi K: Social aspects of shift work in Japan. Int Labour Rev 104:415–433, 1971.
46. Kogi K: Research motives and methods in field approaches to shift work. In Johnson LC, Tepas DI, Colquhoun WP, Colligan MJ (eds): Biological Rhythms, Sleep and Shift Work. New York, Spectrum, 1981.
47. Kogi K: Introduction to the problems of shiftwork. In Folkard S, Monk TH (eds): Hours of Work. New York, John Wiley, 1985, pp 165–184.
48. Kogi K, Ohta T: Incidence of near accidental drowsing in locomotive driving during a period of rotation. J Hum Ergol (Tokyo) 4:65–76, 1975.
49. Lewy AJ, Wehr TA, Goodwin FK, et al: Light suppresses melatonin secretions in humans. Science 210:1267–1269, 1980.
50. Matejecek M, Neff G, Abt K, et al: Pharmaco-EEG and psychometric study of the effect of single doses of temazepam and nitrazepam. Neuropsychobiology 9:53–65, 1983.
51. McGhee JE: An experimental trial to test the efficacy for temazepam to induce sleep and improve subsequent performance during partial sleep deprivation and circadian rhythm desynchronosis. Defense Technical Information Center no. AD-A160795. Presented to the Faculty of The University of Texas Health Science Center at Houston, TX, 1985.
52. Menzel W: Zur Physiologie und Pathologie des Nacht und Schichtarbeiters. Arbeitsphysiologie 14:304, 1950.
53. Menzel W: Menschliche Tag-Nacht-Rhythmik und Schichtarbeit. Basle, Benno Schabe, 1962.
54. Monk TH: Coping with the stress of jet-lag. Work Stress 1:163–166, 1987.
55. Moore-Ede MC, Sulzman FM, Fuller CA: The Clocks that Time Us: Physiology of the Circadian Timing System. London, Harvard University Press, 1982.
56. Nakano Y, Miura T, Hara I, et al: The effect of shift work on cellular immune function. Proceedings of the 6th International Symposium on Night and Shift Work. J Hum Ergol (Tokyo) 11(suppl), 1982.
57. Nicholson AN: Performance studies with diazepam and its hydroxylated metabolites. Br J Clin Pharmacol 8:39–42, 1979.
58. Nicholson AN, Stone BM: Hypnotics and shift work. In Johnson LC, Tepas DI, Colquhoun WP, Colligan MJ (ed): Biological Rhythms, Sleep and Shift Work. New York, Spectrum, 1981.
59. O'Donnell VM, Balkin TJ, Andrade JR, et al: Effects of triazolam on performance and sleep in a model of transient insomnia. Hum Perform 1:145–160, 1988.
60. Penetar DM, Belenky G, Garrigan JJ, et al: Triazolam impairs learning and fails to improve sleep in a long-range aerial deployment. Aviat Space Environ Med 60:594–598, 1989.
61. Petrie K, Conaglen JV, Thompson L, Chamberlain K: Effects of melatonin on jet lag after long haul flights. Br Med J 298:705–707, 1989.
62. Redman J, Armstrong S, Ng KT: Free-running activity rhythms in the rat: Entrainment by melatonin. Science 219:1089–1091, 1983.
63. Reinberg A, Andlauer P, Guillet P, et al: Oral temperature, circadian rhythm amplitude, aging, and tolerance for shiftwork. Ergonomics 23:55–64, 1980.
64. Reinberg A, Smolensky M, Labrecque G: The hunting of a wonder pill for resetting all biological clocks. Ann Rev Chronopharmacol 4:171–208, 1988.
65. Reinberg A, Vieux N, Ghata J, et al: Amplitude of the oral temperature circadian rhythm in relation to the ability to phase shift circadian rhythms of shift workers. Chronobiology 6(suppl 1):57–63, 1979.
66. Rutenfranz J, Colquhoun WP, Knauth P, Ghata JN: Biomedical and psychological aspects of shift work. Scand J Work Environ Health 3:165–182, 1977.
67. Rutenfranz J, Knauth P, Colquhoun WP: Hours of work and shiftwork. Ergonomics 19:331–340, 1976.
68. Rutenfranz J, Knauth P, Kupper R, et al: Pilot project on the physiological and psychological consequences of shiftwork in some branches of the services sector. In The Effects of Shiftwork on Health, Social and Family Life. Dublin, European Foundation for the Improvement of Living and Working Conditions, 1981.
69. Saito H: Rodo jikan, kyukei, kotaisei. Tokyo, Institute for Science of Labour, 1954.
70. Scheving LE, Tsai TH, Scheving LA: Chronobiology of the intestinal tract of the mouse. Am J Anat 168:433–465, 1983.
71. Shift Work Committee, Japan Association of Industrial Health: Opinion on night work and shift work. J Sci Labour Part II:1–36, 1979.
72. Short RV: Method for minimizing disturbances in circadian rhythms of bodily performance and function. U.S. Patent No. 4,600,723 (Jul 15, 1986). Washington, DC, U.S. Patent Office.

73. Short RV, Armstrong S: Method for minimizing disturbances in circadian rhythms of bodily performance and function. U.S. Patient No. 4,665,086 (May 12, 1987). Washington, DC, U.S. Patent Office.
74. Simpson HW: Chronobiotics: Selected agents of potential value in jet lag and other dyschronisms. In Scheving LE, Halberg F: Chronobiology Principles and Applications to Shifts in Schedules. Rockville, MD, Sijthoff and Noordhoff, 1980.
75. Simpson HW, Bellamy N, Halberg F: Double blind trial of a possible chronobiotic (quiadon): Field studies in N.W. Greenland. Int J Chronobiol 1:287–311, 1973.
76. Stepanova SI: Effect of transmeridianal flight on the human body. Kosm Biol Aviakosm Med 8:3–12, 1974.
77. Stepanova SI: Biorhythmic selection of cosmonauts. Kosm Biol Aviakosm Med 9:40–46, 1975.
78. Stepanova SI: Problems of Space Biology: Current Problems in Space Biorhythmology. Moskow, Izdatel'stvo Nauka, 1977. (In Russian)
79. Taylor PJ, Pocock SJ: Mortality of shift and day workers 1956–1968. Br J Ind Med 29:201–207, 1972.
80. Taylor PJ, Pocock CJ, Sergean R: Absenteeism of shift and day workers. Br J Ind Med 29:208–213, 1972.
81. Teleky L: Problems of night work: Influences on health and efficiency. Ind Med Surg 12:758, 1943.
82. Tepas DI: Shiftwork sleep strategies. J Hum Ergol (Tokyo) 11(suppl):325–336, 1982.
83. Tepas DI, Monk TH: Work schedules. In Salvendy G (ed): Handbook of Human Factors. New York, John Wiley, 1987.
84. Van Loon JH: Diurnal body temperature curves in shift workers. Ergonomics 6:267–273, 1963.
85. Van Reeth O, Turek FW: Administering triazolam on a circadian basis entrains the activity rhythm of hamsters. Am J Physiol 25:256–263, 1989.
86. Wever RA: The Circadian System of Man. Results of Experiments under Temporal Isolation. New York, Springer Verlag, 1979.
87. Wever RA: Phase shifts of human circadian rhythms due to shifts of artificial zeitgebers. Chronobiology 7:303–327, 1980.
88. Winget CM, DeRoshia CW, Markley CL, Holley DC: A review of human physiological and performance changes associated with desynchronosis of biological rhythms. Aviat Space Environ Med 55(12):1085–1093, 1984.
89. Wojtczak-Jaroszowa J: Circadian rhythm of biological functions and night work. In Wojtczak-Jaroszowa J (ed): Physiological and Psychological Aspects of Night and Shift Work. Cincinnati, National Institute for Occupational Safety and Health, 1977, pp 3–12.

WILLIAM J. PRICE
DANIEL C. HOLLEY, PhD

SHIFTWORK AND SAFETY IN AVIATION

From the Department of Biological Sciences
San Jose State University
San Jose, California

William J. Price served in the U.S. Navy for 11 years flying long-range, multiengine patrol aircraft, and 9 years as a Navy Reserve Officer flying transport aircraft. He attained the rank of lieutenant commander. Currently he is a captain with a major U.S. airline, where he has 25 years of service, having flown the DC-6, DC-8, B-700, Caravelle, B-727, and B-767/757.

Reprint requests to:
Daniel C. Holley, PhD
Department of Biological Sciences
San Jose State University
One Washington Square
San Jose, CA 95192

Commercial aviation has grown rapidly over the past century. Accidents today, though uncommon, are generally catastrophic, commanding media attention that results in close scrutiny by the public, the government, and various interested components within the industry. Earlier in aviation history, hardware failure was the cause of most accidents. Today, hardware is much more reliable and less likely to be the cause of most accidents. Accidents still happen, however. Attention is now drawn to the role of the human operator in the man-machine system. Human "failure," thus, has become the magnified issue relative to safe aviation systems operations. The emphasis of this chapter is on operator performance as a dependent variable and ultimately on the effects of shiftwork in aviation on safety of operations. It is important to note that the symptom, pilot "fatigue," may be the earliest indicator of a problem that has its etiology in scheduling. Owing to the link between fatigue and resultant performance decrement, we have chosen to consider fatigue reports from a historical viewpoint. We also present an overview of the handling of these issues by various government regulatory agencies, unions, and professional industry associations.

The agencies most concerned with aviation safety are the Federal Aviation Administration (FAA), the National Transportation Safety Board (NTSB), the Air Line Pilots Association (ALPA), the Allied Pilots Association (APA), and the Air Transport Association (ATA). The FAA was mandated by Congress in 1958, succeeding the

Civil Aviation Administration (CAA).[105] It is administered under the Department of Transportation (DOT), and it has greater responsibility than its predecessor, the CAA, to regulate aviation safety. The NTSB is an independent government agency charged by Congress to investigate the probable cause of all transportation-related accidents, including pipeline accidents. The ALPA is the larger of two labor unions representing commercial airline pilots. Its role, however, is not only contract negotiation; it is also heavily involved in accident investigation. ALPA retains its own specially trained investigators and maintains its own specialized equipment, such as audiotape analysis systems. In most accident investigations the NTSB requests the participation of ALPA specialists as well as those from the FAA, the aircraft and engine manufacturers, and the airline involved, among others. The APA is a splinter union representing the pilots of American Airlines solely. The ATA is an organization of management representatives from the various airlines; it retains specialists in many fields of aviation, for example, a vice president for maintenance. Each group noted above has its own legal counsel. Additionally, ALPA, APA, and ATA maintain professional congressional lobbying groups.

The Congress of the United States has made clear who it regards as most responsible for aviation safety. Under the Federal Aviation Act of 1958, Paragraph 1421 (b), it has mandated: "The [Federal Aviation] administrator shall give full consideration to the duty resting upon air carriers to perform their services with the highest possible degree of safety in the public interest." The courts amplified this mandate in *Rauch v. United Instruments, Inc.*[88]: "Congress, through Federal Aviation Act of 1958, in particular para. 601 [49 USCS para. 1421] and other provisions of the Act which are dominated by safety objectives, was seeking to assure personal safety of all persons who are potential passengers or crew members of civil and military aircraft as well as those on the ground whose lives or property might be endangered by accidents resulting from unsafe aircraft or other unsafe flying conditions; no right of action is implied under 49 USCS para. 1421 for violation of safety regulations promulgated by Federal Aviation Administration."

FATIGUE IN AVIATION: HISTORICAL PERSPECTIVE

That flying airplanes is physiologically taxing and might involve "shiftwork" was recorded by Miller in 1936, when he made the following statement to the Eighth Annual Meeting of the Aero Medical Association:[64] "Military aviation does not present as great a field for this study [of fatigue] as commercial air transport operation, which provides: (1) flights of long duration, (2) flights in bad weather over dangerous terrain, (3) extensive night flying, (4) irregular schedules with broken rest periods, (5) prolonged instrument flying and intensive navigation, (6) high total of monthly and yearly hours flown, (7) the additional factor of passenger as well as personal safety, and (8) insecurity of employment and lack of age or disability retirement."

In 1966, S. R. Mohler, then chief of the Aeromedical Applications Division, Office of Aviation Medicine, Federal Aviation Agency, published a detailed review of fatigue in aviation activities.[68] Dr. Mohler cites 106 references in his inquiry. He notes that "serious performance decrement" is likely to result from mental fatigue symptoms, which include irritability, decreased attention span, increased susceptibility to err (therefore of vital consequence in aviation accident causation), decreased libido, increased anxiety, decreased recent memory, increased tendency toward insomnia, decreased cooperativeness, susceptibility to depressive states, decreased acceptance of constructive criticism, increased tendency to withdrawal from avocational social undertakings and hobbies, decreased (paradoxically, sometimes excessively increased) interest in personal care and hygiene, increased tendency to use pharmacological crutches (ethyl alcohol, tobacco, tranquilizers, barbiturates, bromides, nerve tonics), and decreased gastrointestinal efficiency, which may result in indigestion, constipation, or, in some cases, diarrhea (spastic intestinal states).

Beljan et al. in 1972[13] reviewed 3,362 research documents for a report to the National Aeronautics and Space Administration (NASA) to ascertain in part (a) the then current medical and scientific literature on desynchronosis resulting from various environmental changes and (b) to determine whether or not desynchronosis could influence performance and thus represent a medical or behavioral public health problem of significance in aviation. It is important to note that at that time attention was devoted to time zone crossing as a cause of fatigue (i.e., jet lag, desynchronosis). Shiftwork or rotational shiftwork was not considered as important an issue. It is now known that both jet lag and shiftwork can cause circadian system disturbances that may lead to bouts of unacceptable fatigue. The report concluded that (1) human performance efficiency exhibits a circadian periodicity in a normal nychthemeral environment; (2) medical practitioners were not aware of the importance of biological rhythms in considering diagnosis and therapy; (3) a fatigued state reduces the adequacy of human performance; (4) mental fatigue, of primary importance in civil aviation, is caused by stresses acting through psychic factors with possible physical components; (5) the causes of aviation fatigue are monotony and environmental factors such as anxiety, fear, and mental strain, the latter of which are a degree of loading rather than of kind; (6) types of tasks performed are very important when measuring fatigue because simple tasks can usually be performed at great efficiency regardless of fatigue and if fatiguing tasks could be eliminated, performance would become more efficient; and (7) desynchronization from phase shifting of oscillating time cues results in disharmony of human biological rhythms and often in a wide variety of physiological and psychological abnormalities that "can have debilitating effects" on performance efficiency.

On April 27, 1974, a decision was reached by the European Region of the FAA, with the concurrence of the FAA Flight Standards Division and the administrator of the FAA, that accidents and incidents involving Pan American Airways (PAA) justified a special FAA inspection.[50] This action was taken allegedly because of the safety record of the airline. From 1962 to 1974 PAA's fatal accident rate "was 44% higher than the average of the entire U.S. air carrier fleet."[102] Thus began an in-depth, fact-finding mission by seven highly qualified FAA principal operations inspectors and one FAA aviation medical examiner. Of the several deficiencies found, one of special significance regarded human performance. The following observation was reported under the title "Operational Fatigue (Crew Scheduling)": "There is a need for PAA to re-evaluate its flight scheduling patterns to assure that operational fatigue is given serious consideration and preclude this factor from introducing possible cockpit complacency which could ultimately result in an accident or incident. This recommendation also applies to cabin attendants." [A similar warning, in almost identical wording, was included in a letter about the various deficiencies at PAA resulting from the FAA investigations to the chairman of the board and chief executive officer, William T. Seawell, from Clyde W. Pace, Jr., FAA assistant administrator for Europe, Africa, and Middle East (no date)]. Of the eight recommendations made to PAA, the following are pertinent to this review: (a) Provide medical information to airmen including up-to-date information on nutrition, exercise, alcohol, drugs, tobacco, and so forth. (b) Provide medical information to airmen recommending various methods in the art of obtaining sleep and rest on long-range aircraft and at layover points. (c) Investigate the possibility of improving the cockpit humidity through some humidification system, and encourage flight crews to increase fluid consumption on long flights. (d) Investigate reducing B-747 cockpit noise by providing a better seal for the top hatch and other air lock areas. (e) Improve B-747 pilot seat comfort by providing a firmer cushion that does not take a "set" after use. Also, provide a better means of holding the slipcover on the seat than with Velcro. (f) Provide medical information on the best way for flight crewmembers on long-distance flights to be able to stretch their muscles through pull-ups, rubber squeeze balls, etc.

These recommendations would do much to alleviate fatigue on long-haul missions. However, to date, we are unaware that any of them has been adopted by a major U.S. air carrier. In 1975, all notes and written documentation of this FAA committee during its investigation were allegedly destroyed on orders from the FAA administrator (S.R. Mohler, Department of Community Medicine, Wright State University School of Medicine, personal communication, 1989). Two copies of the FAA final report[50] were made, one for PAA and the other for the FAA. The one referenced herein was obtained through the Freedom of Information Act in 1987.

On August 15, 1978, the ATA wrote a 78-page reply (C.F. von Kann, Senior Vice President, ATA, to Office of the Chief Counsel, Rules Docket Section, FAA, August 15, 1978) to an FAA Notice of Proposed Rule Making to modify the FAR section on flight time and duty time limitations and rest requirements for pilots.[30] In this letter the ATA notes that although tests during the circadian nadir in the early hours of the morning indicate human ineptness, the "basic issue under scrutiny when considering fatigue is not whether there are factors that can contribute to a less safe ability to perform, but whether they do in fact generate an unsafe condition—any evidence of which is lacking." It should be noted that the NTSB in its analysis of the 1967 accident in New Orleans cited fatigue as a debilitator in the performance of the captain and thus as the generator of an unsafe condition. The definition of fatigue used by the ATA is, "state of markedly reduced ability to carry out a task and a condition of reduced performance from which there is no certainty that a person can be aroused, even in an emergency, to a full state of operational efficiency."

The letter includes a citation from a review of the literature by Schreuder et al. in 1966[97]: "Finally, it is emphasized that pilot fatigue is a very complex problem; however, it can only be concluded from this study that the occurrence of pilot fatigue as defined is not a common occurrence in the airline pilot, that in the same age bracket, the airline pilot is healthier than the general male population, and that there is nothing to indicate that flying the turbojet is deleterious to health or is conducive to premature aging. It can also be stated that the circadian rhythm is a definite physiological phenomenon but it is believed that there is some adaptation and additionally, a major percentage of the pilot group experience very little difficulty in compensating to this phenomenon." The ATA then concluded, "Though it is recognized that this study covers only the period preceding April 1966, it is most doubtful that its findings and conclusions have changed in the last 12 years."

Although a brief summary of the 78-page letter is difficult, a quote from page 26 may provide an overview of the ATA position: "Extending the minimum rest period will impose a severe economic penalty on the industry which will not go away with rescheduling and redomiciling procedures. Airplanes are not scheduled around rest periods of pilots, they are scheduled to accommodate passengers and cargo." We believe that the Schreuder report of 1966 inaccurately portrayed the effects of circadian desynchrony and shift scheduling on pilot fatigue. In retrospect, a more erudite and accurate account of the data available in 1966 pertaining to this topic was provided in the review by Mohler mentioned above,[67] which was apparently ignored by the ATA.

In 1979 the Association of Sleep Disorders Centers and the Association for the Psychophysiological Study of Sleep published *The Diagnostic Classification of Sleep and Arousal Disorders.*[11] This document is of great relevance; in it a professional health care organization states for the first time that both shiftwork and time zone crossing can lead to clinically defined sleeping disorders. Listed are the following effects of rapid work/sleep shifts: insomnia during the sleep period, gastrointestinal disturbances, chills, lassitude, irritability, desire to nap and difficulties with mental faculties during work hours, severe mood changes and unremitting—or waxing and waning—cognitive difficulties, increased use of hypnotic, analeptic, and tranquilizing drugs as well as alcohol.

During the week of September 19, 1979, the National Institute for Occupational Safety and Health (NIOSH) and the Office of Naval Research (ONR) hosted a symposium, Variations in Work-Shift Schedules: Effects on Health and Performance. Dr. R. L. Masters, medical advisor to ALPA, presented a paper in which he noted that some management, government, and aircrew unions ignore much of the physiological data that are enabling factors for pilots in an aircraft crash. Among these "enabling factors" are fatigue, poor nutrition in the immediate pre-accident time period, and disruption of biological rhythms. He observed that although air carriers cannot begin and end flights at convenient times, it is necessary for safe operations to pay special attention to hours on duty, flight time, rest period, time zone, and diurnal variations. Present rules and regulations, he observed, are arrived at through negotiation and legislation rather than through scientific measurement and fact. Long-haul operations lead to disruption of biological rhythms; short haul constitutes long duty days, with multiple short segments, many takeoffs and landings, high work load in crowded air space, congested airfields and delays. Pilots in both groups work approximately 18 days a month and are away from home for approximately 240 hours a month. Food service and lodging is generally inadequate. Demands of the job are highly tiring because of the attention required and periods of high mental workload. Among the many debilitating factors are diurnal shifts, crossing of five to eight time zones, flights during night and early morning, and being on "reserve" or "on call" all day only to be called at 2100 to fly after midnight to 0800 the following morning. All play a role in a pilot's failure to operate at maximal efficiency when required to perform the most critical functions.[59]

Under direction from Congress in August 1980, NASA conducted a workshop on pilot fatigue and circadian desynchronosis. The goals were to help ascertain whether "the circadian rhythm phenomenon is of concern and to decide whether there is a valid reason to look at it, and what agency should be doing it."[72] Two documents were prepared for the participants of this meeting: (1) a review and an annotated bibliography on this topic,[49] and (2) a special study[58] of safety reports submitted to the NASA Aviation Safety Reporting System (see below). The annotated bibliography began where the Beljan study[13] ended, citing 2,084 research papers that had been published between the end of 1972 and June 1980. Reiterated are the manifestations of fatigue: performance decrements, irritability, restlessness, inability to sleep, decreased attention, slowed or impaired perception, impairment of thinking, and decreased motivation and physical performance. The report suggests that aircrews return to premission, sleep-stabilized sleep/wake patterns to avoid performance decrements resulting from cumulative buildup of sleep loss and disruption. Noted is the possibility that a natural depression of arousal at certain times of day may combine with other causes of performance decrement to form a crucial factor in commercial aviation accidents. It is asserted that transmeridian flights are a source of common sleep disturbances caused by changes in the temporal order of physiological circadian rhythm. The whole of these changes, internal circadian desynchronosis, is characterized by a number of physiological and performance decrements. The report recommends an education program to alert pilots to the importance of maintaining regular habits of sleep and nutrition.

From the study of the NASA Aviation Safety Reporting System (ASRS) data base, Lyman and Orlady[58] derived novel conclusions relative to fatigue in aviation. The ASRS was established in 1975 under a memorandum of agreement between the FAA and NASA. The ASRS collects, analyzes, and responds to aviation safety "incident reports" in order to lessen the likelihood of aviation accidents. ASRS data are intended to be used to identify deficiencies in the National Aviation System (NAS),[26] to support planning and improvements to the NAS, and to strengthen the foundation of aviation human factors safety research. Pilots, controllers, cabin attendants, ground personnel, and others involved in aviation operations can submit anonymous reports to the ASRS when they are involved in, or observe, an incident or situation in which aviation safety was compromised. The system is designed so that they are able to report errors, goofs, and snafus that may have affected safety to a responsible government agency without fear of punishment or retribution. Reports are "sanitized" as to sender and are retained in a computer data base for reference and research. NASA is charged to contact the FAA or other government agencies concerning correction of the reported problems. It should be noted that Lyman and Orlady reviewed 426 ASRS reports describing flight crew performance decrements possibly related to fatigue and analyzed in depth a subset of 77 in which the reporter either explicitly or implicitly associated fatigue with the occurrence. Among their conclusions were the following: (1) fatigue-associated performance decrements do occur; (2) fatigue-associated performance decrements can produce potentially hazardous conditions; (3) failure in monitoring tasks is described frequently in fatigue-associated performance decrement reports; and (4) long duty periods, large numbers of flight segments, and disturbed sleep are frequently reported as the reasons for performance decrements. This report is significant in that it shows specifically that pilot fatigue occurs in relation to the shiftwork environment of commercial aviation.

The final report of the 1980 NASA workshop recognized that air safety could be compromised by pilot fatigue and circadian desynchronosis, among other factors.[72] Fatigue can be exacerbated by sleep loss or alterations and by long duty of 16–18 hours' duration. Desynchronosis is associated with rapid time-zone changes and irregularity of work/rest and sleep/wake cycles. Among the recommendations was acknowledgment that sleep loss plays a role in performance reduction. Thus, scheduling should take into account sleep time relative to the biological clock and should minimize partial sleep loss. Recovery time should take into account the amount of sleep lost. The report recommended advising pilots of cumulative effects of sleep loss on performance—on visual motor skills, ability to receive information, attention span, short-term memory, vigilance, and so forth. It admitted lack of knowledge of performance decrement due to amounts of and periods of sleep or the best strategies for scheduling sleep outside of normal sleep time. The final report to Congress (see above) led to the funding of a research study of commercial airline pilots that is ongoing at the NASA-Ames Research Center, Moffett Field, California, under the stewardship of Dr. R. C. Graeber.

Graeber et al. have presented their findings in a number of reports.[39,40,43–46] Among them are: (1) Long-haul flight crews operate with substantial sleep loss due to (a) circadian disruption of layover sleep, (b) night flying conflicting with sleep, (c) large individual differences in adaptability; (2) difficulties increase with age; (3) the "circadian nadir" reduces alertness substantially despite adequate prior sleep; (4) sleep loss and circadian desynchronization have contributed to serious errors in long-haul flying; (5) safety risks are highest during descent and landing; (6) obtaining less than 4 hours of "anchor sleep" (defined below) produces a greater performance deficit than being "legally drunk"; (7) combining sleep deficit with circadian performance nadir is extremely hazardous; (8) pilots cannot assess accurately their own sleepiness.

At the conclusion of the 1986 annual meeting of the Association of Professional Sleep Societies an ad hoc committee of scientists was formed. Their task was to review recent reports and related information on the role of human sleep and brain clocks in the occurrence of medical and human error catastrophes (e.g., Three Mile Island, Chernobyl, Challenger). Though they do not deal specifically with any given air-related disaster, their findings have significance to the around-the-clock airline industry.[66] The report notes that while the debates of these incidents consistently focus on the extent to which technological failures and high-level policy decisions contributed to the catastrophes, they do not abrogate the responsibility attached to the less obvious factors affecting "individual participants," who are judged afterwards to have contributed significantly to the accident through "human error." The committee suggests that some critical "human errors" have a basis in the brain mechanisms that control sleep and many other oscillatory processes underlying human physiology, behavior, and judgment. It states that "sleep and sleep-related factors appear to be involved in widely disparate types of disaster."

In 1987 ALPA requested that an ad hoc committee investigate current practices involving scheduling of United Airlines crews operating in the Pacific basin. On September 28, 1988, Drs. Graeber (NASA), Kohn (United Airlines, UAL), and Hudson (ALPA) reported on their recommendations for scheduling Pacific flight crews (Captain Richard Brooks, ALPA, UAL Master Executive Council, International (Flights) Chairman Report, on October 2, 1988). The initial recommendations of the ALPA committee were: (1) crews should try to remain on home time; (2) crews should lay over less than 48 hours outside of their home time zone in order to maintain synchronization; (3) crews should be scheduled so that they can obtain a minimum of 4 hours of "anchor sleep" (see below) in the 26 hours before flight; (4) takeoffs and landings should not be scheduled during the period 1 hour before until 1 hour after the circadian nadir, the physiological low point occurring at about 0400 home time in a synchronized person; (5) multisegment duty periods should not be scheduled through the SOT (sleep opportunity time—the 2300–0700 period, based on home time, during which a person who has not experienced desynchronization of his circadian clock can expect the highest probability for "normal" deep sleep with meaningful rejuvenation). It should be noted that some of these recommendations are equally applicable to domestic schedules. "Anchor sleep" is a concept originally proposed by Minors and Waterhouse.[65] Most people obtain their required sleep between 2300 and 0700 in their home time zone. If at least 4 hours of the required approximately 8 hours of sleep is obtained regularly within the "window" of normal sleep time for the person, then serious sleep deficit or degradation of performance is lessened. This 4-hour minimum is referred to as "anchor sleep." It cannot be achieved outside of the normal 2300-0700 window.

In addition, the concept of napping was given special consideration. Naps are short sleep episodes outside of the SOT. Dr. Graeber reported to ALPA that he had obtained FAA approval and the cooperation of UAL and Northwest Airlines (NWA) to do a study of "in the seat napping" as a method for three-pilot 747 crews to improve their performance. As background information he offered: (1) crewmembers do nap in the cockpit during long-haul flights; their napping is often unplanned and uncontrolled; (2) other countries allow limited napping in the cockpit during overwater cruise; (3) the U.S. Air Force Military Air Command allows nonaugmented crews to nap during cruise; (4) high-risk industries are now considering 30-minute naps for control room workers during the nightshift; (5) cruising flight is an opportunity for limited recovery; and (6) current regulations permit the possibility of in-flight structured rest.

It should be noted that Captain Brooks is a former Pan American B-747 pilot with many hours of long-range flying in the Pacific basin. A summary of his observations relating to the clinical analyses of Graeber et al. and the "real world" was included in his report (cited above) and may provide pertinent insight, since operational relevance and theoretical recommendations for improvements often conflict. He noted that attempting to remain on home time in Tokyo for a pilot domiciled in California would have the pilot awake in the early hours of morning in a community that is almost entirely closed down. Entertainment such as television is extremely limited, and restaurants and exercise facilities are closed. In the Pacific, even hotels with such facilities are closed at night. Because of the 8-hour-plus time zone difference and the fact that crews remain in Asia for several days, they are unable to remain on home or domicile time. Further, although napping in flight would be amenable to the three-pilot 747 crews, it is not applicable to the new Boeing 747-400, two-piloted aircraft.

MEDICINE, THE LAW, AND THE PILOT

Commercial pilots are required by law to maintain themselves within stringent physical limits. The FAA requires captains to take a physical examination every 6 months; co-pilots and flight engineers take one annually. Federal law also requires nonpilot, flight-deck personnel,[17] such as navigators and radio operators, and air traffic controllers[18] to take an annual physical examination. To date, no law prevents flight attendants from flying when they are ill or requires them to have periodic physical checkups. Food and Drug Administration (FDA) regulations, however, restrict their preparing, handling, or serving food and beverages aboard an aircraft if they are suspected or known to be in a communicable period of disease, or if they have an open lesion or infected wound on an exposed portion of the body.[19] The pertinent federal aviation regulation (FAR) for pilots, FAR 61.53,[16] states: "No person may act as pilot in command, or in any other capacity as a required flight crewmember while he has a known medical deficiency, or increase of a known medical deficiency, that would make him unable to meet the requirements of his current medical certificate." The regulation receives its power from paragraph 1422 (b) of the Federal Aviation Act of 1958.[105] Under this act Congress directed the secretary of transportation to ensure that all applicants for an airman's certificate should be "physically able to perform" their duties. The courts held that the phrase, "is physically able," as stated in the public law, "must read to mean: is free from significant physical risks."[24]

Unlike military pilots, commercial pilots are not monitored by attending flight surgeons. The FAA authorizes certain physicians, known as aviation medical examiners (AMEs), to perform the required physical examinations. FAR part 67 governs the medical decision of the AME to issue the pilot a medical certificate.[27] This section deals with requirements relative to eye, ear, nose, throat, and equilibrium and to mental, neurological, and cardiovascular status. Part 67.13 (f), general medical condition, provides an overall picture of how the FAA officially views pilot health. Section (2) requires that "No other organic, functional, or structural disease, defect, or limitation that the Federal Air Surgeon finds . . . makes the applicant unable to safely perform the duties or exercise the privileges of the airman certificate that he holds or for which he is applying." These regulations are further defined by the FAA in a document titled *Guide for Aviation Medical Examiners* (cited in Reinhart[89]).

Pilots are not required to consult or see an AME when they are stricken with a "grounding" malady. The only requirement is that the pilot not operate an aircraft. Should he fly when so afflicted, and should the FAA learn of his flying, the pilot's flying license is supposed to be suspended. A few airlines maintain medical departments staffed with FAA-certified AMEs. Several require annual company physical examinations. Generally, the examinations are more thorough than those of the FAA. They usually include chest x-ray, basic blood workup, complete external body examination, electrocardiograms, and a more thorough hearing test and vision test. A pilot who is ill for more than 7 days is required to see a company physician before being released to fly.

Unlike pilots in military aviation, those under instruction in civilian facilities receive very little if any formal instruction in aviation medicine or high-altitude physiology. The FAA provides high-altitude experience and a "ride" in a decompression chamber to 24,000 feet through local air force and naval air station facilities.[34] However, no federal regulations require such training.

The FAA provides some basic medical information in a quarterly document titled *The Airman's Information Manual* (AIM). The stated policy of this document is to provide information only for "a unique situation." The document contains extremely valuable technical information and carries on its cover the label, "Critical to Flying Safety," to ensure prompt perusal. It might be assumed to be an official interpretation of FAA policy and regulations. In Chapter 8, Medical Facts for Pilots, Section 1, Fitness for Flight, the AIM[33] states, under "Medical Certification": "Caution: The FARs prohibit a pilot who possesses a current medical certificate from performing crewmember duties while the pilot has a known medical condition or an increase of a known medical condition that would make the pilot unable to meet the standards for the medical certificate."

Pilots are cautioned that even minor illnesses can degrade performance. "The safest rule is not to fly while suffering from any illness." In regard to fatigue, the AIM admonishes, "Fatigue continues to be one of the most treacherous hazards to flight safety, as it may not be apparent to a pilot until serious errors are made." Fatigue is described as either acute or chronic. Acute is defined as tiredness felt in "normal occurrence in everyday living" resulting from physical and mental strain, strong emotional pressure, and lack of sleep, among other factors. It reduces coordination and alertness "so vital to safe pilot performance" and "is prevented by adequate rest and sleep, as well as regular exercise and proper nutrition." "Chronic fatigue occurs when there is not enough time for full recovery between episodes of acute fatigue. Performance continues to fall off, and judgment becomes impaired so that unwarranted risks may be taken. Recovery from chronic fatigue requires a prolonged period of rest." Both stress and emotion are addressed, and it is noted that "stress and fatigue can be an extremely hazardous combination." Pilots are instructed not to fly until events causing the problems are resolved.

The FAA sells a small text entitled *Medical Handbook for Pilots*, dated May 1974.[28] It includes discussions of alcohol, carbon monoxide, cockpit lighting, and age. "Medical Facts for Pilots"[31] is an 8-page circular distributed free by the FAA that discusses, briefly, general health, hypoxia, hyperventilation, carbon monoxide, drugs, alcohol, fatigue, panic, and scuba diving. Comparing copies distributed in January 1964 and June 1971, we find minor amplifications and additions, but the texts have remained strikingly similar. "Rx: A Few Medical Facts for Pilots"[29] is a free 1-page summary of "Medical Facts for Pilots." A 2-page pamphlet, "Daily Body Rhythms and Flight Safety,"[32] addresses problems of fatigue and alertness affected by circadian rhythms.

The FAA makes clear in both the *Medical Handbook* and "Medical Facts" that the pilot is responsible for not flying when ill or incapacitated. A note in the *Medical Handbook for Pilots*, page 3, states: "The AME can find major problems only when your [medical] certificate comes up for renewal, or when consulted. The rest of the time, you alone must evaluate your flying capabilities. These regulations place the responsibility for determining physical fitness upon the pilot. It is up to you [the pilot] to *know* when a physical deficiency or temporary illness may interfere with aircraft operation." "Medical Facts for Pilots," page 1, paragraph 4: "The pilot himself has the sole responsibility for determining his reliability prior to entering the cockpit for flight." "A Few Medical Facts": "FACT: Your medical certificate is legally invalid during any period of illness that prevents you from performing your flying duties properly."

SHIFTWORK VERSUS JET LAG

Circadian desynchrony (jet lag) induced by transmeridian travel across time zones is reviewed elsewhere in this issue (Chapter 11), and other chapters review the general concepts of shiftwork. However, we believe that a distinction should be made between jet lag and shiftwork as they apply to commercial aviation. Though it is generally accepted that jet lag can be a serious consequence of aviation operations, little attention is devoted to the potentially equally serious issues that may arise from shiftwork scheduling of pilots, for example, sleep disturbances.[25,39,40,81,82,95,96,107] Tables 1 and 2 show representative schedules of relatively senior commercial airline pilots working for major U.S. air carriers in 1990. Table 3 shows a commuter airline schedule flown by a relatively junior

TABLE 1. Representative Long-Range Pacific Three-Pilot* B-747 Crew Schedule Typically Flown 2–3 Times Per Month

Departure	Arrival	F/T	L/O	Notes
LAX 1200	SEL 1720 (0120)	13:20	25:05	Relief pilot aboard
SEL 1825 (0225)	MNL 2105 (0605)	3:40	12:05	Field layover
MNL 0910 (1810)	SEL 1350 (2150)	3:40	5:05	No lounge or rest facilities
SEL 1855 (0255)	TTE 2020 (0520)	2:25	37:30	Hours on duty, 12:40
TTE 0950 (1850)	SEL 1310 (2110)	2:20	5:15	Hotel provided, about 1:30 rest
SEL 1825 (0225)	MNL 2105 (0605)	3:40	12:00	Field layover; on duty, 12:45
MNL 0905 (1805)	SEL 1345 (2145)	3:40	24:55	
SEL 1440 (2240)	LAX 0945	11:05		Relief pilot aboard

F/T—Flight time; L/O—layover time; LAX—Los Angeles; SEL—Seoul, Korea; MNL—Manila, Philippines; TTE—Taipei, Taiwan. The time after the city code is local time; domicile or home time is in parentheses.

* The three pilots are the captain, the first officer or co-pilot, and the second officer or flight engineer.

TABLE 2. Flight Sequence of a Two-Pilot, Large Computer-run Aircraft (e.g., Boeing 767/757 or Airbus 320) Typically Flown Every Fourth Day, Approximately 4–5 Times per Month

Departure	Arrival	F/T	D/T	L/O	Wake-up Time
SFO 0805	JFK 1705 (1405)	5:41	13:11	13:11	0545
EWR 0611 (0311)	ORD 0710 (0510)	1:59		2:50	0100
ORD 1000 (0800)	LGA 1310 (1010)	2:11	8:13	21:17	
JFK 1030 (0730)	SFO 1340	6:13	7:24		0430 (NYC)

FT—Flight time; D/T—duty time; L/O—layover time; SFO—San Francisco; JFK—Kennedy Airport, New York; EWR—Newark, New Jersey; ORD—Chicago; LGA—La Guardia Airport, New York. The time after the city code is local time; domicile or home time is in parentheses. Note: On arrival at JFK on the first day the crew is driven to EWR. Because of heavy traffic, the trip takes about 2 hours.

TABLE 3. Flight Sequence of a Commuter Aircraft (e.g., a Two-Pilot BAC 146), Typically Flown Back-to-Back in a Weekly 4-Day Pattern

Departure	Arrival	F/T	L/O
SFO 1600	SCK 1635	:35	:30
SCK 1705	SNA 1830	1:25	:25
SNA 1855	SCK 2020	1:25	9:00
Report 0545			
SCK 0630	SNA 0755	1:25	:35
SNA 0830	SCK 0955	1:25	:35
SNA 1030	SCK 1155	1:25	:35
SCK 1230	SNA 1355	1:25	1:20 (meal break)
SNA 1515	SCK 1550	:35	

F/T—Flight time; L/O—layover time; SFO—San Francisco; SCK—Stockton, CA; SNA—Santa Barbara, CA.

TABLE 4. Model of a 2:2:1 Air Traffic Control Shiftwork Schedule[63]

Day	Arrive	Depart
Monday	1500	2300
Tuesday	1500	2300
Wednesday	0700	1500
Thursday	0700	1500
Friday	2300	0700

The arrival and departure times may be 1 hour earlier than shown.

pilot. The shifting nature of the work or duty periods is obvious. Others have also published schedules of pilots emphasizing this same concept.[70,84,95]

Studies of the rotating shiftworker are of particular interest to the aviation industry because many of the air traffic control centers,[61–64] airports, and flight crews work rotating shifts or have duty rosters that are shifting in nature (see Table 4 for a schedule currently being used by some air traffic controllers). A continual problem for investigators evaluating data from rotating shiftworkers, however, is the question of "self-selection," that is, those on rotating shift schedules are "survivors" who can take the physiological and social disturbances that may result. According to Rutenfranz et al.,[93] 20% of shiftworkers are unable to continue working shifts and thus drop out (change to dayshifts) or change jobs.

It is not the purpose of this report to either list or discuss all the rhythms in human physiology and psychology. Suffice it to say that it is the exception to find a physiological or psychological parameter that, when sampled with adequate frequency, does not show periodicity. This is the basis for understanding the physiological effects of shiftwork. Under normal day/night and social conditions, a person sleeps during the dark phase of the cycle and is awake during the light phase. His bodily rhythms (both physiological and psychological) are stable and in phase (entrained) with the external environmental time setters (zeitgebers). They are also entrained and in phase with one another (internally synchronized). Under these conditions the human body/mind system functions optimally. Physiological decrements result when deviations from normal rhythmicity are induced.[49] In shiftworkers, especially those on rotating shifts, the sleep/work cycle is often desynchronized from the external day/night cycle and from the prevailing social interaction cycle. When the body rhythms begin to rephase to the new zeitgebers, they do so at different rates.[108] The result is that many rhythms lose their phase relationship with one another, causing internal rhythmic discord or internal desynchrony.[95]

The aviation crews of most major airlines appear to be much like shiftworkers in terms of their chronic exposure to phase alterations. The trip-schedule-bid system based on seniority assures that many of the younger crew members fly less desirable schedules (i.e., night trips). Two schools of thought have polarized, however. One contends that rhythmic inertia makes it desirable to work rapidly rotating shift schedules.[93] The other holds that longer periods (more than 7 days) on a fixed shift are desirable to allow re-entrainment or adaptation to the new sleep/wake schedule.[110] Workers often prefer relatively rapid shift systems.[54] Czeisler et al.,[23] however, have been instrumental in improving worker satisfaction by applying circadian principles to shift schedules. Their initial research indicates that work schedules that rotate by phase delay and include an extended interval between rotations are most compatible with the properties of the human circadian system.

A major difference between the transmeridian traveler and the rotating shiftworker is that the traveler experiences acute phase alteration, whereas the worker experiences repeated, chronic phase alterations. Symptoms reported after transmeridian travel, however, are similar to those reported by shiftworkers.[133,49,109] These include fatigue, insomnia, anxiety, and other sleep/wake disturbances: gastrointestinal dysfunction; and psychosomatic manifestations. Tasto et al.,[99] in a study of approximately 2,000 rotating shift nurses and food processors, found increased incidences of fatigue, digestive troubles, colds, chest pains, menstrual problems, nervousness, use of stimulants, wheezing, alcohol consumption, and leg and foot cramps. They also found that these workers had comparatively less satisfactory psychological health, work performance, and domestic and social life. They concluded that the number of days taken for sickness is not a reliable indicator of health problems. When they looked at the reasons nurses gave for taking sick leave, they found that those on rotating shifts tended to cite more serious medical reasons than did those on fixed shifts.[20]

As noted above, the Association of Sleep Disorders Centers and the Association for the Psychophysiological Study of Sleep published a "Diagnostic Classification of Sleep and Arousal Disorders."[11] This important standardized classification lists disorders of the sleep/wake schedule of both exogenous and endogenous etiology. The report classifies disorders of the sleep/wake schedule as transient (rapid time zone change or jet lag syndrome and simple workshift change in conventional sleep/wake schedule) and persistent (frequently changing sleep/wake schedule). Symptoms of the time zone crossing disorder are sleepiness and fatigue and their mental consequences during the wake period, and insomnia during the sleep period. Symptoms of the shiftwork disorder are similar and include sleepiness and performance decrements during the new work/wake period and disrupted and shortened sleep (which is now scheduled during the former work-wake period, generally in the daytime). The frequently changing sleep/wake schedule is experienced by rotating shiftworkers, flight crews, and regular air travelers, i.e., peripatetic businessmen and international negotiators. The classification states that frequently changing sleep/wake cycles cause a mixed picture of chronic DIMS (disorders of initiating and maintaining sleep) and DOES (disorders of excessive somnolence) distinguished by disrupted and unusually shortened periods of sleep (sometimes occurring several times per day), sleepiness and performance decrements during any scheduled wake period, and difficulty in reestablishing a consolidated sleep period even when circumstances temporarily permit sleep schedule regularity. It is also stated that "among the somatic complications of this syndrome, a tendency for peptic ulcer disease to begin within a few years of starting [rotating] shiftwork is fairly well established."

A major unanswered question in relation to shiftwork, particularly rotating shiftwork, is whether continuous shiftwork affects longevity or general health—for example, psychological stability or resistance to disease or other pathological states. Rutenfranz indicates that some 10–20% of shiftworkers suffer illness, mainly of the gastrointestinal tract, and a large number experience feelings of ill health, principally sleep disorders and food intake disorders.[91] Gordon et al.[42] found that, as compared to men working nonvariable work schedules, those working variable shifts exhibited higher rates of heavy drinking, job stress, and emotional problems. They note that female variable shiftworkers reported higher rates of sleeping pill, tranquilizer, and alcohol use, as well as lower social network scores, more job stress, and more emotional problems. Hyndman,[51] on theoretical grounds, concludes that the role of biological rhythms is maintenance of precise homeostasis. It may be inferred from this that should rhythmic stability be altered on a chronic basis, then *optimal* functioning of a biological system may not be possible. Aschoff[10] has reviewed the properties of circadian rhythms and their relevance for the design of shiftwork scheduling. He states: "The circadian system represents a temporal order that is mediated by the mutual coupling of a variety of oscillators and by the synchronizing effects of zeitgebers." It is likely that the well-being of man depends partly on the maintenance of this order, and that repeated or long-lasting disturbances to it will have harmful effects. Stenova (cited in Doskin and Larrent'yeva[36]) holds that internal synchronization of daily (circadian) rhythms of different physiological functions and biochemical parameters constitutes an *optimal* state of the body and that many disturbances of the body leading to disease start because of disruption of timing of different functions, so-called internal desynchronosis.

Cobb and Rose[15] reported a fivefold increase in risk of blood pressure elevation in air traffic controllers (representing a shiftworker population) as compared to second-class airmen (representing workers on a "regular" schedule). This interpretation may be biased by differences in work loads and responsibilities, however. Taylor and Pocock,[100] using data between 1958 and 1968, investigated 8,603 manual workers from 10 factories in Great Britain. Their objective was to assess the influence, if any, of 10 years or more of shiftwork upon the expectation of life and cause of death. Their conclusion was that shiftwork had no adverse effect upon mortality. Taylor et al.[101] also could not find evidence that any of the shift systems studied adversely affected health. Akerstedt and Torsvall,[4] however, using a questionnaire to sample worker attitude, found a substantial improvement in mental, physical, and social well-being when nightwork was eliminated from a worker's routine.

The circadian rhythmicity of task performance has been well documented.[13,21,49,106] Rutenfranz and Colquhoun[92] found that the performance rhythm is significantly influenced by such factors as fatigue and meal timing and that the preponderance of evidence suggests that the observed fluctuations reflect an underlying 24-hour rhythm analogous to that shown by certain physiological processes that may be closely connected with the cycle of "sleep need." They also state that measures of performance taken during "night" hours are confounded by sleep deprivation or sleep interruption. Nevertheless, their results are of considerable practical interest and clearly have direct application to the problem of the nightshift, on which efficiency is affected not only by daytime sleep duration and quality but also by the phase shifting of the rhythms that occurs during the period of adjustment to the altered rest/activity cycle. Rutenfranz and Colquhoun also noted that changes in performance rhythms in industrial situations are often masked because of motivational and situational factors. For example, workers may mask productivity variations out of fear of changes in piecework wages.

Klein and Wegmann[53] also point out the problems associated with field studies such as work output, frequency of failures, and number of errors. These parameters, in principle, follow the circadian characteristics observed in laboratory research on human performance efficiency. The best performances occur at about 1600–2200, and the poorest performances from 0000 to 0700, as shown in the five examples cited (see also Winget et al.[110]). Folkard and Monk[38] cite six published studies that report relatively continuous, 24-hour "real-life" performance measures. They indicate that the paucity of data on this subject may be due to union or management opposition and to problems in finding appropriate performance measures. In the studies cited, the major impairment of performance occurs during the nightshift. They proposed a description model in which on-shift performance is dependent on the type of task, type of shift system, and type of person and the three factors interact via the worker's various circadian rhythms.

It should be noted that a major factor affecting the shiftworker or the pilot working a nonstable schedule is the resultant sleep disturbance, which may or may not include cumulative sleep loss.[1] This disturbance subsequently predisposes the person to less than optimal performance. Akerstedt et al. investigated more than 2,000 steelworkers, policemen, train drivers, and meteorologists.[2,3,5] They found consistently that nightshifts caused relatively more sleep disturbances than dayshifts. Nightshift workers had difficulties maintaining sleep and feelings of not having been sufficiently "restored." A major correlate is that working during a subjective "sleep time" might result in difficulties maintaining normal wakefulness though the person is supposed to be vigilant and working.[103]

Relatively little recent research has been done on the relationship of shiftwork to accident rates. Rutenfranz et al.,[93] in a review, state that knowledge in this field is conspicuously absent. Some studies on safety records of shiftworkers have correlated time of day with performance decrements. Industrial accidents seem to occur with the greatest frequency between 2200 and 0200 hours.[110] Harris[47] found that most truck accidents occur because of driver error, and many likely were the result of failures in vigilance. Fatigue factors interacting with the circadian variation of arousal reportedly were responsible for the greater number of accidents occurring between 0000 and 0800 hours.

Rutenfranz et al.[94] point out that for the shiftworkers themselves the most important problems are psychosocial ones—for example, the extent to which shiftwork interferes with family and social life. Even if a shift system is planned from a purely physiological point of view it might not be acceptable to the workers. Social interaction (i.e., the social zeitgeber) has been shown to be one of the strongest rhythm entrainers in humans.[10,108,111] Thus, the shiftworker (especially the night and rotating shiftworker) may be faced with conflicting zeitgebers, namely the work/rest cycle that is dictated by his job schedule and the social cycle dictated by activities of friends or family members.

A major difference between the air traveler across time zones and the shiftworker is that the shiftworker is faced with conflicting zeitgebers as outlined above. The air traveler, on the other hand, arrives at a destination where the prevailing social and day/night cycles are not conflicting but are probably relatively similar to the phase relationships at home. Aschoff[10] discussed some quantitative differences in the rates of rephasal of certain physiological and psychological variables after phase shift. He noted that opposite results are observed in terms of rates of rephasal of circadian rhythms after a phase advance of the zeitgeber, as opposed to phase delay of the zeitgeber in isolation studies when compared to actual flight studies. He indicated that these opposite, asymmetrical effects found after zeitgeber shifts in the isolation unit by comparison with those in actual flights across time zones have to be taken into consideration in the analysis of results from shiftwork studies as well as in the design of shift schedules.

Drenth et al.[37] have reviewed some of the psychosocial aspects of shiftwork. They emphasize the unpopularity of shiftwork and also warn of the natural selection process that complicates studies on this subject. They identify five major areas of concern to the shiftworker: (1) social factors—for the most part social life is restricted; (2) home-life factors—sleeping and eating at "abnormal" hours present a range of problems for the spouse and family; (3) health factors—health is an overall reaction to the total situation, and studies showing both impairment and lack of impairment are cited; (4) financial factors—these may be the most important reason for participating in shiftwork; and (5) organizational factors—shiftwork affects work performance, absenteeism, accidents, labor turnover, and other factors. These authors state that the evidence is not good enough to establish differences between shift- and nonshiftworkers in terms of qualitative and quantitative aspects of production. They conclude that one important feature of shiftwork is the influence, predominantly experienced as negative, of the shift rhythm; the interrupted sequence of the evening and night, and the frequent shift change. They go on to say that policy concerning shiftwork has been based on a balanced model. On one side are thought to lie the conveniences and disadvantages, and on the other side so much compensation (and it occurs to few to think of compensation other than in money terms). These factors are adjusted so that the "scale" becomes approximately balanced. From a psychological point of view, it is doubtful whether this approach is correct. In the first place, money has a camouflaging function. The actual objections are not considered, and the sources of inconvenience are left undisturbed. Moreover, the bonus can become a wrong motive for choosing shiftwork. The bonus also has a habituating effect and can result in an unrealistic evaluation of the work situation. We believe that relatively few commercial pilots leave their jobs owing to the rigors of shift scheduling and time zone changes inherent in their work.

Various methods have been suggested to ameliorate the symptoms of jet lag and to facilitate rephasal after arrival in a new time zone. These include the use of diet, drugs, and more recently, phototherapy.[22,109] For various reasons diet and drug intervention may not be practical for the shiftworker or the pilot working a rapidly changing schedule. Recently, interest has focused on the ramifications of bright light as a circadian phase setter in humans.[22] If the human circadian system responds to bright light as does the circadian system of other mammals, then properly timed phototherapy might be a relatively safe and effective method of manipulating the biological clock of the shiftworker or the desynchronized airline pilot. Several laboratories are currently investigating this very exciting area (see p. 261).

CASE HISTORIES IN WHICH PILOT SCHEDULING MAY HAVE CONTRIBUTED TO AIRLINE ACCIDENTS

Delta Airlines DC-8, Flight 9877, Kenner, Louisiana, March 30, 1967[35]

At approximately 0048, Delta Flight 9877, operating as a training flight practicing engine-out approaches, crashed during a landing approach to runway 1, New Orleans International Airport. The fatalities included 5 crewmembers, an FAA observer, and 13 people on the ground. The aircraft, several homes, and part of a motel complex were destroyed. The aircraft had just departed the airport and was in the process of executing a two-engine-out landing. Skies were clear, winds were light, and the visibility was excellent at 5 miles. The NTSB determined that the probable cause was improper supervision by the flight instructor and improper use of the flight and power controls by both the instructor and the captain-trainee during the engines-out simulation.

The board noted the following rigorous schedule of the captain-trainee:

March 28	0800–1700	instruction period
	1800–1900	oral examination
	1900–2300	rest
March 29	(2300)–0150	flight training
	0200–0800	rest
	0800–1700	ground school
	1700–2200	rest
	2300–	flight training
	0048	accident

In its analysis of this schedule, the NTSB noted: "Another factor which probably affected the performance of the captain-trainee is fatigue. In the two days preceding the accident flight he was engaged in intensive ground school and flight training. Presumably because of this workload, part of which was voluntary, and the small rest periods available, he stayed at the motel across the street from the airport during this time. The captain-trainee had a 4-hour rest period from 1900 to 2300 on March 28, a 6-hour rest period from 0200 to 0800 and a 5-hour rest period from 1700 to 2200 on March 29. Considering that these rest periods incorporated travel, bathing, dressing, and other personal activities in addition to study for the training flights, it is obvious that his actual rest was minimal. Although fatigue and its effects are subjective in nature and difficult to assess, the disturbed work/rest cycle superimposed on the natural stresses of the training environment was undoubtedly reflected in the performance of the captain-trainee."[35] Among the signatories of the report was NTSB member Francis H. McAdams, who in 1978 in an NTSB internal memorandum noted that fatigue was due to a number of factors; conspicuously missing from his list were factors associated with work scheduling (see 1978 Pacific Southwest Airlines accident below).

United Air Lines Flight 266, Boeing 727, Los Angeles, January 18, 1969[73]

On the evening of January 18, 1969, Flight 266, a B-727, departed Los Angeles International Airport. The weather was light rain and fog with low cloud cover and 3 miles visibility; the pilot, therefore, was flying almost from the beginning on instruments. The aircraft was dispatched with one generator, in engine number 3, inoperative. (The aircraft has three generators, one in each engine.) Two minutes after takeoff, the crew reported to air traffic control a fire warning in number 1 engine. The engine was shut down, and a request was made to Los Angeles departure control to return to the airport. The voice recorder in the cockpit reveals that the first officer warned the captain that they were now on one generator. Both were aware of the critical electrical overloading of the remaining generator. Although the aircraft has an emergency electrical system, it was not used, perhaps because the flight engineer was relatively inexperienced. He had a total of 40 hours in the B-727, 18 of which were in planes of the same model as Flight 266. The co-pilot or first officer was highly experienced. The aircraft crashed into the water, killing all aboard.[73]

The day before, the captain had returned to Los Angeles from Denver, the location of the company's training center, where he had finished instruction in the operation of a four-engine Douglas DC-8. He had last flown the B-727 on December 2, 1968. The morning of the fatal flight he had observed a DC-8 flight that departed at 0700 from Los Angeles to New York and returned. He lived in

Orange County, approximately 2 hours from Los Angeles Airport. To arrive at the airport 1 hour before departure time would require arising at approximately 0400. The round trip to New York and return would consume about 10 or 11 hours including his 1-hour layover in New York. On arrival in Los Angeles he was informed that he was to fly a B-727 to Denver (Flight 266). He had trained and flew the observation flight with another captain, J. C. Nichols, who confirmed in a November 26, 1981, letter to one of the authors that the early departure of the DC-8 to New York would require an early wake-up, at approximately 0400 or 0500. A letter to one of the authors from the co-pilot of the DC-8 flight crew, now Captain A. L. Pregler, of June 24, 1980, reconfirmed the early departure and the presence of two observing pilots.

Fatigue and the effects of sleep deprivation were not included in the NTSB investigation. It can be ascertained, however, that they may have played a debilitating role. At the time of Flight 266, the co-pilot may have been the only flight member at maximal capability in the aircraft. On lift off, the captain commented that the controls felt "light." The NTSB report commented on the difference between the B-727 and DC-8 control pressures, stating that the DC-8 requires greater pressure. Another observation of the NTSB was that the cockpit could have been in a state of confusion. Mohler in 1966 stated that fatigue can cause a pilot to "fail to respond rapidly and properly in an emergency situation." It is probable that a captain who spent the previous 47 days learning a new aircraft might be confused in attempting to rapidly recall emergency procedures in the old aircraft during a critical flight condition. It should be noted that these procedures were practiced at 6-month intervals and reviewed occasionally in the interim but not practiced. The added debilitation of circadian desynchrony from crossing six time zones in the previous 12 or more hours, the effects of an early arising, and the general effects of a long day would add to a lowered state of mental capacity for the captain. The different "feel" of the aircraft and attempting to rapidly sort out recently learned DC-8 procedures from those for the old B-727 would require a great deal of mental agility. The combined factors noted above, exacerbated by the debilitating effects of sleep loss and fatigue, probably put this captain in a much more dangerous position to handle an emergency than one who was well rested and on regular B-727 duty.

Pan American Airways, Europe, the Pacific, 1969–1975[50,102]

See above, "Historical Perspectives of Fatigue," for an account of the FAA investigation of the PAA long-haul operations scheduling practices.

Eastern Airlines DC-9, September 11, 1974, Charlotte, North Carolina[74]

On the morning of September 11, 1974, an Eastern Airlines DC-9 crashed at Charlotte during a nonprecision-instrument approach, killing 83 people; 10 survived including the co-pilot. The NTSB concluded that the probable cause was the "flight crew's lack of altitude awareness at critical points during the approach due to poor cockpit discipline in that the crew did not follow prescribed procedures." The NTSB reported that the captain "had a rest period of 13½ hours before he reported for the trip. At the time of the accident, he had been on duty about 3 hours."

Using sophisticated tape analysis equipment ALPA investigators found information that revealed serious deficiencies in the NTSB transcription of this accident.[41] They found on the cockpit voice recorder that the captain had complained about being fatigued. He commented, "That's what I need—rest. I don't need all this damn flying. If you fly real hard for about 25 hours, you can see why they have the 30 in 7 rule." [An FAA regulation limits airline pilots to 30 hours of flying in 7 days followed by a required day (24-hour period) off.] After landing at Charlotte he was to fly to Chicago, then Orlando, before being able to rest. He had risen at 0330 the day of the accident for the 0530 takeoff. This was a schedule he had flown 2 days earlier.

Application of the Mohler Physiological Index,[68] a formula to determine degrees of fatigue, shows that the captain's index was 3.27 on the day of the accident and 2.43 during his previous 2 days of flight. Mohler considered 1.75 as acceptable, 1.75–2.30 a high physiological workload, and above 2.30 dangerous.

Other discrepancies were found regarding the crew. They had in fact completed checklists, made required call-outs, had not missed radio transmissions, acknowledged and complied with all instructions, and made aural identification of radio facilities. Although the ALPA petitioned to reopen the investigation (letter and petition from J. J. O'Donnell, President, ALPA, to W. B. Todd, Chairman, NTSB, May 21, 1976), the NTSB refused (H. F. Marthinsen, Manager, Accident Investigators, ALPA, personal communication, 1990).

KLM KL 4805/4806 and PAA 1736, 2 B-747's, March 27, 1977, Tenerife, Canary Islands, Spain[52]

After a bomb explosion on March 27, 1977, at Las Palmas de Gran Canaria Airport (Canary Islands, Spain), inbound aircraft were diverted to Los Rodeos Airport, Tenerife (another Canary Island). Among the many aircraft arriving at the alternate site was KLM 4805 at 1338 zulu (z). It had departed Schipol Airport, Amsterdam, at 0900 z. Local time at Tenerife and Amsterdam is also zulu time.

PAA 1736 departed JFK Airport, New York, at 0742 z [0242 Eastern Standard Time (EST)] and arrived at Tenerife at 1415 z (0915 EST). The crew was based in New York and normally reported to operations 1 hour before departure. No other information is available as to when each member had slept last.

Las Palmas Airport finally reopened to receive traffic. KLM (now flight 4806) was the first aircraft to depart for Las Palmas at 1656 z. PAA 1736 followed at 1702 z (1202 EST), 3 hours after landing. KLM had taxied straight down the runway to the end in fog and light rain. PAA 1736 followed, receiving instructions to turn off the runway at the third exit taxiway. Confusion arose in the PAA cockpit as to whether the controller had said "first" or "third." The co-pilot reconfirmed the third exit taxiway from the tower. Aircraft that had landed at Tenerife filled the taxiway parallel to the runway between exit taxiways 1 and 2, precluding use of the taxiway parallel to the runway. Exit taxiway C-3 required a 135-degree turn because it was designed as a "quick turnoff" for aircraft landing in the opposite direction. Exit taxiway C-4, further down, required only a 45-degree turn. The 747 is a huge aircraft for which large turns are difficult. While taxiing down the runway the crew completed various pretakeoff checklists. For reasons unknown, perhaps poor visibility in some measure, PAA missed exit taxiway number C-3. The tower operator had instructed them to report to the tower upon leaving the runway.[52]

Hartman et al.[48] provide a construct that may provide insight to what followed. They suggest that under adverse conditions people mobilize their resources; they bring all their capacities to bear on the completion of a task. Decrements and impairments in performance may be masked by such mobilization.

Impairments may be unmasked by observing aspects of performance considered unimportant by the individual: (1) loss of flexibility of set—one of the commonly reported characteristics of performance is a loss in the ability to perceive and adjust to new aspects of a task, to shift quickly and effectively from one subpart to another; (2) change in controlling set—performance decrements may be due to reduced levels of aspiration; the individual is satisfied with less adequate performance, and small errors go uncorrected, even though perceived; and (3) increase in conflict—decrements of performance closely correspond to the degree of subjective frustration associated with a task.

The PAA crew may have felt that because they were protected by the controller, it would be easier to turn off at C-4. At this time, they were also concentrating on completing several checklists and taxiing down an unfamiliar runway obscured by fog and rain. They could easily claim that they "missed" seeing the previous taxiway due to the rain and fog. It is suggested that owing to fatigue resulting from a shifted sleep/wake cycle, circadian desynchrony, and sleep deprivation the crew were mobilizing their resources. Not turning off at taxiway C-3 may indicate loss of flexibility of set and change in controlling set, concentrating on checklists and, perhaps, thinking that the tower controller really meant the less difficult exit taxiway, C-4.

KLM, meanwhile, was preparing for takeoff. If the captain exceeded strict Dutch pilot-duty time rules, he could be prosecuted under Dutch law. Interestingly, the time remaining before he was in violation was very short, perhaps a matter of minutes. He had spoken to KLM via shortwave radio about the time limit and was told that if there was a problem, KLM would send a telex to Las Palmas. If the time was exceeded, he would be required to stay at Tenerife, most likely upsetting the company and inconveniencing his passengers. The co-pilot informed the tower that, "We are now at takeoff." The tower returned at time 1706:18.19, "O.K. . . . [1.89-second pause], standby for takeoff. I will call you." After the tower's "O.K.," PAA transmitted that it was still on the runway. The simultaneous transmissions from the tower and PAA apparently caused a loud shrill in KLM's radio receiver (a typical radio interference phenomenon when two units are transmitting on the same frequency). The only recognizable sound on the PAA cockpit voice recorder was, "—k."

As the KLM co-pilot was finishing receiving his clearance from the tower, time 1706:09.61–1706:17.79 z, the captain released the brakes, 1706:11.08, and began adding power to the engines, 1706:13.99, and aligning the aircraft on the runway, 1706:17.17. The final power setting was reached at 1706:19.35. It should be noted that the power can be removed quickly, the engines put into reverse, and maximum braking applied in a few seconds.

The KLM captain, it appears, was under great urgency to depart Tenerife. He had initiated the takeoff roll on hearing his clearance. He completed adding power 1.16 seconds after hearing what he believed was final clearance from the tower, "O.K." The remainder of the message was garbled, perhaps substantiating his belief that he was cleared to take off. The fog and rain prevented his seeing the PAA aircraft in time.

Given the weather conditions, the short amount of time from the garbled transmission, and the rapid takeoff response of the KLM crew, the tower operator was unable to reissue another transmission. In our opinion, it is likely that PAA crew fatigue and stress to facilitate an immediate departure by the KLM crew were exacerbators of this accident.

UAL 2860, DC-8 Freighter, December 18, 1977, near Kaysville, Utah[75]

At approximately 0138 mst on December 18, 1977, near Kaysville, Utah, a UAL DC-8 freighter flew into a 7,665-foot mountain at the 7,200-foot level. The NTSB held that the probable cause was the issuance by the flight controller of imprecise and incomplete holding procedures that the flight crew accepted without question, and imprecise radio communications procedures due to years of bad habits.[75] In 1980, we presented a detailed retrospective analysis of this accident to the 5th International Symposium on Night and Shift Work.[86] We concluded, on the basis of a carefully reconstructed crew work/rest schedule before the accident, that the disaster was in part the result of desynchronosis from work shift and time zone changes and sleep loss due to sleep reversal.

At some time in the flight between San Francisco and Salt Lake, the aircraft sustained an electrical failure, which, unknown to the crew, affected the communications radio and the landing-gear-down light indicators. On arrival into the Salt Lake area the crew lowered the landing gear and found no "down" indication. To diagnose the problem the captain decided not to follow the FAA-approved missed-approach procedure—to climb to 9,000 feet and hold over the Salt Lake. He decided instead to remain at 6,000 feet and hold in a nonstandard holding pattern between Ogden to the northwest and Salt Lake City. He had descended through icing conditions and commented to the controller that he'd "just as soon not get up into it." The controller gave imprecise holding instructions, omitting a critical radial number. The crew acknowledged with a general compass heading, "north" and "northwest." The captain was handling the radios, the co-pilot the flying, and the second officer (flight engineer) was apparently busy checking systems. Although flying the aircraft, the co-pilot may have been mentally absorbed in analysis of the electrical and landing gear problems. This was the procedure taught by UAL at the time. No emphasis was placed in simulator training on flying the aircraft. Emphasis was directed to problem solving. The aircraft was flying 40 knots faster than prescribed and had deviated from the requested holding pattern. This may have been because the co-pilot heard "north" and dialed in 000 degrees in his navigation instrument. The captain had put in the proper 153 degrees but apparently had not cross-checked the co-pilot's instrument. On entering the holding pattern the captain had requested to call company maintenance on their only remaining radio, losing contact with the controller. When the aircraft began to deviate from the prescribed flight path toward the mountains the controller attempted to warn the pilots. The aircraft returned to the controller's frequency, and he issued an emergency climb. The pilots reacted but not with sufficient urgency, and the plane hit the mountain.

In addition to the flight crew, the air traffic controller handling this flight had been working a rotating pattern, the last day of which required arriving at work at 0700, working to 1500, an 8-hour rest period, then returning to work at 2300 (see Table 4). According to the NTSB report, the controller had 2–2½ hours' sleep in a 19-hour period. In our report,[86] we suggested that the physiological stressors of sleep loss and circadian desynchrony, as well as vibration, hypoxia, and short-term nutritional inadequacy for the flight crew, may have played contributing roles in the accident.

The NTSB accident report concerning the air traffic controller noted: "However, fatigue is a subjective physiological reaction since it affects each individual differently. Since the controller denied feeling fatigue, generalizations to the contrary would be speculative at best." Regarding the flight crew, the

NTSB stated: "Possibly fatigue affected the flight crew when the clearance was issued and throughout the remainder of the flight; but there was no evidence that they did not make full use of the 13-hour rest period in San Francisco or of the rest periods afforded them before they reported for duty in Chicago on December 16. If the flight crew made appropriate use of these rest periods, as the evidence indicates they did, fatigue should not have been a factor."

As early as January 1978, a few weeks after the accident, ALPA called for inquiry into the effects on the crew of circadian desynchrony and sleep disruption.[12] The NTSB investigation did not commence until nearly 4 months later because a question arose about a botched toxicological report by the FAA.[55] An interview with the co-pilot's wife, however, indicated that when her husband flew two trips (as noted above) he was tired.

ALPA requested one of us (WJP) to provide a model to demonstrate the possible effects of circadian desynchrony and sleep disruption. The model was developed[85] and later reviewed by M.C. Moore-Ede and C.A. Fuller of the Harvard Medical School.[69] The reviewers confirmed that the data on schedule timing were reasonable and that the review of performance decrement associated with circadian phase shifts in work and sleep schedules was compatible with experimental evidence. They deplored the lack of evidence, easily obtained, from previous work schedules, noting that the lack precluded determination that circadian factors played a role in the accident. They asserted, however, that there was sufficient experimental evidence to indicate that circadian factors could have played a role and that their role must be fully evaluated for the future of aviation safety. They observed that the NTSB statement about the use of rest periods did not take into account the fact that sleep loss occurs when assigned sleep periods are during the subjective day.

Both the model and our accident review[86] were submitted to the NTSB. The board stated in a letter that it had reviewed the work/rest schedules of the crew and considered the evidence insufficient to support fatigue as a causal factor. Subsequent evidence was submitted regarding the tardiness of the NTSB investigation, new evidence on the eating schedule, the air traffic controller's wake/sleep schedule, and the Moore-Ede/Fuller critique. The NTSB acknowledged the letter and provided thanks for "interest in aviation safety." To our knowledge, no subsequent action has been taken.

Anch et al.[7] noted in reference to our analysis "that the lesson to be learned from this and similar tragedies is that there is a greater propensity for an accident to occur during times of diminished physiological and psychological deterioration, resulting from circadian alterations." "This propensity," they added, "can interact with demands of job performance in a synergistic way to compromise the optimum level of performance required for effective management of sophisticated systems."

Pacific Southwest Airlines Flight 182, B-727, and a Cessna 172, N7711G, San Diego, September 25, 1978[76]

At 0901:47 PDT, September 25, 1978, Pacific Southwest Airlines (PSA) Flight 182 collided with a Cessna 172, N7711G, over suburban San Diego. The NTSB determined that the probable cause was failure of the flight crew of Flight 182 to comply with provisions of the maintain-visual-separation clearance rule, including the requirement of informing the air traffic controller when the other aircraft is not in sight.[76] Our analysis of the accident[87] suggests that sleep loss due to the previous night's severely shortened sleep period, possible chronic fatigue due to shortened sleep periods in previous days, and short-term nutritional inadequacy may have hampered alertness and reaction time.

The work/rest schedule of the flight crew was as follows (all cities are in California; the crew was based in San Diego):

Day	Place	Check-in Time	Check-out Time	Place	Off Time
22	San Diego	1530	0015	Oakland	6:30
23	Oakland	0640	0940	San Diego	30:30
24	San Diego	1610	2253	Sacramento	7:07
25	Sacramento	0600	0902		

The rest schedules on 22–23 and 24–25 were extremely short. The NTSB maintains that the 7 hours and 7 minutes on the night preceding the crash, 24–25, was sufficient for adequate sleep. Closer analysis, however, proves differently. The aircrew left the aircraft at 2253 and returned to PSA operations at 0600. Walking to and from the motel, which was located at the airport, undressing and dressing, and attending to personal hygiene could easily consume 2 hours, leaving some 5 hours for sleep. Flight crews universally complain of "spin down," the inability to go to sleep immediately after going to bed soon after flying. They claim they are awake for up to an additional 2 hours. No research data are available on this phenomenon. If the crew of 182 experienced it, sleep time may have been reduced further to approximately 3 hours.

PSA served no food aboard its aircraft and did not provide coffee or sweet rolls before the flight. The only available restaurant at Sacramento Airport had been closed for renovation for several weeks. On the previous night, the crew had flown three legs of approximately 1 hour each with half-hour stops between. There would have been little chance of obtaining food.

The morning of the crash the crew departed Sacramento at 0700 and arrived at Los Angeles at 0805 with a short layover of 25 minutes. During the ground time at Los Angeles a flight attendant came to the cockpit. The following conversation was recorded on the cockpit voice recorder (as confirmed by Dr. Malcom Brenner, Audiology Laboratory, VA Hospital, San Francisco): Attendant: ". . . tired, are you?" Captain: "I'm draggin'!" Co-pilot: "It was a short night."

On departure from Los Angeles PSA 182 followed another PSA flight, 776, a B-727. Nearing San Diego's Lindbergh Field, 2 minutes and 17 seconds before the collision, the air traffic approach controller informed the crew of two Cessnas, one within a mile, another at 3 miles (ALPA research showed this aircraft most likely at 5.7 miles). The crew reported seeing only the nearer Cessna. As they descended and turned to parallel the runway, the controller again reported traffic, but in a very ambiguous manner. He reported an unspecified aircraft straight ahead at 3 miles and "out of one thousand seven hundred." The co-pilot answered, "Got 'em!" The captain reported, "Traffic in sight." At this point they were headed east looking into the bright morning sun. The ambiguous language may have lead the co-pilot to report seeing Flight 776, which was in its final landing approach. It was also in the same general direction as the unseen Cessna. The B-727 is much larger than a Cessna. It was brightly colored with orange stripes. The Cessna was white with a thin mustard stripe, flying much closer to the ground, which is heavily dotted with light-colored buildings. The approach controller turned the flight over to the tower. The tower operator gave them a report, ". . . traffic, 1 mile, a Cessna." Within the cockpit a discussion ensued about what Cessna the tower was referring to. The captain assumed it was the one they had seen and reported earlier, stating that he had seen it "a minute ago," then stating to the tower that it had "passed off to our right." The Cessna they eventually collided with was never on the right of PSA 182. The co-pilot was unsure. He asked, "Are we cleared of that Cessna?" The captain seemed certain; he stated, "Oh, yeah, before we turned downwind, I saw him about one o'clock, probably behind us now!" Twenty-five seconds later, the co-pilot declared, "There's one underneath! I was looking at that inbound there." He had somehow ascertained that the aircraft ambiguously reported by the approach controller was not the other B-727, Flight 776, but a Cessna the crew had not previously seen. They collided 8 seconds later.

Our careful analysis of the flight crew's activities during the previous 57 hours and the transmissions between the aircraft and the controllers before the accident suggests a performance decrement manifest by decreased vigilance and alertness and slowed reaction time during a critical flight phase. These decrements may have precluded the crew from concentrating, remembering, and separating the various subtle but important details of the radio reports. An additional decrement may have been the extended time for the crew to analyze and react to the reports so that by the time they understood that an aircraft was underneath, they had no time to react to the now impending emergency.

The NTSB has to date refused to look for or cite the effects of fatigue in the crash of PSA 182. One month after the accident the board's most senior member, Francis McAdams, stated in a memorandum that the board had "self-imposed restraints in its accident investigation procedures of hidden human factors which cause accidents." He noted: "There is a large body of literature which supports the theory that fatigue, used in the broad sense, is one of the primary causes of human error. Fatigue is generally accepted to result from insufficient rest due to personal or business reasons, personal problems including, among others, marital, alcohol and drug abuse, physical and mental disability that has been hidden or disguised, financial worries, and several others."[60] Sleep deprivation due to scheduling is not mentioned.

The NTSB's Human Factors Group Chairman's Report stated, "The crew checked into the hotel about 2230 and departed at 0700 the next morning. Interviews with hotel and PSA employees who were in contact with the crew indicated nothing irregular or suggestive other than a normal restful night."[83] No mention is made of lack of food or the actual sleep period. An Associated Press news report, September 29, 1978, of interviews with NTSB investigators 4 days after the accident notes that the NTSB was aware of the short layover time and that they had not yet determined how much sleep the crew had. A spokesman for PSA asserted, however, that Federal Aviation Regulations had not been violated because the crew had not flown more than the limit of 8 hours with a 24-hour period. He stated that the crew had less than 5½ hours of flight time in the past 24 hours and "more than enough rest time" under federal regulations.

In January 1981, James B. King, then chairman of the NTSB, wrote a letter to Senator John Heinz of Pennsylvania, who had inquired about crew fatigue. Mr. King stated: "However, up to the present time, there has not been sufficient scientific data developed to properly equate crew fatigue with accident causative or contributory factors. In the instance of the PSA midair collision, the board's investigation examined the issue of fatigue in depth; however, no evidence was developed that would support a finding of crew fatigue."

A former PSA captain, R.P. Chapman, wrote a book about the San Diego accident in 1982.[14] He described fully the working conditions at PSA, stating in essence that the flight sequence of the crew of PSA 182 was the norm rather than the exception. He revealed that PSA had a policy of no food service for flight crews. Citing newspaper articles and internal union and company papers, he showed that the flight crews struck PSA on September 25, 1980, over the working environment, inadequate rest, poor nutrition, and stress.

Using our analysis of the accident and the cockpit voice recorder comments of the crew regarding its loss of sleep, Price wrote to the NTSB and to congressman Thomas Lantos of California. In response, the chairman of the board, James Burnett, wrote that the board routinely inquires into the duty times and activities of operators for the 48–72 hours before an accident to determine adequacy of rest and possible fatigue-related causation. He wrote: "To our knowledge, however, there is no generally accepted means in the scientific community for measuring fatigue or for establishing its effects on crew performance in a particular accident scenario. The Safety Board considers *all* available investigative evidence in determining the probable cause of an accident and, in cases where the evidence has been compelling, has cited fatigue as causal or contributory."

In 1984 Chapman also wrote both the NTSB and the FAA regarding the fatigue issue on PSA 182. Chairman Burnett answered that the NTSB had omitted the comments of the crew concerning its fatigued state. He stated that the Cockpit Voice Recorder Group (an investigative group made up of a safety board investigator and members of PSA management, the air traffic controllers' union, the flight attendants' association, and the pilots' union) had heard the comments, but did not consider them "to have any bearing on the accident." He again reiterated the board's 48–72 hour investigative procedure. He made the following observation about human sleep requirements: "The diversity of sleep requirements among individuals has reduced every attempt to quantify the effects of sleep loss on performance to generalities, i.e., some individuals require 8 hours of sleep or more to function while other individuals function adequately with less. There is no generally accepted means in the scientific community for measuring fatigue or for establishing its effects on crew performance in a particular accident scenario. In the PSA scenario, had the crew been involved in a long-duty day before they became involved in a collision, or had the weather conditions been such as to increase the crew's workload, the safety board could have given some credence to the theory that debilitating fatigue had developed. However, no long-duty period was involved: the crew had been on duty for 3 hours and had flown only a total of 1 hour 36 minutes. The weather was clear with 10 miles visibility. After considering all the factors related to the flight crew performance, the board could not conclude that debilitating fatigue was the cause."

Mr. Burnett stated further that the NTSB would not change its analysis of the fatigue issue unless it had proof that the rest time of one or more flight crewmembers was not spent resting. Interviews with PSA pilots, he wrote, indicated that flight crews normally brought their own food on trips where meals were not available. He mentioned no NTSB interviews with the families of the crew.

Captain Chapman's letter to the FAA observed that most accidents occur within airport control zones and that they can be connected with pilot or controller fatigue. The FAA denied this, stating that after a review of causal factors for Part 121 (scheduled carriers) accidents, the FAA found no connection between accidents within the vicinity of airports and pilot or controller fatigue.

In 1981 the NTSB made an urgent recommendation to the FAA to implement a program to detect the onset of and to alleviate fatigue of air traffic controllers.[8]

The investigation into the causes of the collision of PSA 182 with Cessna N7711G remains closed.

Downeast Airlines, Inc., DHC-6-200, Rockland, Maine, May 30, 1979[77]

At about 2055 EDT, while flying a nonprecision night approach in low clouds and fog, Downeast Airlines Flight 46 crashed into a heavily wooded area 1.2 miles from Knox County Airport, Rockland, Maine. The 2 pilots and 15 passengers were killed; 1 passenger survived. The NTSB determined that the crew descended below legal altitude limits prescribed for the approach. The board believed that the reasons for the illegal descent were inordinate management pressures, the first officer's marginal instrument proficiency, the captain's inadequate supervision of the flight, inadequate crew training, and the captain's chronic fatigue.[77]

The first officer had 2,500 total hours of flight time with approximately 23 hours of actual flying in this aircraft. According to fellow pilots, he was not up to the rigors of a night instrument approach. The NTSB report noted that the decision to fly by both captain and first officer was due to the vile temper of the owner. Written testimony indicated that the owner had coerced pilots to fly illegally lower than FAA minimums, had fired a pilot who judged a flight unsafe because of less than minimal weather, and had intimidated weather observers to report the weather better than it really was.

The captain was also the chief pilot. Weeks before the accident he complained of loss of appetite, exhaustion, preoccupation, chest pain, and difficulty breathing. Witnesses stated he felt he had no real authority and was continually being chastised and criticized by the owner. He feared for his job.

According to the NTSB the captain reportedly had 8 hours of sleep the night before the accident. He arrived at work at 1200 and was on duty to 2055, the time of the crash. The NTSB surmised that although his flight time had been less than 3 hours, the day's work and his distress may have increased his fatigue.

The original studies from Great Britain of Bartlett et al. (cited in the NTSB accident report[77]) show that as fatigue increases, people become increasingly willing to accept lower standards of accuracy and performance. According to these studies, fatigued pilots neglect to integrate data from the flight instruments and respond only to the instruments that have their attention at the time. Fatigued pilots also overlook activating important controls. In these experimental studies, evidence also indicates that errors increase at the end of a flight. Performance deteriorates and pilots relax because the flight is about to end. These studies are dated 1947, 1943, 1947, 1940, and 1948.

Using these data, the NTSB speculated that owing to his fatigued state, the captain may have concerned himself more with looking outside for the runway than with his second responsibility of monitoring and cross-checking the co-pilot's progress on the flight instruments.

Relative to this accident and the issue of fatigue, the latest studies referenced by the NTSB are dated 1948. The Beljan literature search of 1972 found 3,362 citations relating to human performance in aviation; many of these sources deal with fatigue, and some date to 1972. The work of Hartman et al.[48] was completed in 1974 and has 238 references. It seems that much work on fatigue and sleep disturbance was available yet was not considered by the NTSB to provide further insight into how fatigue due to shiftwork might have affected the captain's capacity.

Air New England, Inc., DeHavilland, DHC-6-300, Hyannis, Massachusetts, June 17, 1979[78]

The NTSB abstract states: "About 2248 EDT, on June 17, 1979, Air New England, Inc., Flight 248 crashed into a heavily wooded area about 1.5 nautical miles northeast of Barnstable Municipal Airport, Hyannis, Massachusetts. The crash occurred during an instrument-landing-system approach to runway 24 in instrument meteorological conditions. Of the eight passengers and a crew of two aboard, the captain was killed, the first officer and six passengers were injured seriously, and two passengers received minor injuries. The aircraft was destroyed.

"The NTSB determines that the probable cause of the accident was the failure of the flight crew to recognize and react in a timely manner to the gross deviation from acceptable approach parameters, resulting in a continuation of the descent well below decision height during a precision approach without visual contact with the runway environment.

"Although the board was unable to determine conclusively the reason for the failure to recognize and react to the gross deviation, it is believed that the degraded physiological condition of the captain seriously impaired his performance. Also, the lack of adequate crew coordination practices and procedures contributed to the first officer's failure to detect and react to the situation in a timely manner."[78]

The original schedule called for the flight crew to report at 0845 and to finish at 1831 and included 12 legs to various New England cities. Weather, equipment, and company personnel problems caused changes in the schedule. On arrival that evening at the end of the scheduled sequence, the crew was told to fly two more flights of two legs each, which annoyed the captain. During one of the ensuing legs, the captain misconfigured his instruments for an instrument approach. The first officer saw this and alerted the captain. The accident occurred about 2248, after 9 hours and 16 minutes of actual flight time, during the 15th approach for landing, at the end of a 12-hour day, in an aircraft known for its dark, noisy cockpit. The weather was a 200-foot ceiling and ¾-mile visibility in fog and drizzle. The captain's only known food intake during the 14-hour workday was a Danish pastry and a cup of coffee taken during the late afternoon while on the ground between flights.[78]

Mitsubishi MU-2 N873Q, Nashville Airport, November 1, 1979[56,57]

At 2141 local time on November 1, 1979, a Mitsubishi MU-2 crashed into a lake adjacent to Nashville Airport. The reported weather was "clear sky, 3 miles visibility in ground fog."[56,57] The NTSB report indicated that both engines, all electronics, and all instruments were working. The only information available concerning the crew's duty schedule was provided by the chief pilot:

Time	Depart	Arrive
0520	Fayetteville, TN	Houston, TX
1030	Houston	Bay City, TX
1630	Bay City	Baton Rouge, LA
?	Baton Rouge	Chattanooga, TN
?	Chattanooga	Nashville
2141	Crash at Nashville	

The aircraft was originally scheduled to return to Fayetteville, approximately 70 miles from Nashville, after dropping a passenger at Nashville.

According to the NTSB investigation report,[57] "The schedule being flown on the day of the accident was not unusual and was generally flown with one pilot. The aircraft was scheduled to depart from Fayetteville, Tennessee, early the next morning with the same pilot." There is no mention of investigation as to whether the pilot had flown this schedule the day before as well. By our estimations, using the crash time as an approximate landing time, then calculating time for taxi in, passenger drop, clearance receipt, taxi out, flight to Fayetteville, taxi in, parking procedures, travel to a near hotel, and bed preparation time, the pilot would not have been in bed until nearly midnight. A departure time of 0520 requires being at the airport at about 0420. Awakening, lavatory requirements, dressing, and travel to the airport would require from 1 to 1½ hours. Bed time, thus, could have been no more than 3 hours if the previous day's schedule was the same.

The NTSB appears not to have investigated what rest facilities may or may not have been provided for the crew at its layover in Bay City, Texas, after arrival at approximately 1100 CST (1200 domicile time). The maximum free time would be about 4½ hours. Time for eating and lavatory requirements could be about 1½ hours, leaving 3 hours for rest during the time of day when the body is most alert.

Flight time from Fayetteville to Bay City via Houston was about 6 hours 10 minutes with an added two stops. Assuming that the crew had completed its flight to Fayetteville, it would have been on duty for more than 20 hours with a 3-hour rest period. The NTSB notes that the single pilot would have then repeated the same flight schedule the following day.

It is highly probable that the pilot had suffered a sleep deficit before embarking on this lengthy duty day. Fatigue resultant from a long, busy day of flying with a minimal rest period at the destination could have exacerbated poor judgment and reduced ocular acuity. The observations of Hartman et al.[48] listed above would then be relevant.

The pilot reported having the runway in sight. He descended too low, striking power lines located well beneath the normal glide slope. Had he used the electronic Instrument Landing System glide slope, he would have remained well above the power lines. He apparently chose not to use the glide slope and relied on visual clues alone, bearing out the concept that fatigue makes it difficult to shift to a new task. The fog in the area may have subjected him to the "black hole effect," an illusion that causes pilots to think they are higher than they really are because of lack of peripheral visual clues.[6,90] The illusion again may have been exacerbated by Hartman's second concept, inability to correct small errors though they are recognized. The urge to sleep may have further driven the pilot to get home as soon as possible so that he might get to bed. He knew that tomorrow he would have to repeat the same grueling schedule.

China Airlines, B-747SP, N4522V 300 Nautical Miles Northwest of San Francisco, California, February 19, 1985[79]

A China Airlines 747 had engine failure en route to Los Angeles. None of the crew noticed the slowing airspeed until the aircraft entered a spin and plummeted 31,500 feet off the California coast, injuring two passengers seriously and causing major structural damage to the aircraft. According to R.C. Graeber, NASA-Ames Research Center, the pilots had not been watching the airspeed at all during the flight. "That's typical behavior of a person with sleep deprivation or a circadian low. I am convinced that fatigue played a significant role." Although an NTSB investigator urged the board members to list fatigue as a probable cause, the board refused.[98]

Aloha Airlines Flight 243, B-737-200, Kahuluhi Airport, April 28, 1988[80]

While climbing through approximately 24,000 feet on its way from Hilo, Hawaii, to Honolulu, Oahu, the top, front half of the fuselage of an Aloha B-737-200 tore loose. A flight attendant was blown overboard; the remaining 5 crew and 89 passengers survived. The aircraft made an emergency landing at Kahuluhi, Maui.

Investigation by the NTSB found that the fuselage fasteners had been examined under an FAA Airworthiness Directive in November 1987. Cracks found were repaired. Aloha management stated that an eddy current inspection of rivets had also been accomplished. No mention of such inspection was found in the maintenance records. Visual examination by the NTSB of the rivet holes revealed detectable fatigue cracks. Laboratory analysis showed the presence of many more cracks that would have been uncovered by normal eddy current testing.

It was found that the majority of Aloha's maintenance was conducted at night because the airline's schedule required full aircraft utilization during the day. Such intense utilization places a great deal of pressure on maintenance personnel to get the aircraft flying as soon as possible except in the most critical cases.

The NTSB acknowledged the adverse effects of circadian rhythm, sleep loss, and irregular work and rest schedules on inspectors and mechanics. In the case of the FAA requirement, the inspectors were to closely examine nearly 1,300 rivets and eddy current 360 rivets per panel. To perform this work necessitated climbing scaffolding and walking along the upper fuselage carrying a bright light. The eddy current inspectors carried a probe, meter, and light. At times, the inspectors were attached to ropes hanging from rafters to prevent falling. Each rivet, then, was inspected for cracks although the aluminum skin of the aircraft was covered by several layers of paint.[9]

The physiological and psychological stress on inspectors and mechanics under normal day-wake/night-sleep conditions can be readily understood. What further toll is taken as a result of the added debilitations of disturbed circadian rhythm and disturbed sleep/wake cycles can only be guessed. Airline management nonetheless still schedules heavy maintenance during late hours of the night and early morning in order to have aircraft ready for a full day's flying.

CONCLUSIONS

A plethora of scientific research data show that sleep deprivation and circadian desynchrony due to rapidly rotating shift schedules, rapid time zone changes, and unorganized sleep/wake cycles can result in severe performance decrement. Nevertheless, responsible government agencies and the airline industry fail to address these issues adequately. Congress has made clear its intent to keep aviation safe, and the courts have concurred. The Federal Aviation Administration has provided some regulations that attempt to address the issues, but it does not appear enthusiastic in enforcing these regulations or bringing regulations into accord with the large body of accumulating data.

The National Transportation Safety Board is charged with finding reasons why accidents occur. Scientific evidence explaining the effects of sleep loss, circadian desynchrony, and the concomitant deleterious effects of fatigue is mounting. From an examination of its own reports and documents, the NTSB appears to shy further from the issues of scheduling and sleep- or fatigue-related accident causation as the scientific data mounts. It prefers instead to apply the euphemism, "pilot error," to accidents where sleep deprivation due to rapidly rotating shiftwork and circadian desynchrony may have played a role.

The aviation industry has entered the era of the two-pilot, computer-controlled aircraft. After data are entered into computers on the ground, the pilots become systems managers in flight, only occasionally interacting with the aircraft by entering data into its computers. A major concern is ensuring that both pilots are fully informed of every action or activity—of every movement of a control, entering the computer data, or pressing a button. Much greater crew coordination and verbal communication between pilots are needed than were necessary in older, conventional aircraft.[38a,50a] As reported by Mitler et al.,[66] regarding the loss of the space shuttle Challenger, the effect of irregular working hours and insufficient sleep on senior project managers of Morton-Thiokol may have "increased judgment errors [and] prevented effective communication and exchange of information." With the advent of the B-747-400, it is not uncommon for aircraft to remain aloft over 12–16 hours. Even with augmented crews, rapidly changing time zones and sleep/wake cycles affect the human components of the system. The accounts of how these factors may have debilitated crews of earlier, shorter-range aircraft and may have played a role in their demise have been largely ignored, and valuable data have been overlooked.

The chronohygiene of the human component in the man-machine loop must be considered when optimal functioning of the system is mandated. No longer should we limit duty time simply on the basis of length of time a person has been on duty or has been flying. We should also consider the times of day allocated for duty and sleep. Should off-duty sequences conform to a time other than the person's normal sleep time, then it should be considered that sleep quality and length will probably be impaired. One way to alleviate some of this problem is to limit duty time that overlaps with normal "subjective" sleep times. It also should be considered that sleep quality and length are decreased during rest (off duty) periods that coincide with a person's normal waking hours. It is also clear that, in regard to rotating schedules or schedules that change often (e.g., the "bid" system), an attempt should be made to alter the worker's off-duty/work structure to preclude the abrupt scheduling of flying during normal sleep times. To cover early duty periods, schedules can be devised that consider human physiology and employ sound chronobiological principles. Heeding the recent studies of chronobiologists,[23] pilots might benefit by schedules that rotate in a phase-delayed manner and allow adequate recovery when work occurs during subjective sleep time. As new strategies and methods to cope with shiftwork are developed, the airline industry must become more involved and be more aggressive at implementation so that flight crews can perform their jobs efficiently, healthfully, and *safely*.

We must re-evaluate mishaps and accidents where sleep deprivation and circadian desynchrony are suspected contributing factors, then dissect out as much information as possible. The recommendations of the Sleep Research Society subcommittee[66] can provide a basis for chronohygiene within not only the aviation industry, but all industries where people are required to conform to shiftwork schedules. Both occupational medical practitioners and company management must recognize that human beings are not machines that can be "plugged in" to perform highly cognitive jobs at any time of day. Sleep loss and indiscriminate rotating of shift take a toll. On the ground, the operator may pay the price with an injury or an error, or the customer might receive poor service or defective merchandise. In the air, such errors can kill hundreds of human beings both in the aircraft and on the ground where the pieces finally come to rest. Recalling the words of Santayana, "One who does not know history is bound to repeat it."

Acknowledgment. The authors sincerely thank Jill A. Erickson for her superb, untiring bibliographical and technical support in preparation of the manuscript.

REFERENCES

1. Akerstedt T: Sleepiness in shiftwork: A review with emphasis on continuous monitoring of EEG and EOG. Chronobiol Int 4:129–140, 1987.
2. Akerstedt T, Gillberg M: Sleep disturbances and shift work. In Night and Shift Work: Biological and Social Aspects. Proceedings of the Fifth International Symposium on Night and Shift Work, Rouen, 12–16 May 1980. Oxford, UK, Pergamon Press, 1981, pp 127–137.
3. Akerstedt T, Gillberg M: Displacement of the sleep period and sleep deprivation: Implications for shift work. Hum Neurobiol 1:163–171, 1982.
4. Akerstedt T, Torsvall L: Experimental changes in shift schedules: Their effects on well-being. Ergonomics 21:489–856, 1978.
5. Akerstedt T, Torsvall L, Gillberg M: Sleepiness and shift work: Field studies. Sleep 5:S95–S106, 1982.
6. Alkov RA: What you see is not always what you get. Approach, February 1983.
7. Anch AM, Browman CP, Mitler MM, Walsh JK: Sleep: A Scientific Perspective. Englewood Cliffs, NJ, Prentice-Hall, 1988, pp 76–77.
8. Anonymous: The national transportation board urges lessened controller workload. Aviat Wk Space Technol October 9, 1981, p 27.
9. Anonymous: Safety board urges FAA to revamp maintenance, inspection training. Aviat Wk Space Technol 131(17):77–78, 1989.
10. Aschoff J: Features of circadian rhythms relevant for the design of shift schedules. Ergonomics 21:739–754, 1978.
11. Association of Sleep Disorders Centers, the Sleep Disorders Classification Committee: Diagnostic classification of sleep and arousal disorders. Sleep 2:1–137, 1979.
12. Babcock G: Air Line Pilot Association Memorandum to Captain Bob Patterson, Chief Accident Investigator, Re: United Airlines, Inc., DC-8F Accident December 18, 1977, near Kaysville, UT, Dated January 17, 1978.
13. Beljan JR, Rosenblatt LS, Hetherington NW, et al: Human Performance in the Aviation Environment: Final Report. National Aeronautics and Space Administration. Contract No. NAS2-6657, 1972.
14. Chapman RP: Pilot Fatigue—A Deadly Cover-up. Smithtown, NY, Exposition Press, 1982, pp 118, 124–153.
15. Cobb S, Rose RM: Hypertension, peptic ulcer and diabetes in air traffic controllers. JAMA 224:489–492, 1973.
16. Code of Federal Regulations, Title 14, Federal Aviation Regulations, section 61.53, Operations during medical deficiency.
17. Code of Federal Regulations, Title 14, Federal Aviation Regulations, section 63.19, Operations during physical deficiency.
18. Code of Federal Regulations, Title 14, Federal Aviation Regulations, section 65.49(d).
19. Code of Federal Regulations, Title 21, section 1250.35(a,b).
20. Colligan MJ, Frockt IJ, Tasto DL: Frequency of sickness absence and worksite clinic visits among nurses as a function of shift. Appl Ergonom 10:79–85, 1979.
21. Colquhoun WP: Biological Rhythms and Human Performance. London, Academic Press, 1971.
22. Czeisler CA, Kronauer RE, Allan JS, et al: Bright light induction of strong (type o) resetting of the human circadian pacemaker. Science 244:1328–1333, 1989.
23. Czeisler CA, Moore-Ede MC, Coleman RM: Rotating shift work schedules that disrupt sleep are improved by applying circadian principles. Science 217:460–463, 1982.
24. Day v. National Transportation Safety Board. 414 F.2d 950 (CA5, 1969).

25. Dement WC, Seidel WF, Cohen SA, et al: Sleep and wakefulness in aircrew before and after transoceanic flights. Aviat Space Environ Med 57(Suppl):B14–28, 1986.
26. Department of Transportation, Federal Aviation Administration Advisory Circular: Aviation Safety Reporting Program AC No 00-46C, Dated February 4, 1985.
27. Department of Transportation, Federal Aviation Administration Form 8500-9, October 1973.
28. Department of Transportation, Federal Aviation Administration: Medical Handbook for Pilots AC67-2. Washington, DC, US Government Printing Office, May, 1974, Stock No 050-007-00254-8.
29. Department of Transportation, Federal Aviation Administration, Civil Aeromedical Institute: Rx (a few medical facts for pilots). June, 1975, Aviation Medical Education Series No 1A.
30. Department of Transportation, Federal Aviation Administration Docket No 17669; FAA Notice 78-3, 78-3A, 1978.
31. Department of Transportation, Federal Aviation Administration: Medical Facts for Pilots. July, 1983, AFO-800-0783, FAA-P-8740-41.
32. Department of Transportation, Federal Aviation Administration: Daily Body Rhythms and Flight Safety. October, 1984, AFO-800-1084, FAA-P-8740-46.
33. Department of Transportation, Federal Aviation Administration: Airman's Information Manual: Official Guide to Basic Flight Information and ATC Procedures. Washington, DC, May 3, 1990 (printed quarterly).
34. Department of Transportation, Federal Aviation Administration: Physiological Training Form OMB No 2120-0101.
35. Department of Transportation, National Transportation Safety Board: Aircraft Accident Report SA-397 (File No 1-0003), Delta Air Lines, Inc., DC-8 N802E, Kenner, Louisiana, March 30, 1967. Adopted December 20, 1967.
36. Doskin VA, Lavrent'yeva NA: Pressing problems of space biorhythmology. Book review of Stepanova SE: Aktual'nye Problem Kosmicheskoy Bioritmologii. Kosm Biol Aviakosm Med 13(5):88–90, 1979.
37. Drenth PJ, Hoolwerf G, Thierry H: Psychological aspects of shiftwork. In Personal Goals and Work Design. New York, John Wiley, 1976, pp 209–223.
38. Folkard S, Monk TH: Shiftwork and performance. Hum Factors 21:483–492, 1979.
38a. Foushee HC: The role of communications, sociopsychological, and personality factors in the maintenance of crew coordination. Aviat Space Envrion Med 53(11):1062–1066, 1982.
39. Gander PH, Graeber RC: Sleep in pilots flying short-haul commercial schedules. Ergonomics 30:1365–1377, 1987.
40. Gander PH, Myhre G, Graeber RC, et al: Adjustment of sleep and the circadian temperature rhythm after flights across nine time zones. Aviat Space Environ Med 60:733–743, 1989.
41. Glines CV: Probable cause: Pilot fatigue? Air Line Pilot 45(11):19–21, 47, 1976.
42. Gordon NP, Cleary PD, Parker CE, Czeisler CA: The prevalence and health impact of shiftwork. Am J Pub Health 76:1225–1228, 1986.
43. Graeber RC: Alterations in performance following rapid transmeridian flight. In Rhythmic Aspects of Behavior. Hillsdale, NJ, Lawrence Erlbaum, 1982, pp 173–211.
44. Graeber RC: Dimensions of flight crew performance decrements: Methodological implications for field research. In Breakdown in Human Adaptation to Stress: Towards a Multidisciplinary Approach (Volume I, Part 2, Human Performance and Breakdown in Adaptation). Boston, Martinus Nijoff, 1984, pp 584–605.
45. Graeber RC: Crew Factors in Flight Operations. IV. Sleep and Wakefulness in International Aircrews. National Aeronautics and Space Administration, February, 1986, Technical Memorandum 88231.
46. Graeber RC, Lauber JK, Connell LJ, Gander PH: International aircrew sleep and wakefulness after multiple time zone flights: A cooperative study. Aviat Space Environ Med 57(suppl):B3–9, 1986.
47. Harris W: Fatigue, circadian rhythm and truck accidents. In Vigilance: Theory, Operational Performance, and Physiological Correlates. New York, Plenum Press, 1977, pp 133–146.
48. Hartman BO, Storm WF, Vanderveen JE, et al: Operational Aspects of Variations in Alertness. NATO Advisory Group for Aerospace Research and Development, 1974, AGARD-AG-189, pp 1–2.
48a. Hawkins FH: Human Factors in Flight. Brookfield, VT, Gower Technical Press, 1987, pp 45, 158–161, 169–178, 181–183, 248–254.
49. Holley DC, Heinhold MP, Edgar DM, et al: Effects of Circadian Rhythm Phase Alterations on Physiological and Psychological Variables: Implications to Pilot Performance. National Aeronautics and Space Administration Technical Memorandum 81277, 1981.

50. Hudson JW, Bell HJ, Mayfield RL, et al: Pan American World Airways 1975 Final Report. Federal Aviation Administration, June 13, 1975, p 26.
51. Hyndman BW: The role of rhythms in homeostasis. Kybernetik 15:227–236, 1974.
52. Joint Report on KLM-PAA Accident, March 27, 1977, Los Rodeos Airport, Tenerife, Canary Islands, Spain (translated from Spanish). Report of the International Investigating Teams of Spain, the Netherlands, and the United States of America. December 7, 1978.
53. Klein KE, Wegmann HM: Circadian rhythms of human performance and resistance: Operational Aspects. In Sleep, Wakefulness and Circadian Rhythm. Neuilly-Sur-Seine, NATA Advisory Group for Aerospace Research and Development, 1979, AGARD LS 105, pp 2–17.
54. Knauth P, Kiesswetter E: A change from weekly to quicker shift rotations: A field study of discontinuous three-shift workers. Ergonomics 30:1311–1321, 1987.
55. LeRoy CH: Addendum to Human Factors Group Chairman's Factual Report. National Transportation Safety Board, Bureau of Technology, 1978, DCA 78-AA-005.
56. Lipscomb JC: National Transportation Safety Board Notification of Transportation Accident, NTSB Form 6102.19. Dated November 19, 1979.
57. Lipscomb JC: History of Flight. National Transportation Safety Board Accident No IAD80-F-A007, November 21, 1979, p 3.
58. Lyman GE, Orlady HW: Fatigue and Associated Performance Decrements in Air Transport Operations—An Aviation Safety Reporting Systems Study. Batelle Columbus Laboratories, ASRS Office, Mountain View, CA, Contract No. NAS2-10060, 1980.
59. Masters RL: Shift work research in aviation: An operational perspective. In Biological Rhythms, Sleep and Shift Work. Advances in Sleep Research, Vol 7. New York, SP Medical and Scientific Books, 1981, pp 329–333.
60. McAdams F: Human error in air carrier accidents. National Transportation Safety Board Memorandum, Notation 2297—Special Study, October 23, 1978.
61. Melton CE: Physiological Responses to Unvarying (Steady) and 2-2-1 Shifts: Miami International Flight Service Station. Federal Aviation Administration, Office of Aviation Medicine, February 1985, Report No AD-A155751, FAA-AM-85-2.
62. Melton CE, Bartanowicz RS: Biological Rhythms and Rotating Shift Work: Some Considerations for Air Traffic Controllers and Managers. Federal Aviation Administration, Office of Aviation Medicine, January, 1986, Report No AD-A168742, DOT/FAA/AM-86/2.
63. Melton CE, McKenzie JM, Smith RC, et al: Physiological, Biochemical, and Psychological Responses in Air Traffic Control Personnel: Comparison of the 5-day and 2-2-1 Shift Rotation Patterns. Federal Aviation Administration, Civil Aeromedical Institute, December, 1973, Report No FAA-AM-73-22.
64. Miller WH: Fatigue: Some special effects and tests. J Aviat 7:162–166, 1936.
65. Minors DS, Waterhouse JM: Anchor sleep as a synchronizer on abnormal routines. Int J Chronobiol 7:165–188, 1981.
66. Mitler MM, Carskadon MA, Czeisler CA, et al: Catastrophes, sleep and public policy: Consensus report. Sleep 11:100–109, 1988.
67. Mohler SR: Fatigue in aviation activities. Aerospace Med 37:722–732, 1966.
68. Mohler SR: A physiological index as an aid on pattern construction. Interim Supplemental Operational Fatigue Report. Washington, DC, Federal Aviation Administration, Aeromedical Applications Division, Office of Aviation Medicine, July 8, 1974, pp 1–9.
69. Moore-Ede MC, Fuller CA: Evaluation of aircraft accident reports. Forum 13:13–15, 1980.
70. Moore-Ede MC, Sulzman FM, Fuller CA: The Clocks that Time Us: Physiology of the Circadian Timing System. Cambridge, MA, Harvard University Press, 1982, p 448.
71. Narrative Statement of Pertinent Facts, Conditions and Circumstances. National Transportation Safety Board Form 6120.4, Investigation 1, Section 1.8, 1979, p 8.
72. National Aeronautics and Space Administration: Pilot Fatigue and Circadian Desynchronosis, Report of a Workshop Held in San Francisco, California on August 26–28, 1980. NASA Technical Memorandum 81275, Dated 1980.
73. National Transportation Safety Board: Aircraft Accident Report SA-413 (File No 1-0004), Report No NTSB-AAR-70-6, United Air Lines, Inc., Boeing 727-22C N7434U, Near Los Angeles, CA, January 18, 1969. Adopted March 18, 1970.
74. National Transportation Safety Board: Aircraft Accident Report No NTSB-AAR-75-9, Eastern Air Lines, Inc., Douglas DC-9-31 N8984E, Charlotte, NC, September 11, 1974. Adopted May 23, 1975.
75. National Transportation Safety Board: Aircraft Accident Report No NTSB-AAR-78-8, United Airlines, Inc., Douglas DC-8-54 N8047U, Near Kaysville, UT, December 18, 1977. Adopted July 27, 1978.

76. National Transportation Safety Board: Aircraft Accident Report No NTSB-AAR-79-5, Pacific Southwest Airlines, Inc., Boeing 727-214 N533PS, and Gibbs Flight Center, Inc., Cessna 172 N7711G, San Diego, CA, September 25, 1978. Adopted April 20, 1979.
77. National Transportation Safety Board: Aircraft Accident Report No NTSB-AAR-80-5, Downeast Airlines, Inc., DeHavilland DHC-6-200 N68DE, Rockland, ME, May 30, 1979. Adopted May 12, 1980.
78. National Transportation Safety Board: Aircraft Accident Report No NTSB-AAR-80-1, Air New England, Inc., DeHavilland DHC-6-300 N383 EX, Hyannis, MA, June 17, 1979. Adopted January 3, 1980.
79. National Transportation Safety Board: Aircraft Accident Report No NTSB-AAR-86-3, China Airlines, Boeing B-747SP N4522V, 300 Nautical Miles Northwest of San Francisco, California, February 19, 1985. Adopted March 29, 1986.
80. National Transportation Safety Board: Aircraft Accident Report No NTSB-AAR-89-3, Aloha Airlines, Inc., Boeing B-737-200 N73711, Kahuluhi Airport, Maui, April 28, 1988. Adopted June 14, 1989.
81. Nicholson AN: Duty hour and sleep patterns in aircrew operating world-wide routes. Aerospace Med 43:138–141, 1972.
82. Nicholson AN: Pascoe PA, Spencer MB, et al: Nocturnal sleep and daytime alertness of aircrew after transmeridian flights. Aviat Space Environ Med 57(suppl):B43–B52, 1986.
83. Petrakis JJ: Human Factors Group Chairman's Factual Report. National Transportation Safety Board, November 2, 1978, Docket No 6A-466, Exhibit No 6A.
84. Preston FS, Ruffell Smith HP, Sutton-Mattocks VM: Sleep loss in air cabin crew. Aerospace Med 44:931–935, 1973.
85. Price WJ: Model of probable fatigue factors involved in United Airlines flight #2860 accident. Forum: The International Society of Air Safety Investigators 13:11–12, 1980.
86. Price WJ, Holley DC: The last minutes of flight 2860: An analysis of crew shift work scheduling. In Night and Shift Work, Biological and Social Aspects. Proceedings of the Fifth International Symposium on Shift Work, Rouen, 12–16 May 1980. Oxford, UK, Pergamon Press, 1981, pp 287–294.
87. Price WJ, Holley DC: Sleep loss and the crash of flight 182. J Hum Ergol 11(suppl):291–301, 1982.
88. Rauch v United Instruments, Inc, 548 F.2d 452 (CA3 Pa, 1976).
89. Reinhart RO: The Pilot's Manual of Medical Certification and Health Maintenance. Osceola, WI, Specialty Press, 1982.
90. Roscoe SN: Landing airplanes, detecting traffic, and the dark focus. Aviat Space Environ Med 53:970–976, 1982.
91. Rutenfranz J: Shift work and biological rhythms. Arzneimittelforschung 28:1867–1872, 1978.
92. Rutenfranz J, Colquhoun WP: Circadian rhythms in human performance. Scand J Work Environ Health 5:167–177, 1979.
93. Rutenfranz J, Colquhoun WP, Knauth P, Ghata JN: Biomedical and psychosocial aspects of shift work: A review. Scand J Work Environ Health 3:165–182, 1977.
94. Rutenfranz J, Knauth P, Colquhoun WP: Hours of work and shiftwork. Ergonomics 19:331–340, 1976.
95. Samel A, Wegmann HM: Desynchronization and internal dissociation in aircrew. Ergonomics 30:1395–1404, 1987.
96. Sasaki M, Kurosaki Y, Mori A, Endo S: Patterns of sleep-wakefulness before and after transmeridian flight in commercial airline pilots. Aviat Space Environ Med 57(12, Suppl):B29–B42, 1986.
97. Schreuder OB, Lederer LG, Cullen JK, et al: Medical aspects of aircraft pilot fatigue with special reference to the commercial jet pilot. Aerospace Med 37(4):i–iv, 1–44, 1966.
98. Stoller G: Fatigue in the cockpit: A growing concern. Conde Nast's Traveler:21–26, June 1988.
99. Tasto DL, Colligan MJ, Skjei EW, Polly SJ: Health Consequences of Shift Work. Menlo Park, CA, SRI International, 1978, URU-4426.
100. Taylor PJ, Pocock SJ: Mortality of shift and day workers, 1958–1968. Br J Ind Med 29:201–207, 1972.
101. Taylor PJ, Pocock SJ, Sergean R: Absenteeism of shift and day workers: A study of six types of shift system in 29 organizations. Br J Ind Med 29:208–213, 1972.
102. Thomas DD, Marcum J, Malcom W, et al: Flight safety in Pan Am. A Report by the Operations Review Group of Pan American World Airways, Pan Am Building, 200 Park Ave, New York, New York 10166, April 23, 1974.
103. Torsvall L, Akerstedt T, Gillander K, Knutsson A: Sleep on the night shift: 24-hour EEG monitoring of spontaneous sleep/wake behavior. Psychophysiology 26:352–358, 1989.

104. United States Code Service, Title 49, Federal Aviation Act, section 1421, 1958.
105. United States Code Service, Title 49, Federal Aviation Act, section 1422(b), 1983.
106. Webb WB: Biological Rhythms, Sleep, and Performance. New York, John Wiley, 1982.
107. Wegmann H-M, Gundel A, Naumann N, et al: Sleep, sleepiness, and circadian rhythmicity in aircrews operating on transatlantic routes. Aviat Space Environ Med 57(suppl):B53–B64.
108. Wever R: The Circadian System of Man: Results of Experiments under Temporal Isolation. New York, Springer-Verlag, 1979.
109. Winget CM, DeRoshia CW, Markley CL, Holley DC: A review of human physiological and performance changes associated with desynchronosis of biological rhythms. Aviat Space Environ Med 55(12):1085–1096, 1984.
110. Winget CM, Hughes L, LaDou J: Physiological effects of rotational work shifting: A review. J Occup Med 20:204–210, 1978.
111. Winget CM, De Roshia CW, Ogawa KH, Holley DC: Significance of light and social cues in the maintenance of temporal organization in man. Physiologist 32(1):594–595, 1989.

H. DONALD KENNEDY, JR, MPH, JD

SHIFTWORK AS RELATED TO STRESS CLAIMS UNDER WORKERS' COMPENSATION STATUTES

Head, Occupational Health and Preventive Medicine
Naval Medical Command
Southeast Region
Jacksonville, Florida

The views expresed in this article are those of the author and do not reflect the official policy or position of the Department of the Navy, Department of Defense, or the U.S. Government.

Reprint requests to:
H. Donald Kennedy, Jr., MPH, JD
Occupational Health and Preventive Medicine
Naval Medical Command
Southeast Region
Jacksonville, FL

STRESS IN THE WORKPLACE

Stress in the workplace is hardly new, but compensating employees for stress-related mental and emotional disabilities is a rapidly growing trend that deeply concerns both public and private employers. Employers are increasingly concerned about stress claims by employees and the potentially broad exposure for employer liability. Some employers are reluctant to discipline employees for fear of incurring the financial risks of stress-related claims. Statistics on a national basis are limited, but one study revealed that insurance claims for mental stress injuries more than doubled between 1980 and 1982, whereas claims for other disabling work injuries decreased during that period. Mental stress claims accounted for 11% of all occupational disease claims during the study period.[1]

Stress claims will probably increase in the years ahead if for no other reason than that the pool of potential claimants has become enormous. Not everyone does work that could result in a bad back or black lung disease, but nearly everyone faces stress. Across the country, employees are filing stress claims, generally through the workers' compensation system rather than through tort action. However, with our recognition of workplace stress, attention has been focused on the court, as well as on the workers' compensation system. This focus has obscured, but not diminished, the economic impact of on-the-job stress from other causes such as lost time due to stress-related illness, absenteeism, and accidents, as well as increased medical insurance premiums. Stress on the job is frequently cited as a leading cause of problem drinking and drug use. The cost of alcohol and drug abuse in the workplace is substantial; some sources put it as high as $100 billion per year in lost productivity, medical costs, absenteeism, and accidents. Stress may play a key role in employee factors such as job turnover and low productivity. Stress may also be a factor in both mental and physical illness; consequently, the workplace costs of illness can be in part attributable to stress. Commonplace complaints related to muscle tension, such as headaches and backaches, are often related to job stress and result in considerable lost time to employers. Work-related stress may also lead to fatigue, insomnia, gastrointestinal disorders, and anxiety.

A growing body of medical evidence implicates stress as an important factor in cardiac and gastrointestinal disease, in resistance to and recovery from oncological and immunological disorders, as well as in psychological disorders. Medical disease alone costs employers billions of dollars in workers' compensation awards; however, it is difficult to ascertain the percentage for which job stress alone is accountable. For example, numerous factors other than stress are involved in heart disease; on-the-job stress may be only an aggravating factor, making it impossible to determine the amount of workers' compensation awards for heart disease that is directly attributable to work-related stress.

Most accidents are due to human error, and two major sources of human error in workplace accidents are stress and a lack of safety consciousness. Although stress has been linked to accident-prone behavior, firm numbers for percentages of accidents caused by stress have not been established. While all workers experience stress, some react in ways that make them more accident prone. Stressed workers are less attentive and more likely to disregard safety precautions. They are also more likely to become confused, exhibit poor judgment, daydream, and become absentminded. The reaction to stress may be to become frustrated and take unnecessary risks. In a stress-accident cycle, one behavior increases the likelihood of another. Once under stress, an employee becomes more easily fatigued and experiences slower reaction time, unclear thinking, and impaired physical coordination. Muscles tense and are more prone to strain and tears. When an accident occurs, it creates even more stress for the employee, who becomes even more likely to cause another accident.

Shiftwork has been found to contribute significantly to work-related stress for many people. It has been associated with an increased incidence of some specific medical disorders, including ischemic heart disease and peptic ulcers, as well as with general complaints of fatigue, malaise, anxiety, and sleep deprivation. The reader is referred to Chapters 6 and 7 in this issue for discussions of the medical and psychological effects of shiftwork. The recognition that working the nightshift is frequently associated with sleep deprivation may lead to citations of schedule-related decreased vigilance and alertness as a factor in on-the-job accidents. Desynchronosis has been implicated as a major factor in aviation accidents attributed to human error (see Chapter 10).

This chapter traces the origins of workers' compensation, reviews the general requirement of a causal connection between the employment and the injury or disability, and discusses the analytical framework in which courts have considered whether and under what circumstances workers' compensation benefits may be awarded for mental, nervous, and emotional disorders allegedly induced by work-related emotional stimuli, and, finally, examines a few shiftwork cases.

ORIGINS OF WORKERS' COMPENSATION LEGISLATION

Workers' compensation is a mechanism for providing, through the medium of insurance, cash wage benefits and medical care to victims of work-connected injuries and for passing on the cost of insurance premiums to the consumer in the price of the product.[3] The necessity for workers' compensation legislation arose out of the sharp increase in industrial accidents that paralleled the rise of the factory system and the simultaneous decrease in the employee's common law remedies for his injuries.[4] At common law, an injured employee faced virtually insurmountable odds in trying to obtain damages from an employer.[5] The employee's sole recourse was to bring suit against the employer for negligence. At common law, an employee won a negligence suit only if the employer failed to provide reasonably safe machines, equipment, or appliances in the workplace. Clearly, these circumstances levied a heavy burden of proof on the injured worker.

To make matters even worse, the employer was entitled to three extremely potent defenses. First, an injured employee who was contributorily negligent in any degree could not recover, even if the employer was also negligent. This defense based on "contributory negligence" was recognized by the courts in 1809.[6]

The second defense available to the employer was established in 1837.[7] Under this "fellow servant" defense, an employer could refuse to indemnify an injured employee if it could be shown that the negligence of a fellow employee caused the injury.

The third defense, "assumption of the risk," was established in 1842 by the statement, "The servant is not bound to risk his safety in the service of his master, and may, if he thinks fit, decline any service in which he reasonably apprehends injury to himself."[8] The implication of this statement was that a worker who was free to avoid a hazardous work area would have no standing to sue when injury occurred, even if the worker did not know the area was hazardous.

These three common law doctrines were entitled the "unholy trinity" defenses. Dean Prosser described the basis of these judge-made laws by declaring, "The cornerstone of the common law edifice was the economic theory that there was complete mobility of labor, that the supply of work was unlimited, and that the worker was an entirely free agent, under no compulsion to enter into the employment."[9] Under this socioeconomic philosophy very few workers injured by industrial accidents were able to recover any type of compensation.

As the full impact of the "unholy trinity" defenses became apparent to the common law courts, new efforts were made toward reforming this judicially created imbalance between the rights of employers and employees. Although judicial exceptions afforded some relief to the injured worker, interest in imposing liability upon the employer only began to gain momentum with the creation of "employers' liability statutes."[10] Many of these individual state statutes abolished the fellow servant rule, reduced the emphasis on contributory negligence to comparative negligence, and reclassified working conditions that applied to assumption of the risk. Although these first legislative efforts were not very successful, they served as experimental models from which initial compensation legislation evolved.

The employers' liability laws, however, were soon found to be inefficient and unsatisfactory. They still suffered from the inherent weaknesses of the common law methods: the injured employee still had to bring suit against the employer; the employers' defenses, although limited somewhat, still hindered the injured employee's ability to recover; the costs of litigation were still borne by the injured employee; and the injured employee still had to fear losing job security because of a vengeful employer.

Where did workers' compensation legislation begin? Anglo-Saxon common law would seem to suggest that it was developed by judicial decree. However, this clearly was not the case. In fact, the seeds of modern workers' compensation law were sown by sociopolitical thought in nineteenth-century Prussia.[11] In 1838, just 1 year after English courts created the fellow servant rule and only 4 years before they adopted the assumption-of-risk doctrine, the civil code of Prussia adopted law that made railroads liable for the injuries of their employees and passengers.[12] This was just the beginning, for in 1854 the Prussians made certain manufacturers pay up to one-half of all workers' sickness costs, and in 1884 Germany passed the world's first workers' compensation law. This historic socioeconomic legislation became the law of Germany some 13 years before Great Britain, 25 years before the first American state, and 65 years before the last American jurisdiction adopted workers' compensation legislation.

Scholars who have researched the history and origins of workers' compensation believe philosophers and politicians, particularly socialists, had a tremendous influence on its thought and development. Although the prominent social philosophers wielded significant influence, it was the powerful political figures of nineteenth-century Germany who made it a reality. Indeed, the great Prussian Emperor Frederick the Great once said, "It is the duty of the state to provide sustenance and support of those of its citizens who cannot provide sustenance for themselves,"[13] and the founder of workers' compensation is believed to be Chancellor Otto von Bismarck.

It may be of interest to note that some evidence points to Bertha von Krupp of the famed German munitions and steel manufacturer, Krupp Works, as the founder of workers' compensation. Evidently, she cared very much for the injured workers at her family's plants and succeeded in persuading her husband Albert that "taking care of workers was not only good charity but also good business."[14] Furthermore, it is alleged that the Krupps persuaded Bismarck that "it was not only good business but good politics."[15]

While scholars may dispute the identity of the true founder of workers' compensation, there seems to be little doubt as to the reason why the chancellor supported it. Following the German victory over the French in the Franco-Prussian War of 1870–1871, Bismarck's concern about the mounting Marxist-socialist political movement developing in the Second Reich increased. Bismarck believed that giving workers more economic security through workers' compensation would cause the German worker who was leaning toward socialism to reconsider. One commentator has gone so far as to label the German Workers' Compensation Act a "Gift from the Throne."[16] This "gift," in fact, has been labeled an essential component of Bismarck's antisocialist plan. It has been theorized that after Germany suppressed trade unions and the Socialist party as illegal, workers' compensation became the "carrot" that steered the working class away from socialism. There is no doubt that politics played a major role in the inception and adoption of German compensation law, but it must be realized that the primary purpose of the law was to alleviate the burden of socioeconomic injuries.

The British Workers' Compensation Act of 1897 was the legislative model that the majority of American jurisdictions duplicated and enacted in the early

1910s. The British experiment provided the basic statutory scheme, which still exists in today's American statutes. Similar to its German counterpart, the British Workers' Compensation Act was due to the combined efforts of philosophers and politicians. In fact, in Great Britain politics played an even larger part in the adoption of workers' compensation law than it had played in Germany.

The most important issue of the 1895 election was workers' compensation. The conservative Tories, led by Joseph Chamberlain, allied themselves with the minority liberal Unionists. With the adamant Chamberlain leading the fight in the House of Commons, it was only a matter of time before the British Workers' Compensation Act became a reality. One of Chamberlain's most impassioned pleas for workers' compensation gave rise to the famous quotation describing injured workers as "the wounded soldiers of industry."[17] The Workers' Compensation Bill was announced in the House of Commons on May 3, 1897. By this time support for it was so widespread that the opposing Liberals could hardly enter an objection to its introduction and passage. The bill was quickly approved by the House of Commons, sent to the House of Lords, and passed there 3 days later.

To characterize the passage of the British Workers' Compensation Act as revolutionary is a serious understatement. It marked one of the most significant developments in Anglo-Saxon jurisprudence. In short, it created an entirely new legal relationship between employer and employee. The principle that "the cost of the product should bear the blood of the worker"[18] was emphatically proclaimed during this initial developmental period and later became a standard theme for early workers' compensation arguments in court.

As one would expect, workers' compensation laws in the United States were a direct response to both the German and the British compensation acts. The early employers' liability statutes attempted to expand the liability of the employer, but they suffered from inherent deficiencies, which were the direct result of their reliance on the tort theories of recovery. It was apparent that a new legal principle was required.

The impetus for the creation of this new principle came in the form of an exposé of the Prussian system by John Graham Brooks. This publication, better known as the Fourth Special Report of the Commissioner of Labor, initiated legislative studies across the nation.[19] By 1910, workers' compensation commissions had been set up by Congress in the states of Massachusetts, Minnesota, New Jersey, Connecticut, Ohio, Illinois, Wisconsin, Montana, and Washington.[20] These commissions had the unenviable task of framing an effective compensation statute that could pass judicial review. The difficulty of the task was all too apparent: each of the state compensation acts before 1911 had been stricken on grounds of an unconstitutional taking without just compensation.

Finally, in late 1911, the constitutional barrier to state workers' compensation acts was overcome. The Wisconsin Workers' Compensation Act of 1911 was upheld as constitutional.[21] One by one other state compensation statutes were constitutionally upheld and by 1920, all but eight states had adopted compensation acts.[22]

THE COMPENSATION PRINCIPLE

The ultimate social philosophy behind compensation liability is the belief in the wisdom of providing, in the most efficient, dignified, and certain form, financial and medical benefits for the victims of work-connected injuries, which an enlightened community would feel obliged to provide in any case in some less satisfactory form, and the wisdom of allocating the burden of payment to the most appropriate source, the consumer.[23] To be sure, it must be emphasized that doctrines of tort, and fault in particular, are of no consequence, and therefore cannot affect the result of workers' compensation adjudications. The test is not who or what caused an event, but whether the event was related to employment. Simply put, there are but two relevant issues to be decided in a workers' compensation proceeding: did the employee suffer a work-related injury, and, if the answer to the first question is yes, did the employee receive compensation?

Workers' compensation payments are based on a test of work-relatedness between employee and injury. Principles of tort center on the individual's righting of an individual wrong. Workers' compensation is concerned with the benefits derived from collective social involvement and protection. In essence, workers' compensation was developed in order to alleviate a grave socioeconomic infirmity. Its fundamental goals included: providing adequate and punctual monetary benefits to an injured worker, regardless of fault; reducing unnecessary and expensive litigation; releasing both public and private sectors from the financial burden of industrial accidents; encouraging employers to upgrade safety equipment and procedures; and promoting continued studies to aid in the reduction of industrial accidents and injury.[24]

Under all compensation acts it is generally essential that there be some substantial causal relationship between the employment and the injury or disability. The form of expression commonly used in compensation statutes to describe this relationship is, "arising out of and in the course of the employment," although there is considerable variance. The words, "arising out of," involve the idea of causal relationship between the employment and the injury, or inquiry into the character of origin of the risk, whereas the term, "in the course of," relates more particularly to the time, place, and circumstances under which the injury occurred.

Workers' compensation benefits are payable under two broad coverage categories: injury (or accident), and occupational disease. The vast majority of workers' compensation claims have been for injuries or accidents, which, until recently, generally were taken to mean physical disabilities or deaths that resulted from single incidents. Occupational disease claims, on the other hand, are claims for deaths or disabilities resulting from illnesses that are "peculiar to" an industrial trade or process, such as coal miners' pneumoconiosis or black lung disease. Some courts have emphasized duration of onset in distinguishing occupational diseases from injuries. Occupational diseases are said to be of "slow and gradual development," whereas accidents or injuries "can always be traced from a definite time, place, and cause." Normally, there are three ways a disease can be considered occupationally related:

1. By exposing a worker to an injurious substance that is unique to the work done, an employment may increase the worker's risk, compared to the general public's, of contracting the disease.

2. An employment may expose a worker to an increased risk of contracting a "disease of ordinary life." Thus, if a hospital worker is exposed to patients with tuberculosis and subsequently contracts that disease, the tuberculosis is considered an occupational disease. A cold contracted at work would not be considered occupational in nature unless statistics indicate that fellow employees have above-average numbers of colds. In short, the workplace must increase the employee's risk of developing the disease.

3. Finally, if a traumatic injury at work aggravates a disease of ordinary life, the resulting disability is occupational in nature. A worker suffering from heart disease is subjected to stress at work and is stricken with a heart attack. The heart attack would be considered of occupational origin, despite the fact that the underlying disease—arteriosclerosis—is nonoccupational.

Most occupational diseases are dose related; that is, the more intense or the longer the duration of exposure to the harmful stressor, the greater the possibility that the worker will develop the disease. An individual susceptibility also plays an important, yet undefinable, part in determining which workers develop the disease. A worker exposed to low levels of asbestos for 10 years may develop asbestosis; yet another exposed to higher concentrations for 20 years may show no untoward effects. Adding to the contradictions is a generally embraced scientific belief that no level of exposure is guaranteed safe. In other words, not all occupational diseases are dose related; at least in theory, brief exposure to asbestos fibers could cause mesothelioma, a fatal cancer of the lung lining.

An additional complication in the evaluation and understanding of occupational disease is that most occupational diseases are characterized by long latency periods. They do not manifest themselves at the time of exposure; instead, 10–30 or more years may pass between the injurious exposure and the manifestation of the disease. During the latency period, although the disease is present in the body, the clinical symptoms have not yet appeared, or the disease may not actually develop until the injurious substance has been lying dormant in the worker's body for years. In either case, cessation of exposure to the injurious substance does not eliminate the possibility that the worker may develop the occupational disease in the future. Indeed, this characteristic latency period explains why a substance may be used in industry for many years before anyone realizes that it is hazardous.

Compensable traumatic injuries usually produce physical impairments that obviously are the result of an accident at the workplace. Occupational diseases, however, present greater problems of diagnosis. The initial question is whether the worker actually has a disease. If so, then a physician must determine which disease the worker has and what the cause of the disease may have been. Finally, the worker's level of impairment must be determined.

When the physician diagnoses a particular disease, its etiology may be unknown or the subject of controversy. Determining which stressor, if any, caused the disease in a particular worker may be impossible. Finally, ascertaining the exact nature of a diseased worker's physical impairment may be difficult.

ANALYSIS OF STATE LAW AS IT PERTAINS TO STRESS-RELATED CLAIMS

There is little federal involvement in stress-related workers' compensation claims. Most stress-related claims are resolved through state workers' compensation boards and state appeals courts. The result is an assortment of constantly evolving standards. A claim compensated in one state may not even be considered in another. Companies doing business in several states are faced with varying degrees of risk regarding stress-related claims. For example, an employee of a Cincinnati firm cannot seriously consider filing a claim based on mental stress unless a physical injury accompanies the claim. On the other hand, just across the river in Kentucky, stress-related claims for mental disabilities are treated like any other work-related claim.

From coast to coast, states differ on what types of mental disability claims may be compensated through worker's compensation. Most states recognize the compensability of claims where job stress causes a heart attack or ulcers. These claims are called mental-physical claims because the source of the injury is mental even though the disability is physical. The question in these claims is whether the workplace was the primary source of stress. Also, most states recognize physical-mental claims, when, for example, a back injury leads to depression. The mental disability is compensable because it involves a physical injury.

If an employee says that job stress led to a nervous breakdown and depression, this is called a mental-mental claim because there is no physical corroboration for either the source of the claim or the disability. At this point the states sharply differ. Some states do not recognize mental disability claims at all unless some type of physical injury is involved. Other states allow awards for mental disorders due to job stress. Mental disabilities are treated no differently than any other claim in these states.

As one may expect, this area of the law makes insurance companies nervous. Of primary concern are the mental-mental claims because the standards are so different from state to state. There appears to be a liberal trend in state case law favoring compensation of mental stress claims. Although these claims were virtually unheard of 15 years ago, the cost associated with them could soon reach $50 million annually. This trend is viewed as a further expansion of workers' compensation coverage to include awards for nervous breakdown, anxiety, and other mental disabilities due to pressure at the job. The greatest source of concern for the insurance industry, however, is the size of the pool of potential stress-related claimants. Traditional back injuries were largely confined to those doing heavy work, but stress is a condition that almost all workers are subject to.

Although it is generally accepted that workers' compensation benefits may be awarded for work-related mental or nervous disorders resulting from physical impact or physical injuries, there is less agreement concerning the compensability of mental or nervous disorders resulting from work-related emotional stimuli.

A number of courts have taken the position that a disabling mental disorder resulting from a work-related emotional stimulus may properly be considered an accidental injury or disease within the meaning of workers' compensation statutes. These courts have reasoned that there is no valid justification for distinguishing between mental disorders resulting from a physical impact or injury, the compensability of which is generally recognized, and mental disorders caused or aggravated by emotional stimuli, particularly in view of the policy of workers' compensation statutes to provide coverage for work-related disabilities in general.

Under this most liberal standard, mental disability claims are treated like any other claim, and no threshold requirement is specified for the stress that caused the disability. The compensability of such claims seems to turn on whether the workplace or an off-the-job problem is the primary source of the stress. For example, it was held that a psychogenic disability precipitated by employment was compensable within the meaning of the statute defining a compensable injury as one suffered "by accident arising out of and in the course of the employment or by disease proximately caused by or resulting from the nature of the employment."[25] Reasoning that the definition reflected a statutory policy indemnifying employees for all infirmities resulting from employment, the Supreme Court of Hawaii said that compensation could be awarded if the injury reasonably appeared to have flowed from the conditions under which an employee was required to work. Pointing out that the statute made no distinction between organic and psychic injuries, the court said that the legislature chose to treat all work-related injuries as a cost of production to be borne by industry and, ultimately, the community in general. The court added that mental disabilities resulting from employment are as much a cost of production as are physical injuries.

Some courts have taken the position that a disabling mental disorder induced by a work-related sudden emotional stimulus may properly be considered an accidental injury or disease within the meaning of the workers' compensation statutes. In Illinois,[26] for example, a successful mental disability claim requires the source of mental stress to be a sudden, severe, emotionally shocking event. The Illinois court reversed a judgment denying compensation benefits to a claimant who suffered a psychological disability as a result of viewing a co-worker's severed hand, which had been caught in a punch press. The claimant fainted after helping the victim and was hospitalized for treatment of anxiety reaction. The court held that an employee may be awarded compensation for a psychological disability produced by a sudden, severe emotional shock that is traceable to a definite time and place and to a readily perceivable cause, even though the employee suffered no physical trauma or injury. The court reasoned that there was little justification for a rule permitting payment of benefits to one suffering from a psychological disability caused by a minor physical injury and yet denying compensation to an employee with a similar psychological disability caused by a sudden, severe emotional shock.

A number of courts have reasoned that a disabling mental disorder induced by a work-related nonsudden emotional stimulus may properly be considered an accidental injury or disease under workers' compensation statutes. Although these courts do not require a single shocking event for mental injury, the source of stress should be unexpected, unusual, or extraordinary. Explaining that a nontraumatically caused mental injury is compensable only if it results from mental stresses and tensions that are of greater intensity than those experienced on a daily basis by employees generally, a Wisconsin court[27] reasoned that there was ample credible evidence to support a finding that a claimant, the purchasing agent for a mail-order cheese company, was exposed to work stresses that were out of the ordinary. These stresses resulted from the company's volume of business, the existence of deadlines, and problems caused by machine breakdowns and merchandise losses. There was also mention that medical evidence had established a causal connection between the employee's mental condition and the job and that work stress was the principal cause and major factor in the breakdown.

Some courts have taken the position that a disabling mental disorder resulting from a work-related emotional stimulus may not properly be considered an accidental injury or disease within the meaning of workers' compensation statutes. They have generally reasoned either that an emotional stimulus may not properly be considered an "accident" or that a mental disorder may not properly be considered an injury within the meaning of the compensation statutes. These courts rely on specific statutory language saying that any injury must be a physical one or at least have a physical element. In some cases, a physical disability caused by a stressful event, such as a heart attack, might be compensable, or a mental disability might be compensable if caused by a physical accident, such as depression from a broken back, but in no case would a nervous breakdown be compensated when the source is limited to job stress alone. Explaining that a psychic trauma was not a compensable accident, a Louisiana court[28] denied compensation benefits for a newspaper circulation representative who suffered a mental breakdown as the result of work-related demands and pressure, the accumulated fatigue of lengthy workdays, and considerable tension. The court pointed out that no single physical incident of trauma precipitated or contributed to the breakdown, which was possibly due to the effects of constant fatigue of several months' duration.

In summary, many cases support the view that such disorders are compensable accidental injuries or diseases within the framework of workers' compensation statutes, where the disorders are induced by emotional stimuli generally or by sudden or nonsudden emotional stimuli. Moreover there is authority that a mental or nervous disorder resulting from a work-related emotional stimulus may be compensable as an occupational disease. Courts recognizing the right to compensation generally have reasoned that compensability should not be made to depend on the nature of the cause of the disorder, and that mental or nervous disorders, whether they result from physical or emotional stimuli, are equally compensable.

However, a number of cases support the contrary view that mental or nervous disorders induced by work-related stress are not compensable accidental injuries or diseases. Courts taking this view have generally reasoned that such disorders could not be said to have been caused by "accident" or "injury" within the meaning of their compensation statutes.

A few work-related stress cases are categorized as shiftwork claims. In Tennessee an employee brought suit contending that the long hours and irregular shifts that he was required to work caused a disabling chronic anxiety reaction with hypertension and related complications.[29] He complained that his nerves were giving him difficulty and that he was not able to work shifts. He then worked regular hours without experiencing any difficulty until a strike occurred that required supervisory personnel, including himself, to work long hours (for about 1 month). During and after the strike his physical and mental condition deteriorated; he had difficulty sleeping, loss of appetite and weight, moodiness, and increased hypertension. His wife testified that he was short with his family and did not especially enjoy their company. He was directed to work the various shifts for less than the normal weekly duration of a shift, but the stress made him so nervous that he could not do the work. He subsequently quit when his supervisor told him it was not possible to give him a job with constant hours. Three doctors (psychiatrists) were of the opinion that shifting caused the difficulty, and the employee was advised to stop work. The Tennessee court was not prepared to hold that shiftwork or a requirement that supervisory personnel work long hours during a strike is a "risk connected with employment." These conditions are not present in any peculiar or increased degree in the employment in question, by comparison with employment generally. Furthermore the court pointed to the implication for business concerns engaging in shiftwork.

More recently, the Tennessee Supreme Court[30] denied compensation to a freight clerk in the trucking industry who claimed that his depressive disorder was aggravated when he was switched from the evening to the 2300–0730 shift. He could not sleep during the day and claimed that this inability worsened his depressive condition. The court reversed a state court's allowance of the claim, stating both that inability to sleep during the day was not an injury by accident and that the inability to sleep was not in the course of employment and was a hazard incidental to employment.

Although Tennessee courts appear to require a sudden emotional stimulus and therefore would likely deny recovery under a shiftwork theory, states such as Hawaii and California liberally interpret their workers' compensation statutes so as to permit recovery.

CONCLUSION

Until recently, most courts and legislatures required that workers' compensation claimants establish not only that their injuries were caused at work, but also that their injuries were "accidents" or "accidental in character." Physical trauma often was said to be a necessary cause of a compensable injury, and physical disability was sometimes said to be a necessary effect. Thus under the early workers' compensation laws of most states, for an incident to be compensable, both the cause of a medical condition and the medical condition itself must have been physical in nature. Current thinking in the field, on the other hand, emphasizes causal connection or work-relatedness. If a claimant can show that a medical condition was, in fact, caused by work, the requirements for workers' compensation probably are satisfied. Rules precluding recovery because an injured worker fails to show an accident are said to frustrate the basic purpose of workers' compensation.

A few state statutes appear to preclude compensability of psychiatric or emotional conditions that result from allowed injuries or occupational diseases. But, in general, there seldom has been a legal impediment to coverage of mental disabilities that result from the initial accident or occupational disease in already allowed claims. But any review of the history and development of workers' compensation law in most states reveals the novelty of compensability for mentally stressful incidents that give rise to solely psychic disabilities. In some states it took decades to decide that such a clearly work-related physical condition as a low-back strain caused by lifting ordinary weight should be treated as a compensable injury. The theory of recovery in such cases—now a thing of the past—is that, since the incident giving rise to the medical condition was not itself "external" or out-of-the-ordinary or physically traumatic, the claim was not compensable. The general rule regarding workers' compensation—that an employer takes its employees as it finds them, with all their weaknesses, diseases, and infirmities—apparently also applies to emotional weaknesses, diseases, and infirmities.

Cracks in the walls of noncompensability—particularly in regard to injury claims—have been growing rapidly in recent years, and in some states, the wall has tumbled down. The trend in the courts has been to permit recovery for stress-related claims. There appears to be an opposing trend within the state legislatures, on the part of the insurance lobbies, to limit or exclude recovery for stress-related injuries and diseases. Due to the vast numbers of potential claimants in this area of the law, it is not easy to predict outcomes. Individuals involved in stress-related claims should contact their state compensation offices and seek the advice of attorneys practicing in what is becoming a very specialized field of law.

REFERENCES

1. Stress Management in Work Settings, NIOSH publication no. 87-111, (1987).
2. Deleted.
3. Larson, The Nature and Origins of Workers' Compensation, 37 Cornell Law Quarterly 206 (1952).
4. Larson, Workers' Compensation Law 15 (1984).
5. D. Owen, Prosser A. and Keeton on the Law of Torts (5th ed. 1984).
6. Larson, The Law of Workers' Compensation 39 (1964).
7. Larson, supra note 3, at 17.
8. Id. at 17–18.
9. Prosser, supra note 5, at 569 (1984).
10. Larson, supra note 3, at 226.
11. Larson, supra note 4, at 33.
12. Id. at 33.
13. Id. at 34.
14. Wisconsin Department of Industry, Labor and Human Relations, Workers' Compensation Division, 100th Anniversary of the Department (1983).
15. Id.
16. L. White, Human Debris: The Injured Worker in America (1983).
17. D. Hanes, The First British Workers' Compensation Act, 1897 (1968).
18. Prosser, supra note 5, at 573.
19. Larson, supra note 4, at 37.
20. Id.
21. 147 Wis. 327, 133 N.W. 209 (1911).
22. Larson, supra note 3, at 233.
23. Larson, supra note 4.
24. U.S. Chamber of Commerce, Analysis of Workers' Compensation Laws (1987). Published by U.S. Chamber of Commerce, Washington, D.C.
25. Royal State National Insurance Co. v Labor & Industrial Relations Appeal Board, 53 Hawaii 32, 487 P2d 278 (1971).
26. Pathfinder Co. v Industrial Commission 62 Ill 2d 556, 343 NE2d 913 (1976).
27. Swiss Colony, Inc. v Dept of Industry, Labor and Human Relations, 72 Wis 2d 46, 240 NW2d 128 (1976).
28. Johnson v Hartford Accident & Indemnity Co. 196 SO 2d 635 (La. App, 1967).
29. Lawson, Employers Insurance of Wausau, 330 F. Supp. 321 (D.C. Tenn. 1971).
30. Henley v Roadway Express 699 SW2d 150 (Tenn. 1985).

ROGER R. ROSA, PHD
MICHAEL H. BONNET, PHD
RICHARD R. BOOTZIN, PHD
CHARMANE I. EASTMAN, PHD
TIMOTHY MONK, PHD
PATRICIA E. PENN, PHD
DONALD I. TEPAS, PHD
JAMES K. WALSH, PHD

INTERVENTION FACTORS FOR PROMOTING ADJUSTMENT TO NIGHTWORK AND SHIFTWORK

For authors' affiliations and acknowledgment of source, see p. 415.

Reprint requests to:
Roger R. Rosa, PhD
National Institute for Occupational Safety and Health
Division of Biomedical and Behavioral Science
Cincinnati, OH 45226

Many human physiological and psychological functions follow a 24-hour cycle related to a diurnal, or daytime, activity pattern. This is true of several processes as diverse as respiration rate, urine excretion, cell mitosis, blood pressure, adrenal hormone production, enzyme activity, and even behavioral output such as short-term memory function and reaction time. A good example of a physiological process showing a circadian rhythm is body temperature—an index of basal metabolic rate. In humans, body temperature reaches a high point in late afternoon (1600–1800) and a low point in early morning (0400–0600). Body temperature may be influenced by activity, but it is not controlled by it.[7] Changes in the activity cycle do not readily result in changes in circadian rhythms, although these rhythms can adjust to a different activity cycle after a period of several days.[2] The relative intransigence of circadian rhythms has important implications for work scheduling. Shiftworkers are often required to work at night before their circadian rhythm has adjusted to a nighttime schedule.

Continuous operations are a fact of life in numerous industries. Critical industries operating continuously include public services such as police and fire protection, hospital staffing, and public utilities. Other industries require continuous processing, such as steel and petrochemical production. Consequently, shiftwork must be recognized as an inevitable part of the job for a significant segment (approximately one-fourth) of the American work force.[27]

In the simplest terms, shiftwork periodically forces workers to be awake at times when they would normally be asleep. They must be active at times of low physiological arousal and sleep at times of high physiological arousal. This inversion of the sleep/wake pattern results in the dissociation of several physiological, psychological, and social rhythms. It is not unreasonable, then, to construe this disruption as a fatiguing, stressful state for the worker experiencing it, and even for the family experiencing it through the worker.

The disruptions caused by night and rotating shiftwork potentially have both short-term and long-term consequences. In the short run, the safety of both the workers and the public who might be dependent on them could be compromised by reduced worker alertness, which increases the potential for accidents and operational errors. In the long run, workers' health may be compromised if they do not readily adapt to shiftwork or cannot eventually move into a strictly daytime job.

Reduced worker alertness on the nightshift is a function of inadequate day sleep and also of reduced physiological arousal attributed to the circadian rhythm. Many studies of day sleep after nightshift have demonstrated that day sleep is shorter and lighter and beset with many more interruptions than night sleep.[91] Thus, day sleep is less restorative than night sleep; it therefore further compromises an already reduced arousal governed by the circadian rhythm. Time-of-day differences in errors and accidents attributable to lack of alertness have been demonstrated in a variety of contexts. For example, meter-reading errors at a Swedish gas works and single-vehicle accidents judged to be fatigue related were both shown to be most frequent in the late night and early morning hours.[57]

Time of day also has been implicated in some notable individual cases of disaster-related human error.[57] At the Three-Mile Island nuclear reactor, shiftworkers failed to correct a stuck valve. This error of omission was judged a significant factor in the near-meltdown. The Chernobyl catastrophe, reported to have been the result of human error, began shortly after 0100. Poor judgment related to sleep loss and shiftwork was also cited as a factor in the report of the Presidential Commission on the Space Shuttle Challenger Accident. Another near-accident in a NASA launch was attributed to error by operators who had been on duty for 11 hours during their third night of 12-hour shifts.

In addition to the general malaise from sleep disruptions, shiftwork has been associated with long-term health consequences including gastrointestinal and cardiovascular disorders.[61] The gastrointestinal problems are mostly general discomfort and nausea, but peptic ulcer disease has also been reported.[4] The mechanisms linking shiftwork, disruption of circadian rhythms, and gastrointestinal problems are not clear. It has been shown, however, that secretion of intestinal enzymes follows a circadian rhythm,[86] and shiftworkers consistently report disrupted eating schedules.

A number of studies have identified a higher incidence of cardiovascular disease in rotating shiftworkers despite their tendency to leave nightwork if they experience poor health. The most elegant study of cardiovascular disorders in shiftworkers is from Knutsson et al.[44] Researchers traced the medical histories of shiftworkers in one small city over a period of 15 years. A threefold higher risk of contracting cardiovascular illness was demonstrated in shiftworkers, independent of age and smoking history.

While we have been concentrating on the physiological stress of circadian rhythm disruption, we should also emphasize the psychological stress produced by disruption of familial and other social rhythms.[94] Workers sometimes rate the loss of family and other social contacts as the most important disadvantage of rotating shifts. In fact, workers are sometimes willing to increase their physiological cost (by sacrificing sleep, for example) to maximize social gain. The social and personal cost of working shifts has become even higher in the 1970s and 1980s because there are more single-parent families or families with two parents employed.

It is clear that the 24-hour workday has both psychological and physiological costs for the worker and the family. Moreover, the need for 24-hour staffing of factories, hospitals, safety, and support services will probably increase. Thus, we will continue to be faced with conflicts between the work hours required of our 24-hour society and the diurnal nature of human physiology and psychology. In view of recent fatigue-related transportation accidents and nuclear power catastrophes, it is critical that the scientific community look for ways to foster adjustment to, or ways of coping with, shiftwork. Better adjustment to shiftwork will benefit not only the worker's safety and health, but also the public's safety and health.

The present report is a first step toward developing interventions with potential for minimizing excessive fatigue and promoting adjustment to nightwork and extended workshifts. Several physiological and behavioral factors are considered for possible control and manipulation to reduce fatigue and enhance alertness. Review of these factors is aimed at proposing directions for research into the most feasible intervention areas. The reviewed factors include: (1) **work schedule design,** aimed at redesigning schedules to allow more rapid adjustment of biological rhythm or longer recovery periods; (2) **rest/sleep scheduling** directed toward timing rest or sleep periods to minimize or counteract bouts of fatigue; (3) **environmental stimuli,** focused on controlling stimuli to promote alertness or adjustment to new work hours; (4) **physical activity and conditioning,** aimed at controlling physical activity and improving conditioning to resist fatigue; (5) **pharmacological aids,** directed toward using drugs to induce sleep or promote alertness at unusual times; (6) **diet,** focused on developing regimens to potentially improve alertness or relaxation; and (7) **individual behavioral techniques,** pointed toward better personal control of fatigue, alertness, and stress.

WORK SCHEDULE DESIGN*

Work schedules necessarily conform to the need to deliver a product or service in an efficient and timely manner. The schedule adopted by a particular organization is some combination of precedent and current practical concerns. When the schedule involves nightwork or extended workshifts, however, it might or might not account for the psychophysiological demand placed on the worker. Recent alternatives to commonly used work schedules have potential for lessening physiological and psychological stress on the worker. Lowering stress

---

* Information in this section is based on Monk.[58]

should translate not only into improved job efficiency, but into better safety and health. Considered in this section are design factors pertaining to shift rotation and length of workday and workweek as they affect the worker.

Shift Rotation Factors

One of the most commonly used shift schedules in the United States requires the worker to rotate weekly from day to night to evening shifts.[87] This pattern has been designated a "backward" rotation because its direction is counterclockwise, or backward in time. The backward rotation is sometimes preferred by shiftworkers because it is usually structured to provide a "long change" between nightshift and evening shift.[92] In the long change, 2 or 3 nonworking days occur after nightshift, followed by more free time during the day before return to the evening shift.

Biological rhythm research has suggested that the weekly backward rotation may not be the most adaptable pattern for shiftwork. Two characteristics of the human circadian rhythm contribute to this suggestion. One characteristic is its tendency to adapt quite slowly—usually taking 2–3 weeks—to nighttime activity.[2] The other characteristic is its endogenous period, or time to complete a cycle. At 25 hours, it is slightly longer than the 24-hour day.[100]

The first characteristic, slow adaptation, means that a weekly rotation is too short to allow full adaptation of the circadian rhythm. A maladapted rhythm affects both the ability to remain alert while awake and the ability to obtain rest and recovery through adequate sleep.[2] Consequently, researchers[25] have argued that very long rotations (3–4 weeks), or permanent nightshifts, are desirable to allow full circadian rhythm adaptation for certain tasks. For other tasks, very rapid rotations (shift changes every 2 days) are desirable so that the circadian rhythm never diverges from its daytime orientation.

Both slow and fast rotations have advantages and disadvantages. The theoretical advantage of slow rotation is complete inversion of the circadian rhythm to a nighttime activity pattern. For a slow rotation to work best, however, the worker must remain on a night schedule on nonwork days, but social and other personal pursuits may make a daytime nonwork schedule more attractive. Fast rotations have the advantage of keeping the circadian rhythm in a daytime orientation, which tends to maximize waking alertness and restful sleep on day and evening shifts. The circadian rhythm is not in a constant state of disruption from partial adaptation to different day and night orientations. It has also been suggested that a stable circadian rhythm minimizes stress and thus carries fewer long-term health consequences, such as cardiovascular disease.[43] Two disadvantages of rapid rotations, however, are very low nighttime alertness and poor daytime sleep because of the day orientation of the rhythm.

The other characteristic of the circadian rhythm opposing backward weekly rotation is its 25-hour endogenous period. Under normal conditions, external cues (zeitgebers) force the rhythm into a 24-hour period. Under isolated laboratory conditions, where the individual is allowed to "free-run" without time cues, however, an approximately 25-hour circadian period is observed.[100] During free-running at the endogenous circadian period, sleep times occur later and later with respect to clock time. This forward-moving tendency of the circadian rhythm makes it easier for people to stay awake later, but more difficult to fall asleep earlier, than the normal bedtime.

Some researchers[17] have argued that shift schedules should be designed to move clockwise in time to take advantage of the forward-moving tendency of the circadian rhythm. In such a design, the shiftworker would start on dayshift, move forward to evening shift, then to nightshift, which would be followed by rest days before the return to dayshift. Theoretically, the forward-rotating schedule allows the worker to gradually move sleep times progressively later with respect to clock time so that it is easier to fall asleep. The backward rotation forces the worker to try to sleep earlier, which is more difficult because it is contrary to the endogenous tendency of the circadian rhythm.

As stated above, the advantage of the backward rotation is the "long change" from nightshift to evening shift and the extra rest potentially provided. From the biological rhythm perspective, however, the forward rotation and its potential for quicker adaptation is favored by most researchers. It is not clear, however, whether a forward rotation consistently results in well-adapted sleep times. Turek's hypothetical analysis[93] of sleep opportunities on both backward and forward rotations suggests that neither schedule permits sleep to rotate consistently in one direction or another.

Direct comparisons of fast versus slow, or forward versus backward, rotations are rare. One study[17] introduced two forward rotations to subgroups of workers at a plant originally on a backward weekly rotation. One forward rotation was slow, changing every 21 days. The other forward rotation was weekly. Compared to the original schedule, worker satisfaction improved with the 21-day shift schedule, and overall plant productivity increased. It is not clear, however, whether these improvements were due to the rate or the direction of rotation because both were changed simultaneously.

Three other studies considered the effects of speed of rotation on different variables. In one study, Knauth and Rutenfranz[42] measured adaptation of the body temperature circadian rhythm during permanent nightshift versus rapidly rotating shift systems. Body temperature in permanent nightworkers never fully adapted even after 21 nights. Body temperature in rapidly rotating shiftworkers barely deviated from the daytime rhythm orientation. On the basis of these results, the researchers advised the rapid rotation. In another study, Pocock et al.[73] measured absenteeism on a backward weekly rotation compared to a forward, 2- to 3-day rotation. Absence due to illness was more frequent after changing to the rapid rotation. The authors concluded that rapid rotation, while popular, was more demanding for the worker. As discussed above, the lack of adaptation to nightshift could be a factor contributing to this demand. In a third study, Williamson and Sanderson[102] compared responses from several self-report questionnaires obtained from workers on a weekly forward rotation to the same measures obtained after 5 months on a 2- to 3-day forward rotation. Significant improvements in subjective health, well-being, and satisfaction were observed after the change to the rapid shift rotation.

In summary, we have considered two work schedule design factors as potential interventions to alleviate the fatigue and stress of night and shiftwork. One factor involves the speed of shift rotation, and the other factor, the direction of shift rotation. With respect to direction, forward rotation seems more desirable on the basis of deductions from biological rhythm research. With respect to speed, slow rotation is warranted if circadian adaptation to nightwork is desired, and fast rotation if lack of adaptation to nightwork can be tolerated.

Compressed Workweeks

Recent research at NIOSH has been concerned with an innovation in work schedules called the compressed workweek. The compressed workweek requires more hours of work per day in exchange for fewer days of work per week. Typical schedules include a 4-day workweek at 10 hours per day, or an alternating schedule of 3 days on, 4 days off, 4 days on, 3 days off at 12 hours per day.[90] For shiftworkers, it is hoped that more days off will allow better recovery from nightwork and also allow larger blocks of time for social contact and leisure pursuits. One 12-hour schedule, for example, allows for every other weekend off. This schedule is quite popular because it allows more frequent social contact on weekends.

The benefit to the worker of more days off with compressed workweeks must be balanced against the risk of greater fatigue and less alertness from the extended workshifts required under that schedule. Recall that the shiftworker may already be experiencing reduced alertness, and these deficits might get worse with a longer workshift, especially a longer nightshift. NIOSH studies[80] of compressed workweeks using 12-hour workshifts have verified increased fatigue and decreased alertness on these shifts compared to 8-hour shifts. We have demonstrated that these effects are especially acute at night, when the fatigue of hours of work exacerbates the low point in circadian arousal. The shorter workweeks (2–4 days in our studies), however, did appear to offset some of this fatigue.

The popularity of compressed workweeks at the worksites we studied suggests that these schedules will persist as alternatives to typical shift rotations. The fatigue and stress of nightshifts remain, however, and may be compounded by such schedules. Thus, measures in addition to the schedule change should be introduced to attempt to counteract some of the nightwork effects.

SLEEP SCHEDULING DURING SHIFTWORK*

Shiftwork necessitates changes in habitual sleep/wake rhythms, often resulting in appreciable sleep loss. Because of the circadian rhythm, decreased alertness and performance is more likely during nocturnal workshifts, especially after sleep loss. In general, sleep loss produces more fatigue as the duration of a task increases, as physical or mental workload increases in difficulty, and as memory demand increases. Sleep loss also produces more fatigue when the task is newly acquired or the pace is set externally.[38] Sleep reverses degradations in performance and alertness better than rest without sleep.[51] Therefore, optimizing sleep is a priority for the shiftworker. However, as discussed earlier, shiftworkers often find it difficult to sleep during the day after nightwork. Internal circadian rhythm cues signaling arousal and external noise from an active household and neighborhood combine to make day sleep difficult. For this reason, short naps are often taken to supplement longer periods of day sleep. They are often taken to bring total sleep time closer to the 8-hour average. In our worksite study of rotating shifts,[80] for example, napping after nightshifts occurred 29% of the time, bringing total sleep time to 7.4 hours.

The advantages of napping have not been systematically studied in civilian shiftwork operations requiring 8–12 hours of work per day. Almost all nap

---

* Information in this section is based on Bonnet.[9]

studies[18,64,65] have been conducted on people in extended operations requiring constant work, with very little sleep, for periods of 2–3 days. Acute bouts of extended operations, simulating those required in defense, public safety, and medical emergencies, are not directly applicable to chronic periods of nightwork and sleep loss experienced by the civilian shiftworker. Studies of chronic nightwork and napping would be most relevant to the population served by NIOSH. Nonetheless, studies of napping during acute periods of extended work do point to potential beneficial effects.

Most of the extended operation studies begin with a normal night of sleep and interject 2- to 4-hour sleep periods at various times during the continuous vigil. Psychomotor performance, alertness, mood, or performance at various job simulations are measured at intervals during the operation. The timing of the nap designates whether it is intended to prevent anticipated fatigue and alertness loss (*prophylactic* naps) or to compensate for experienced fatigue and alertness loss (*replacement* and *maintenance* naps).

Prophylactic Naps

One group of studies has examined what have been called prophylactic naps.[18] These are naps taken before a period of sleep loss and intended to enhance performance during the extended work period. In these studies, subjects are given extra sleep ranging from 1 to 4 hours during the day preceding an initial nocturnal work period.[5,10,18,26,66] Without naps, all of these studies demonstrated a substantial decrease in performance and alertness after a night of total sleep loss. With 1- to 4-hour naps on the preceding day, morning performance was clearly improved compared to the total sleep loss condition in each experiment. These studies provide evidence that a nap before an all-night workshift or continuous operation can be effective in alleviating fatigue.

Replacement and Maintenance Naps

Replacement naps compensate for previous loss of sleep. Their assumed benefits for the shiftworker have not been documented. In extended vigils, however, such naps helped either to maintain alertness levels or to delay their decline.[18,51] More importantly, naps were clearly more effective than rest without sleep at those times.

Maintenance naps are a special case of replacement naps. They would occur on the job, *during* the workshift. These naps could compensate for daytime sleep deprivation or, in the absence of significant sleep loss, they could serve as a bridge over the nighttime low point in circadian alertness and arousal. Many Japanese 24-hour industries have provided the option of a sleeping break at work to their employees. They have even provided sleeping rooms for this purpose.[69] In his survey of Japanese napping practices on nightshift, Kogi[45] reported that 40–50% of the workers napped at night and that their naps lasted 2–3 hours. We know of no systematic practice of maintenance napping in the United States.

There is only one demonstration of the effectiveness of maintenance napping as it might apply to the civilian shiftworker. Gillberg[26] let subjects sleep for 1 hour in the middle of a one-night vigil in the laboratory and demonstrated improved alertness compared to resting while awake in the middle of a vigil. Napping over several successive nightshifts has never been tested.

Napping as an intervention for reducing the fatigue of shiftwork raises several empirical questions. Some of these questions are encountered in studies of extended operations over a period of 2–3 nights. Such questions address how long the nap should be, at what time it should occur, how long a person needs to "wake up," and what kinds of work napping affects.

Specific to the shiftworker are questions about the longer-term influences of napping on adaptation to nightwork. In the short run, the present evidence suggests that naps would facilitate adaptation to nightwork. Napping before or during the first 1–2 nightshifts should help maintain alertness and ease the transition from a day or evening shift. No data are available, however, on how napping affects adaptation to long-term nightwork. Over several nights, napping could either help or hinder adaptation. Napping could help adaptation by maintaining alertness, by bridging low points in arousal, and by providing better recovery than rest (without sleep). Napping could hinder adaptation by providing an excuse for sacrificing regular sleep, by making a person too drowsy upon awakening, or by slowing the inversion of the circadian rhythm. The latter possibility is based on a study[54] that showed sleep to be an "anchoring" or synchronizing point for circadian rhythms. As such, naps could keep circadian rhythms in a daytime orientation. This might be beneficial to workers on rapidly rotating shifts but detrimental to those on slowly rotating shifts or permanent nightshifts.

In summary, naps have good potential as an effective intervention for reducing fatigue and promoting adaptation to nightshifts. Their long-term effects need systematic study in terms of their interactions with other sleep, circadian rhythms, and rate of adaptation to different shift schedules.

ENVIRONMENTAL STIMULI

Manipulating environmental stimuli such as temperature and light would be an unobtrusive way to influence adaptation to night and shiftwork. If effective parameters can be established, environmental conditions promoting adaptation could be established at the workplace and in the home. With minimal effort, the worker could be exposed to these stimuli and could possibly accomplish other tasks at the same time. However, environmental stimuli can also have detrimental effects.

Ambient Temperature*

Intuitively, it appears that ambient temperature would have a significant impact upon adjustment to various shift schedules. Clearly, temperature varies in importance with the type of work being performed, the time of day, and the season. Therefore, it is not unusual, for example, that 61% of iron and steel workers rated the afternoon shift the most tiring in the summer, and 92% rated the nightshift the most tiring in the winter.[67] Few studies, however, have looked at the complex interactions of time of day, length of work period, time at task, physical condition of workers, and number of days or weeks on a shift as a function of temperature. No references could be found examining the effects of low temperatures on shiftwork. The lack of studies on cold effects is surprising considering the number of people who must work in cold or inclement weather.

With respect to higher temperatures, one study examined the interactive effects of shiftwork, heat, and task complexity.[70] Subjects did desk work at either

---

* Information in this section is based on Bonnet.[9]

23.4 or 27.7°C (74.1 or 81.9°F) for a week of dayshifts or a week of nightshifts. It was concluded that during the dayshift, heat made the subjects less flexible in dealing with a complex task. During the night, subjects generally performed more poorly, but differences as a function of temperature were not found. Heat during the day slowed reaction times to levels seen during nightwork, but, again, heat did not cause further reductions at night. No clear interaction with heat and time on shift was seen. Adaptation effects over the week were not reported. In a companion study,[82] no difference in circadian rhythms of adrenaline or potassium excretion were observed as a function of the interactive effects of heat and shiftwork. The lack of remarkable effects for temperature in these studies is not surprising given the limited range of temperature examined.

Pokorski et al.[74,75] examined the interactive effects of heat (no temperatures reported) and energy expenditure on heart rate and subjective ratings of fatigue in four groups of shiftworkers. Heat resulted in higher heart rates and reports of greater fatigue in some groups despite a lower energy expenditure than other groups.

Several studies have documented circadian rhythms in skin temperature, deep body temperature, and sweating. In a circadian study of sweating, Little and Rummel[50] found a peak in water loss at 2000 and a trough at 1200. They also found some decline in the amplitude of the body temperature curve. It is unclear, however, how these circadian changes interact with ambient temperature in affecting the ability to work.

While these few studies suggest that heat can increase the stress of work, they are insufficient to address the issue of heat as a control factor in adjustment to shiftwork. Temperatures, however, are normally lower at night than during the day. Thus, it can be presumed that heat exposure would be lower on nightshift, and this might offset some heat-related physiological decrements. In cold environments, however, the worker might be forced to expend more energy (and become more fatigued) at night than in the day owing to a lower nighttime body temperature.

In summary, ambient temperature affects the ability to work, but there are no studies actually manipulating temperature to reduce fatigue or to improve nighttime alertness.

Bright Light*

Recent studies have reported manipulating exposure to light to change circadian rhythms.[16,20,23,36,48,101] Development of these techniques in the workplace is promising because many of the problems of shiftwork can be attributed to poorly adapted circadian rhythms.

As discussed earlier, it is difficult for circadian rhythms to adjust to the nightshift. Consequently, some experts recommend rapidly rotating shift systems that do not disrupt circadian rhythms. With a minimal number of consecutive nightshifts, the concomitant sleep loss is minimized. Such schedules, however, force people to work at the low arousal point of the circadian cycle, when efficiency may be decreased and accident risk increased.

An alternative to requiring work at the circadian low point is to induce a shift in circadian rhythms. Nightworkers would then enjoy better daytime sleep

---

* Information in this section is based on Eastman.[22]

after work and greater alertness while at work. This strategy requires better control over the zeitgebers (external controls or time cues) that determine the phase of circadian rhythms. A problem with developing such a strategy, however, is that the relative importance for human circadian rhythms of various zeitgebers (sleep schedule, meal schedule, knowledge of time of day, social cues, light/dark cycle, etc.) is unclear. The light/dark cycle, however, is one zeitgeber that has recently shown some promise of promoting circadian rhythm adjustment.

It was once thought that the light/dark cycle was not an important zeitgeber for humans because they, in otherwise constant conditions, "free-ran" (did not entrain) to a 24-hour light/dark cycle.[100] Social and other time cues seemed to be of greater importance because removing them through temporal isolation of the subject resulted in altered circadian rhythms. Lewy et al.,[49] however, suggested that very bright light might be an effective zeitgeber for man. They demonstrated that very bright light altered certain endocrine circadian rhythms that are not affected by ordinary indoor light. Their discovery triggered several lines of research on the influence of bright light on several human biological rhythms. One line of research is evaluating bright light as an antidote for winter depression. Another line of research is determining the parameters of bright light that will shift normal human circadian rhythms.

In animals, it is well established that controlled light exposure (even ordinary room light) can shift the phase of free-running circadian rhythms.[72] The direction (advance or delay) and magnitude (number of hours) of the shift depend on *when* the light is applied within the circadian cycle. This relationship is specified by a phase response curve.

In applying the principles derived from animal experiments, we expect morning light to advance rhythms (make them peak earlier) and evening light to delay rhythms (make them peak later). Lewy et al.[48] used these techniques to demonstrate advances with morning light and delays with evening light in patients with winter depression. However, significant phase shifts in the normal control subjects were not observed. Honma et al.[36] were able to advance free-running rhythms with morning light but did not find delays with evening light. Czeisler et al.[16] produced a large phase delay with evening light in one woman with unusually advanced circadian rhythms.

In general, the results of the few studies completed so far are consistent with the concept of a human phase response curve to bright light. However, because the expected shifts cannot always be demonstrated, research is needed to determine the optimal parameters of light (timing, intensity, duration, etc.) to produce a desired phase shift.

If future research confirms that the light/dark cycle is a powerful zeitgeber for man, then we may be able to manipulate that cycle to ameliorate the problems of shiftwork, jet lag, and some circadian rhythm-based sleep disorders. (The use of light to shorten the duration of jet lag is further addressed in Chapter 9.) The treatment itself would be relatively easy and inexpensive. It only requires exposing the person to bright light, produced by banks of artificial light, at an appropriate time of day. It is more difficult, however, to block out light that might impinge upon the person at an inappropriate time of day. For example, if bright light were used in the evening to delay circadian rhythms, inadvertent exposure to morning sunlight could advance the circadian rhythm and cancel the effect of the evening light. This is not a problem in experiments performed in temporal isolation units, but it would affect practical situations such as shiftwork. Much additional work is necessary to determine how much sunlight should be blocked (e.g., with window shades, dark glasses, etc.) to prevent unwanted phase shifts. Even if the total bright-light exposure pattern could be successfully controlled, we do not know the extent to which other 24-hour zeitgebers would interfere with attempts to shift circadian rhythms.

Eastman[21] has recently proposed light-work-sleep schedules for shiftworkers that are expected to shift circadian rhythms so that sleep and work will always occur at appropriate phases of the circadian cycle. These schedules employ strategically placed sequences of a gradually shifting sleep/wake schedule (e.g., a 26-hour schedule) coupled with bright light exposure patterns produced with light banks, welder's goggles, and other means. She has been testing components of these schedules on normal volunteers and has been able to shift circadian rhythms in some people, despite other conflicting 24-hour zeitgebers.[20,21,23] Future work is aimed at shiftworkers to determine the optimal light-work-sleep schedules required to improve sleep, reduce fatigue, and maintain alertness.

PHYSICAL ACTIVITY AND CONDITIONING*

Ability to adapt to, or withstand, extended workshifts and rotating shift schedules could depend on the physical work load demanded of workers and on their physical ability to respond to that demand. It seems plausible that manipulation of both the physical demand and the fitness of the worker to withstand that demand should foster adaptation to a work schedule. However, factors such as the time of day of work and the length of the work period have rarely been measured directly in studies of physical work or the physical condition of workers. This section will review each of these variables and attempt to synthesize findings about them where possible.

Time of Day of Work

Because physical work involves the production of energy, changes in the relationship of cardiac and respiratory variables in conjunction with metabolic variables dictate the ability to perform work. Important circadian rhythms for the production of work include sympathetic activity and the production of glucocorticoids, catecholamines, and pituitary hormones. Activity in all of these systems is typically reduced at night, and decreased availability of glycogen and lipids at night should limit the ability to perform long bouts of strenuous exercise. At night, there is also a decrease in respiratory frequency coupled with a reduction in tidal volume, vital capacity, and alveolar ventilation.[53] Cardiac changes that accompany the nocturnal respiratory changes include decreased arterial systolic pressure, pulse pressure, and (usually) heart rate.[41,103]

Physical fitness and work capacity is typically measured by VO_2 max (maximal volume of oxygen), which is based on the relationship between heart rate and oxygen uptake during increasing levels of work. However, formulae developed for the calculation of VO_2 max have been based on the results of daytime studies[103] and are not directly comparable to measures of nightwork. Heart rate, for example, starts at a lower level and increases more slowly in response to increasing work load at night.[103] This lower level may make subjects

---

* Information in this section is based on Bonnet.[9]

appear more fit, especially for very short work periods. Consequently, VO_2 max at night should be determined directly, not from existing formula.

Wojtczak-Jaroszowa[103] compared VO_2 max in a group of 24 subjects starting at either 0100 or 0900. When measured directly, 83% of subjects had a lower VO_2 max at night compared to daytime values (3.6 L/min vs 3.8 L/min). There was no significant difference for the calculated values (3.8 L/min vs 3.7 L/min). These data indicate that there is about a 5% decrease in the ability to perform work at night. Clearly, this decrease interacts with other variables to further degrade performance until circadian rhythms adjust to the shift schedule.

Length of Work Period

Historically, it was common to observe tasks for 20- to 25-minute periods and to use values found to predict performance over 8-hour workdays. This procedure often led to an overestimation of the amount of work performed in 8 hours. Similarly, using 8-hour models to predict production over longer workshifts overestimates the ability to do physical work.

One of the most quantified variables for examining the length of the work period is lifting capacity.[55,56] Studies of standardized, prolonged lifting show that an average male tolerates lifting a 19.64-kg box for 25 minutes (perhaps 50% VO_2 max)[56] and that his ability to lift declines over time, even with normal breaks. By the end of an 8-hour shift, he would only be able to lift about 12.99 kg for 25 minutes. From these and other data, a 30% VO_2 max load is frequently accepted as the limit for prolonged physical effort.[47] This limit constrains box weight to about 16.31 kg throughout an 8-hour shift. If the workday is extended to 12 hours, there is an additional weight decrease of 12–22% per lift.[55] By the end of 12 hours, workers may be willing to lift only 11.62 kg (or 15.63 kg averaged across the shift).

The above data only apply to dayshift workers. Wojtczak-Jaroszowa[103] examined shiftworkers in a glass factory before work and at four points during each of the three daily shifts. The work required 25–30% of each worker's VO_2 max. The results indicated that pulmonary ventilation, oxygen uptake, and energy expenditure were significantly higher during the nightshift than in all other shifts. Although the speed of work on the nightshift was slightly slower, the energy expenditure was about 10% higher. These results were replicated in a laboratory study of young adult male and females who rode on a bicycle ergometer at about 30% VO_2 max for 8 hours (with frequent rest periods) during day, evening, and night hours. Results indicated a characteristic increase in pulse rate across the 8-hour work period and a tendency for pulse rate to start at lower values during nightwork. Pulse rate rose more quickly at night so that it was higher at the end of that shift compared to the other shifts.

The implications of these data are clear. The 5% decrease in ability to perform work at night is magnified when a full 8-hour shift is examined, so that overall nighttime performance loss is greater. The increasing popularity of 12-hour shifts will again magnify these effects. Thus, it is important to assess lifting capacity (and other physical tasks) not only during the day, but also during the night, so that separate standards for nightshifts can be established.

Physical Condition of Workers

Physical condition directly affects major physiological variables such as heart rate and VO_2 max, which normally are used to measure work tolerance and circadian effects on work tolerance. Consequently, physical condition has a clear and direct impact on the amount of physical work that can be accomplished. Of particular interest for this review are studies suggesting that improved physical condition can either increase tolerance to shiftwork or increase rate of adjustment to shiftwork. Only a few studies, all by one research team, demonstrate these effects.

Harma et al.[32] found that physically fit dayworkers had lower heart rates, less perceived exertion, and faster recovery of heart rate during both day and night than workers of average fitness. These differences, coupled with a larger amplitude circadian rhythm, led these investigators to conclude that physically fit people can tolerate shiftwork better than less fit people.

In follow-up studies, Harma et al.[30,31] examined the effects of a physical training program on the mood, sleep, and performance of a group of three-shift nurses. After 4 months of two to six training sessions per week, the exercise group had a 5-beat decrease in heart rate and a 5% increase in VO_2 max. The control group had no such changes. The exercise group also reported decreased general fatigue (particularly during the nightshift), decreased musculoskeletal symptoms, and increased sleep length after the evening shift. The nocturnal decrease in subjective fatigue was considered most important, because fatigue is usually highest at night. On the basis of these studies, Harma et al.[28] suggested that the most important factors in determining tolerance to shiftwork in women were maximal oxygen consumption (VO_2 max) and muscle strength.

One study did not find conditioning beneficial. Moog and Hildebrandt[59] attempted to determine if physical conditioning during a workshift increased speed of adaptation to the workshift. Training consisted of 30 minutes of riding a bicycle ergometer at 0300. Changes in sleep and body temperature rhythms were used as indices of adaptation. No differences in these rhythms were observed between exercising subjects and nonexercising controls.

These studies suggest that there are beneficial effects of physical training, but that these effects may be limited to overall increases in strength and more positive subjective reports. It is not clear whether physical activity (either self-scheduled or work-scheduled) increases adjustment to shiftwork. While this conclusion may be disheartening to proponents of physical training, it is clear that important variables remain to be examined such as the amount of training and the exact circadian placement of the exercise in relationship to the work/rest cycle. Such studies should also control the placement of sleep and rest periods to further facilitate the readaptation of the circadian rhythm.

Summary

These studies suggest that a 5–10% decline in work capacity is likely to occur during nocturnal work periods compared to daytime work periods. This decline is a result of a decrease in VO_2 max interacting with the 8-hour nocturnal work-shift. The ability to perform work declines as time on task and length of work period increase, and these effects are more pronounced at night. In general, fatigue increases most rapidly as energy expenditure increases above 50% VO_2 max. It is not clear whether exercise and physical fitness promote adaptation to nightwork. However, experiments that place different amounts of physical activity at carefully chosen points in the circadian cycle have not been reported and should be undertaken.

PHARMACOLOGICAL AIDS*

Two principal complaints of nightworkers involve insufficient or substandard sleep and impaired alertness during working hours. The degree to which these problems can be alleviated with pharmacological aids is the focus of this section.

Prescription Sedative-Hypnotics, Daytime Sleep, and Nocturnal Alertness

For people working nights, the primary abnormality of sleeping during the day is a reduction in total sleep time. Initial ability to fall asleep is not a frequent problem. Awakenings after sleep onset, however, are more frequent and longer during the day. Sleeping more than 5 or 6 hours per day is often quite difficult. The reduction and disruption of sleep appears to worsen with age,[3,96] and adaptation appears to be minimal. Even long-term nightworkers show sleep patterns indicating little evidence of adaptation to daytime sleep.[98]

The efficacy of sedative-hypnotic medication in the treatment of insomnia associated with nightwork has not been extensively studied. Compounds of interest include both benzodiazepines and over-the-counter compounds. Barbiturates and other older hypnotics (e.g., chloral hydrate, ethchlorvynol, glutethimide) will not be considered here because they play a limited role in the management of insomnia.[33]

Benzodiazepines appear to increase total sleep time and decrease awakenings reliably during daytime sleep. The short-acting compound triazolam improved sleep both in subjects on simulated shiftwork regimes[10,97] and in actual shiftworkers.[96] Flurazepam, a long-acting benzodiazepine, has also been shown to improve daytime sleep after a 12-hour sleep/wake phase reversal.[76,83] However, Seidel et al.[83] found evidence of sedation during waking hours after sleep induced by flurazepam. In the same study, triazolam produced as much improvement in sleep as flurazepam without carryover sedation. The effects of other benzodiazepines (i.e., midazolam and oxazepam) upon day sleep in nightworkers have also been investigated. The studies are of limited value, however, because the investigators limited sleep time to 5 hours and did not test waking function at night.[82]

Whether drug-induced improvements in daytime sleep lead to better alertness and less fatigue at night is a separate question. Bonnet et al.[10] found a statistically significant trend for daytime sleep with triazolam to improve performance and alertness at night. However, this study included only one simulated nightshift. A study of triazolam-aided daytime sleep across five consecutive nightshifts showed no significant beneficial effect on nighttime function.[97]

Benzodiazepines have also been studied for the treatment of sleep disturbance associated with jet lag. These paradigms are somewhat similar to shiftwork studies in that sleep is temporally displaced relative to the normal sleep/wake cycle. The results, however, may not be directly comparable. Transmeridian travel produces daylight, time, and social cues (zeitgebers) that are congruent with the desired sleep/wake schedule. These zeitgebers promote adjustment of the internal sleep/wake rhythm. During shiftwork, the temporal relationship between these external cues and the desired sleep/wake schedule is in conflict. If daylight and other zeitgebers do not shift to be compatible with the desired

---

* Information in this section is based on Walsh.[95]

sleep time, adaptation is likely to be retarded. Therefore, jet lag studies are not particularly helpful for the assessment of pharmacotherapy for shiftwork-related sleep/wake disturbance. (A discussion of the use of pharmacological aids for jet lag is included in Chapter 9.)

Over-the-Counter Sedative-Hypnotics

There are few laboratory studies of current over-the-counter sleeping medications, and none that look specifically at the benefit of these medications for shiftworkers. Kales et al.[39] reported no significant hypnotic effect of diphenhydramine on the nocturnal sleep of four normal sleepers. Roehrs et al.[79] reported that 50 mg of diphenhydramine taken three times a day reduced time taken to fall asleep relative to a placebo condition. Deeper sleep, however, was not increased. Although these studies do not represent an adequate test of hypnotic efficacy, neither study suggests significant promise for conventional over-the-counter medications as hypnotics for enhancing day sleep.

Side Effects and Abuse Potential of Sedative-Hypnotics

The major side effect of benzodiazepine sedative-hypnotics is sedation at undesired times. Sedation is particularly evident for longer-acting substances with elimination half-life greater than 10 hours. Because of these effects, shorter-acting compounds are generally preferable. They would be particularly desirable in a shiftwork situation because alertness during required hours of wakefulness may already be suboptimal. Abuse potential is rather low with benzodiazepines, particularly if they are prescribed for only the first two to four days on nightshift. More frequent use of sedative-hypnotics is rarely justified as the sole course of treatment for sleep disruption of any etiology, including shiftwork, because these medications provide only symptomatic relief. Chronic use also increases the likelihood of tolerance, increased sleep disturbance or "rebound insomnia,"[40] or heightened anxiety[1] upon abrupt discontinuation.

Prescription Central Nervous System (CNS) Stimulants

Little systematic research of CNS stimulant effects on alertness and performance at night has been conducted despite the well-known performance enhancement effects of these agents during daytime administration.[99] In fact, some measures of performance can be normalized by stimulants even after 3 days of total sleep loss.[46] Borland et al.[13] have demonstrated some tendency for caffeine to improve performance on the nightshift, when circadian rhythm declines in performance are typically observed. No other studies are available. It should be noted, however, that nightworkers and rotating shiftworkers report more use of "pep medication" than dayworkers.[88]

The judicious short-term use of CNS stimulants to combat sleepiness on nightshift needs further exploration. Specifically, caffeine, pemoline, methylphenidate, and the amphetamines could be studied. Any potential benefits would have to be weighed against the side effects and the potential for abuse, which are not trivial for the prescription stimulants.

Pharmacological Manipulation of the Circadian Sleep/Wake Cycle

Recent studies suggest that some pharmacological compounds may directly influence the endogenous sleep/wake rhythm. Considerable research, however, is needed before use of these compounds becomes a viable treatment for shiftwork-related sleep/wake disorders. Lithium appears to lengthen the human circadian temperature rhythm.[37] Theophylline may delay the sleep phase of humans.[68] Bicuculline may prevent phase delays of circadian rhythms, but not phase advances.[77] Melatonin administration purportedly has a direct effect on endogenous circadian phase.[6,62] (The effects of melatonin are further discussed in Chapter 9.)

The possibility of specific pharmacological control of circadian rhythms is intriguing but speculative at the present time. A somewhat related issue is the relative hypnotic potency of any drug at different times of administration. No systematic studies address this issue. There is substantial evidence, however, that other nonhypnotic drugs have circadian variations in effectiveness.[60]

Summary

The degree to which sedative-hypnotics can be helpful for nightworkers must be established in terms of both improved sleep and improved alertness during times of desired wakefulness. Benzodiazepines, particularly the shorter-acting compounds, are the drugs of immediate availability and interest, and effective dosages for daytime sleep need to be established. Similarly, the relative absence of significant research employing CNS stimulants to combat the profound circadian sleepiness of the early morning hours of nightshift is surprising. Further work is needed in this area as well.

DIET*

Changes in meal times are associated with nightwork, and most nightworkers sleep through at least one daytime meal. Nightworkers eat during their shift, when dayworkers are asleep. These obvious differences in the *timing* of eating and drinking behavior may not be the only significant dietary changes. Nightworkers may also change *what* they eat and drink. This possibility raises a number of questions, such as whether the eating and drinking times of nightworkers simply mimic the meal timing of dayworkers, and whether there are significant changes in food and drink consumed by nightworkers. If consumption differences exist between dayworkers and nightworkers it is not known whether they are reflections of different energy-expenditure requirements. It must also be asked whether the stress of working nights promotes abusive eating and drinking habits. Finally, we should consider whether eating and drinking habits can be manipulated to improve the ability of workers to adjust to nightwork.

Changes in Eating and Drinking Behavior

Survey and diary studies in the United States and Europe indicate that nightworkers differ from dayworkers in the number of meals eaten per day.[14] Nightworkers also report a dissatisfaction with their eating habits. However, both increases and decreases in caloric intake have been associated with nightwork, as have differences in relative nutrient intake. Overall, these differences suggest that nightworkers tend to nibble or eat more frequently. Because several European studies report that nightworkers are frequently obese, it is difficult to argue that nightwork increases the energy requirement of the body to a point where consumption fails to maintain normal body weight.

---

* Information in this section is based on Tepas.[90]

Contrary to folklore, experienced nightworkers do not necessarily report elevated levels of ethanol or caffeine consumption.[78] When elevated use of these substances is observed, it is probably a manifestation of age differences or of subject sampling errors, and perhaps indicates the need for objective urine or blood testing. U.S. nightworkers are, on average, younger than dayworkers, and older workers, in most cases, consume less ethanol and caffeine. It may well be that many or all of the dietary differences reported are simply a function of the age of the subjects studied.

Some studies have reported a high incidence of gastrointestinal complaints in nightworkers.[61] It is often assumed that these complaints are produced by the psychological stress of working nights. The quality of the food services provided nightworkers, however, is frequently inferior to that provided dayworkers. It is quite possible that a major cause of nightworkers' gastrointestinal disturbances is poor food services or bad eating habits. Additional research is needed to resolve this issue.

Economic, social, and cultural factors also influence eating and drinking habits. For example, a worker in eastern Europe may have soup and cheese for breakfast, whereas an American worker may start the day with a bowl of sugar-coated cornflakes. Commuting schedules and religious practices are other factors that may change the timing or content of meals. Given these differences, it may not be appropriate to generalize findings from different geographical locations and cultural areas. Such differences make it difficult to establish a link between eating and drinking habits and deteriorated health or workplace performance.

Manipulating Eating and Drinking Behavior

A number of authors have proposed diet regimens or dietary restrictions as aids in coping with nightwork. Some of these authors simply recommend eating and drinking changes that promote, rather than prevent, normal sleep.[85] Other authors assume that nightwork is easier when circadian biological rhythms are phase-shifted so they are in synchrony with nightwork hours.[24] They further assume that special dietary regimens induce fairly rapid chronobiological rhythm shifts.

The proposal that meal timing and diet content can produce fairly rapid shifts in chronobiological rhythms appears to be based mainly on the results of experimentation with animals.[78] Many studies have demonstrated rapid shifts in circadian rhythms produced by appropriate manipulations of laboratory animal eating and drinking behavior. Unfortunately, there are no definitive studies of shiftworkers showing that manipulation of diet produces circadian rhythm shifts making it easier to cope with nightwork. However, modest laboratory and field data suggest that humans, in general, are *less* sensitive to food and drink manipulations than are laboratory animals.[78] Human research also has demonstrated that laboratory studies of diet may not generalize to field manipulations of diet in a social or work environment. It is quite possible that enthusiastic nonexperimental reports of the success of these diet regimens may be artifacts of the expectations of those promoting the regimens. Definitive research using experienced shiftworkers is needed to test these interesting speculations.

Authors who promote eating and drinking habits said to be conducive to sound sleep hygiene may be working from a more solid base. Many of their recommendations appear to be based on recommendations made by sleep disorder centers to patients seeking treatment.[34] Those recommendations are usually restricted to avoidance of caffeine near sleep time and avoiding greasy foods that might cause indigestion and disturb sleep. Much of this advice, however, may not be needed by shiftworkers if, as the research suggests, they do not (as a group) exhibit unusual eating and drinking habits. For example, if experienced nightworkers do not have elevated caffeine consumption levels, one must ask if there is any real reason to warn them about consuming too much caffeine. One must also ask whether dietary education of this sort has any long-term effects on worker habits; the difficulty in maintaining special dietary rules for long periods is well known.

Summary

Nightwork does change the timing of meals and probably changes what people eat and drink. There is little evidence to support the suggestion that these changes, as practiced by the typical experienced shiftworker, have either a positive or a negative effect on performance or how well they cope with shiftwork. Furthermore, there is little evidence from human research to support the hypothesis that change or manipulation of eating or drinking habits can improve the ability of the average shiftworker to cope with nightwork. There is reason to suggest that the findings of animal or clinical research cannot be directly extrapolated to shiftworkers. This does not mean, however, that the eating and drinking habits of shiftworkers are unrelated to their ability to cope with nightwork. Since there is a significant public interest in this problem, research on experienced nightworkers is needed to substantiate claims that have evolved without benefit of definitive human laboratory and field testing.

INDIVIDUAL BEHAVIORAL TECHNIQUES*

Some techniques described in the general literature of applied psychology should be considered for ameliorating the effects of shiftwork. The following interventions are drawn from industrial performance studies, the stress management literature, vigilance studies, sleep studies, and the broader psychological literature.

Because many deleterious effects of shiftwork are the result of sleep deprivation, sleep hygiene is of major importance in coping with shiftwork. Previously developed procedures for establishing and maintaining effective sleep habits, such as stimulus control instructions,[11] could be adapted for shiftworkers.[71] Stimulus control instructions are a set of procedures for optimizing the bedroom for sleep by removing all distracting stimuli. If family members are also instructed in these procedures, they can understand and cooperate with the worker's needs. Time management training for shiftworkers and their families can also help with sleep and social scheduling.

Stress reduction techniques have been useful for a number of work-related stresses. These methods include relaxation training, biofeedback, some applications of hypnosis, and cognitive skill training. Relaxation training has the broadest applicability and may be used for general stress reduction, autoregulation of specific physiological systems, enhancing the recuperative value of rest breaks, and an aid to sleep onset. Biofeedback requires greater equipment and personnel expenses than relaxation training and has produced mixed results.[63] For some

* Information in this section is based on Bootzin and Penn.[12]

shiftworkers, training in hypnosis or self-hypnosis could aid sleep induction or promote arousal and relaxation at work. Cognitive skill training may be a particularly important area for investigation because expectancy can be a powerful mediator of the effects of stress. Several strategies for improvement of self-efficacy[8] could help workers cope with stress, improve self-esteem, and enhance task performance.

Other behavioral techniques may be useful for specific purposes. For example, behavioral methods demonstrated to be effective for diet and weight regulation, smoking cessation, and substance abuse could similarly be used by shiftworkers. Family counseling for shiftworkers appears to be a neglected area. Because family life has a major impact on adaptation to shiftwork, the development and evaluation of family interventions should be given high priority.

Social activity during work breaks is another method of increasing arousal at work. This may be particularly useful for shiftworkers who have reduced social opportunities away from work. Social activity, however, can also distract workers from the task at hand. Consequently, studies are needed on the optimal arrangements for social activity during work.

Several types of self-regulation and electroencephalogram (EEG) biofeedback techniques have been studied for their potential in enhancing alertness and performance,[19] in addition to reducing stress. Learned suppression of theta EEG can lessen performance decrements caused by fatigue. The increased production of negative slow-wave potentials may enhance performance above normal levels.[19] The long- and short-term effects of EEG regulation could be studied for shiftworkers, but its implementation may be less cost effective than other methods. For example, controlling respiration may enhance alertness[35] and requires no special equipment.

Cognitive strategies for remaining alert are potentially applicable to shiftwork. Several reviews indicate that visualization or mental practice can lead to gains in sports performance and academic activities.[52] Hypnosis and attention focusing can also be explored as means of increasing alertness and sustaining performance.

Incentives are likely to play an important role in the successful adaptation to shiftwork. Relatively greater financial rewards are frequently given to shiftworkers, and these incentives are often the motivation for working the nightshift. For many workers, however, other incentives, such as more time off duty, may be valued more than additional money. An effective strategy for increasing motivation may be to provide a menu of incentives for shiftworkers,[15] including compensations that reduce the stress of shiftwork.

In summary, a variety of behavioral methods from various areas of psychology have considerable potential for reducing fatigue and enhancing performance. Some of the most effective techniques may involve interventions that deal with the worker's family and with activities away from work.

CONCLUSION

A broad range of factors has been reviewed that, if controlled, might promote adaptation to nightwork, shiftwork, and extended workshifts. In general, most of these factors have not been systematically applied to the civilian shiftwork population, and the relative merits of one approach over another have yet to be established.

Systematic study has at least been begun in four of these areas: work schedule design, napping, bright light stimulation, and drugs. With respect to work schedule design, a small number of consultants in this country are now working with various industries to devise more "biocompatible" schedules for the worker. The long-term effectiveness of these new schedules, however, has not been reported. Napping has been considered in military applications, but not in the types of schedules required of the civilian shiftworker. Bright light exposure has been successful in shifting rhythms in controlled laboratory situations, but workplace studies have yet to be conducted. Pharmacological studies of the shiftworker are gaining support from drug manufacturers. All of those studies, however, have been in acute laboratory situations. Long-term studies have not been reported and are clearly needed because of the side effects and abuse potential of drugs.

Physical activity, ambient temperature, diet, and a host of individual behaviors have been studied only superficially in terms of the shiftworker. Work should be attempted in these areas, however. From this review, it is clear that numerous applications to the shiftworker are possible.

The relative merits of these interventions need to be considered and a balance found between their effectiveness at improving safety, health, and well-being, and their practicality. Initial effectiveness should be measured by improved alertness and performance (on and off the job), improved sleep (if applicable), and better satisfaction and well-being. Long-term effectiveness should be measured by reduced accident outcomes, improved health or maintenance of sound health, and increased productivity.

The practical burden on the worker and the organization should also be evaluated. An intervention will not be attempted or, if attempted, will not succeed if too much energy or too many resources are required of the worker or the organization. If the intervention burden is high in comparison to the reward, the worker will view the intervention as just another chore added to an already burdensome work environment. And the organization will view the intervention as too costly, unless reduced costs can be demonstrated in other areas (such as reduced attrition or absenteeism).

REFERENCES

1. Adam K, Oswald I: Can a rapidly eliminated hypnotic cause daytime anxiety? Pharmacopsychiatry 22:115–119, 1989.
2. Akerstedt T: Adjustment of physiological circadian rhythms and the sleep-wake cycle to shiftwork. In Folkard S, Monk TH (eds): Hours of Work: Temporal Factors in Work Scheduling. New York, John Wiley, 1985, pp 185–198.
3. Akerstedt T, Torsvall L: Age, sleep and adjustment to shiftwork. In Koella WP (ed): Sleep 1980: 5th European Congress on Sleep Research. Basel, Karger, 1981, pp 190–195.
4. Angerspach D, Knauth P, Loskant H, et al: A retrospective cohort study comparing complaints and diseases in day and shift workers. Int Arch Occup Environ Health 45:127–140, 1980.
5. Angiboust R, Gouars M: Tentative d'evaluation de l'efficacité operationelle du personnel de l'aeronautique militaire au cours de veilles nocturnes. In Colquhoun WP (ed): Aspects of Human Efficiency. London, English Universities Press, 1972, pp 151–170.
6. Arendt J, Aldhous M, Wright J: Synchronization of a disturbed sleep-wake cycle in a blind man by melatonin treatment. Lancet April: 772–773, 1988.
7. Aschoff J: Circadian rhythms: Interference with and dependence on work-rest schedules. In Johnson LC, Tepas DI, Colquhoun WP, Colligan (eds): The Twenty-four-Hour Workday: Proceedings of a Symposium on the Variations of Work-Sleep Schedules. DHHS (NIOSH) publication no. 81-127, 1981, pp 13–50.
8. Bandura A: Self-efficacy mechanism in human agency. Am Psychol 37:122–147, 1982.
9. Bonnet MH: Dealing with shiftwork: Physical fitness, temperature, and napping. Paper presented at the 32nd Annual Meeting of the Human Factors Society, Anaheim, California, October, 1988.

10. Bonnet MH, Dexter JR, Gillin JC, et al: The use of tirazolam in phase-advanced sleep. Neuropsychopharmacology 1:225–234, 1988.
11. Bootzin RR, Nicassio PM: Behavioral treatment for insomnia. Prog Behav Modif 6:1–45, 1978.
12. Bootzin RR, Penn PE: Behavioral techniques for enhancing alertness and performance. Paper presented at the 32nd Annual Meeting of the Human Factors Society, Anaheim, California, October, 1988.
13. Borland RG, Rogers AS, Nicholson AN, et al: Performance overnight in shiftworkers operating a day-night schedule. Aviat Space Environ Med 57:241–249, 1986.
14. Cervinka R, Kundi M, Koller M, et al: Shift related nutrition problems. Paper presented at the International Research Workshop on Psychological Approaches to Night and Shiftwork, Edinburgh, July 19–23, 1982.
15. Colquhoun WP: Shiftwork discussion and conclusions. In Johnson LC, Tepas DI, Colquhoun WP, Colligan MJ (eds): The Twenty-four Hour Workday: Proceedings of a Symposium on the Variations of Work-Sleep Schedules. DHHS (NIOSH) publication no. 81-127, 1981, pp 755–761.
16. Czeisler CA, Allan JS, Strogatz SH, et al: Bright light resets the human circadian pacemaker independent of the timing of the sleep-wake cycle. Science 233:667–671, 1986.
17. Czeisler CA, Moore-Ede MC, Coleman RM: Rotating shift work schedules that disrupt sleep are improved by applying circadian principles. Science 217:460–463, 1982.
18. Dinges DF, Orne MT, Whitehouse WG, Orne EC: Temporal placement of a nap for alertness: Contributions of circadian phase and prior wakefulness. Sleep 10:313–329, 1987.
19. Druckman D, Swets JA: Enhancing Human Performance. Washington, D.C., National Academy, 1988.
20. Eastman CI: Bright light improves the entrainment of the circadian rhythm of body temperature to a 26-hour sleep-wake schedule in humans. Sleep Res 15:271, 1986.
21. Eastman CI: Bright light in work-sleep schedules for shift workers: Application of circadian rhythm principles. In Rensing L, Heiden U, Mackey MC (eds): Temporal Disorders in Human Oscillatory Systems. New York, Springer-Verlag, 1987, pp 176–185.
22. Eastman CI: A critical review of the circadian rhythm and bright light literature with recommendations for shift work. Paper presented at the 32nd Annual Meeting of the Human Factors Society, Anaheim, California, October, 1988.
23. Eastman CI: Field studies of humans following 26-hour bright light and sleep-wake schedules. Abstracts, Soc Res Biol Rhythms, p 66, 1988.
24. Ehret CF: New approaches to chronohygiene for the shift worker in the nuclear power industry. In Reinberg A, Vieux N, Andlauer P (eds): Night and Shift Work: Biological and Social Aspects. New York, Pergamon, 1981, pp 263–270.
25. Folkard S: Shiftwork and performance. In Johnson LC, Tepas DI, Colquhoun WP, Colligan MJ (eds): The Twenty-four Hour Workday: Proceedings of a Symposium on the Variations of Work-Sleep Schedules. DHHS (NIOSH) publication no. 81-127, 1981, pp 347–374.
26. Gillberg M: The effects of two alternative timings of a one-hour nap on early morning performance. Biol Psychol 19:45–54, 1984.
27. Gordon NP, Cleary PD, Parker CE, Czeisler CA: The prevalence and health impact of shiftwork. Am J Pub Health 76:1225–1228, 1986.
28. Harma MI, Ilmarinen J, Knauth P: Physical fitness and other individual factors in explaining the shiftwork tolerance of women. In Oginski A, Pokorski J, Rutenfranz J (eds): Contemporary Advances in Shiftwork Research: Theoretical and Practical Aspects in the Late Eighties. Krakow, Medical Academy, 1987, p 99.
29. Reference deleted.
30. Harma MI, Ilmarinen J, Knauth P, et al: Physical training intervention in female shift workers. I. The effects of intervention on fitness, fatigue, sleep, and psychosomatic symptoms. Ergonomics 31:39–50, 1988.
31. Harma MI, Ilmarinen J, Knauth P, et al: Physical training intervention in female shift workers. II. The effects of intervention on the circadian rhythms of alertness, short-term memory, and body temperature. Ergonomics 31:51–63, 1988.
32. Harma MI, Ilmarinen J, Yletyinen I: Circadian variation of physiological functions in physically average and very fit dayworkers. J Hum Ergol 11(suppl):33–46, 1982.
33. Harvey SC: Hypnotics and sedatives. In Gilman AG, Goodman LS, Gilman A (eds): The Pharmacological Basis of Therapeutics. New York, Macmillan, 1980, pp 339–375.
34. Hauri P: The Sleep Disorders. Kalamazoo, Upjohn, 1982.
35. Heil J: Imagery for sport: Theory, research and practice. In Straub WF, Williams JM (eds): Cognitive Sport Psychology. New York, Sport Science Associates, 1984.

36. Honma K, Honma S, Wada T: Phase-dependent shift of free-running human circadian rhythms in response to a single bright light pulse. Experientia 43:1205–1207, 1987.
37. Johnson A, Pflug B, Engelmann W, Klemke W: Effect of lithium carbonate on circadian periodicity in humans. Pharmakopsychiatr Neuropsychopharmakol 12:423–425, 1979.
38. Johnson LC, Naitoh P: The operational consequences of sleep deprivation and sleep deficit. AGARDograph no. 190, North Atlantic Treaty Organization, 1974.
39. Kales A, Malmstrom EJ, Tau TL: Drugs and dreaming. In Abt E, Riess BF (eds): Progress in Clinical Psychology. New York, Grune & Stratton, 1969, pp 154–167.
40. Kales A, Soldatos CR, Bixler EO, Kales JD: Early morning insomnia with rapidly eliminated benzodiazepines. Science 220:95–97, 1983.
41. Klein KE, Wegmann HM, Bruner H: Circadian rhythm in indices of human performance, physical fitness and stress resistance. Aerospace Med 512–518, 1968.
42. Knauth P, Rutenfranz J: Experimental shiftwork studies of permanent night and rapidly rotating shift systems. In Colquhoun WP, Rutenfranz J (eds): Studies of Shiftwork. London, Taylor & Francis, 1980, pp 81–93.
43. Knauth P, Rutenfranz J: Development of criteria for the design of shiftwork systems. J Hum Ergol 11(suppl):337–367, 1982.
44. Knutsson A, Akerstedt T, Jonsson BG, Orth-Gomer K: Increased risk of ischaemic heart disease in shift workers. Lancet July:89–92, 1986.
45. Kogi K: Comparison of resting conditions between various shift rotation systems for industrial workers. In Reinberg A, Vieux N, Andlauer P (eds): Night and Shift Work: Biological and Social Aspects. New York, Pergamon, 1981, pp 417–424.
46. Kornetsky C, Mirsky AF, Kessler EK, Dorff JE: The effects of dextroamphetamine on behavioral deficits produced by sleep loss in humans. J Pharm Exp Therapy 127:46–50, 1959.
47. Kozlowski S: Physiology of physical work. Warsaw, PZWL, 1970. (In Polish)
48. Lewy AJ, Sack RL, Miller S, Hoban TM: Antidepressant and circadian phase-shifting effects of light. Science 235:352–354, 1987.
49. Lewy AJ, Wehr TA, Goodwin FK, et al: Light suppresses melatonin secretion in humans. Science 210:1267–1269, 1980.
50. Little MA, Rummel JA: Circadian variation in thermal and metabolic responses to heat exposure. J Appl Phys 31:556–561, 1971.
51. Lubin A, Hord DJ, Tracy ML, Johnson LC: Effects of exercise, bedrest and napping on performance decrement during 40 hours. Psychophysiology 13:334–339, 1976.
52. Mahoney MJ: Cognitive skills and athletic performance. In Straub WF, Williams JM (eds): Cognitive Sport Psychology. Lansing, Sport Science Associates, 1984.
53. Malinowski A: The influence of shift work on some morphofunctional features. Zdrowie Publ 84:73, 1973. (In Polish)
54. Minors DS, Waterhouse JM: Anchor sleep as a synchronizer of rhythms on abnormal routines. In Johnson LC, Tepas DI, Colquhoun WP, Colligan MJ (eds): The Twenty-four Hour Workday: Proceedings of a Symposium on the Variations of Work-Sleep Schedules. DHHS (NIOSH) publication no. 81-127, 1981, pp 493–516.
55. Mital A: Maximum weights of lift acceptable to male and female industrial workers for extended work shifts. Ergonomics 11:1115–1126, 1984.
56. Mital A: Prediction models for psychophysical lifting capabilities and the resulting physiological responses for work shifts of varied durations. J Safety Res 17:155–163, 1986.
57. Mitler MM, Carskadon MA, Czeisler CA, et al: Catastrophes, sleep, and public policy: Consensus report. Sleep 11:100–109, 1988.
58. Monk TH: The relationship of chronobiology to sleep schedule and performance demands. Paper presented at the 32nd Annual Meeting of the Human Factors Society, Anaheim, California, October, 1988.
59. Moog R, Hildebrandt G: Effects of physical training on adaptation to night-work. In Oginski A, Pokorski J, Rutenfranz J (eds): Contemporary Advances in Shiftwork Research: Theoretical and Practical Aspects in the Late Eighties. Krakow, Medical Academy, 1987, pp 81–85.
60. Moore-Ede MC: Circadian rhythms in drug effectiveness and toxicity in shiftworkers. In Rentos PG, Shepard RD (eds): Shift Work and Health. DHEW (NIOSH) publication no. 76-203, 1976, pp 140–144.
61. Moore-Ede MC, Richardson GS: Medical implications of shiftwork. Ann Rev Med 36:607–617, 1985.
62. Murakami N, Hayafuji C, Sasaki Y, et al: Melatonin accelerates the re-entrainment of the circadian adrenocortical rhythm in inverted illumination cycle. Neuroendocrinology 36:385–391, 1983.

63. Murphy LR: Occupational stress management: A review and appraisal. J Occup Psychol 57:1–15, 1984.
64. Naitoh P, Angus RG: Napping and human functioning during prolonged work. In Dinges DF, Broughton RJ (eds): Sleep and Alertness: Chronobiological, Behavioral, and Medical Aspects of Napping. New York, Raven, 1989, pp 221–248.
65. Naitoh P, Englund CE, Ryman D: Restorative power of naps in designing continuous work schedules. J Hum Ergol 11:259–278, 1982.
66. Nicholson AN, Pascoe PA, Roehrs T: Sustained performance with short evening and morning sleeps. Aviat Space Environ Med 56:105–114, 1985.
67. Oginski A, Oginski H, Pokorski J: Impact of seasons on individual shift preferences. In Oginski A, Pokorski J, Rutenfranz J (eds): Contemporary Advances in Shiftwork Research: Theoretical and Practical Aspects in the Late Eighties. Krakow, Medical Academy, 1987, pp 435–442.
68. Okudaira N, Kripke DF, Mullaney DJ: Theophylline delays human sleep phase. Life Sci 34:933–938, 1984.
69. Omoto A: Personal communication from U.S. representative of Tokyo Electric Power Company, 1988.
70. Ottman W, Plett R, Knauth P, et al: Combined effects of experimental shiftwork and heat stress on cognitive performance tasks. In Haider M, Koller M, Cervinka R (eds): Night and Shiftwork: Long-term Effects and Their Prevention. New York, Peter Lang, 1985, pp 362–368.
71. Pearce JW, Crowell DH, Kapuniai LE: Coping with Night Work and Shift Work. Honolulu, Sleep Disorders Center of the Pacific, 1987.
72. Pittendrigh CS: Circadian systems: Entrainment. In Aschoff J (ed): Handbook of Behavioral Neurobiology. Vol. 4. Biological Rhythms. New York, Plenum, 1981, pp 95–124.
73. Pocock SJ, Sergean R, Taylor PJ: Absence of continuous three-shift workers: A comparison of traditional and rapidly rotating systems. In Colquhoun WP, Rutenfranz J (ed): Studies of Shiftwork. London, Taylor & Francis, 1980, pp 391–398.
74. Pokorski J, Oginski A, Knauth P: Work physiological field studies concerning effects of combined stress in morning, afternoon and night shifts. In Haider M, Koller M, Cervinka R (eds): Night and Shiftwork: Long-term Effects and Their Prevention. New York, Peter Lang, 1985, pp 369–376.
75. Pokorski J, Oginski A, Kuleta J, et al: Physiological response to shiftwork in blast-furnace workers. In Oginski A, Pokorski J, Rutenfranz J (eds): Contemporary Advances in Shiftwork Research: Theoretical and Practical Aspects in the Late Eighties. Krakow, Medical Academey, 1987, pp 355–364.
76. Pollak C, McGregor P, Weitzman E: The effect of flurazepam on daytime sleep after acute sleep-wake cycle reversal. Sleep Res 4:112, 1975.
77. Ralph MR, Menaker M: Bicuculline blocks circadian phase delays but not advances. Brain Res 325:362–365, 1985.
78. Reinberg A: Chronobiology and nutrition. In Reinberg A, Smolensky MH (eds): Biological Rhythms and Medicine: Cellular, Metabolic, Physiopathologic, and Pharmacologic Aspects. New York, Springer-Verlag, 1983, pp 265–301.
79. Roehrs TA, Tietz EI, Zorick FJ, Roth T: Daytime sleepiness and antihistamines. Sleep 7:137–141, 1984.
80. Rosa RR, Colligan MJ, Lewis P: Extended workdays: Effects of 8-hour and 12-hour rotating shift schedules on performance, subjective alertness, sleep patterns, and psychosocial variables. Work Stress 3:21–32, 1989.
81. Rutenfranz J, Neidhart B, Ottman W, et al: Circadian rhythms of physiological functions during experimental shift work with additional heat stress. In Haider M, Koller M, Cervinka R (eds): Night and Shiftwork: Long-term Effects and Their Prevention. New York, Peter Lang, 1985, pp 347–359.
82. Scollo-Lavizzari G: Hypnotic efficacy and clinical safety of midazolam in shift-workers. Br J Clin Pharmocol 16:73s–78s, 1983.
83. Seidel WF, Roth T, Roehrs T, et al: Treatment of a 12-hour shift of sleep schedule with benzodiazepines. Science 224:1262–1264, 1984.
84. Reference deleted.
85. Spring B: Effects of foods and nutrients on the behavior of normal individuals. In Wurtman R, Wurtman J (eds): Nutrition and the Brain. Vol 7. New York, Raven Press, 1986, pp 1–47.
86. Suda M, Saito M: Coordinative regulation of feeding behavior and metabolism by a circadian timing system. In Suda M, Hayaishi O, Nakagawa H (eds): Biological Rhythms and Their Central Mechanism. New York, Elsevier, 1979, pp 263–271.

87. Tasto DL, Colligan MJ: Shift Work Practices in the United States. DHEW (NIOSH) publication no. 77-148, 1977.
88. Tasto DL, Colligan MJ: Health consequences of shift work. DHEW (NIOSH) publication no. 78-154, 1978.
89. Tepas DI: Flextime, compressed workweeks, and other alternative work schedules. In Folkard S, Monk TH (eds): Hours of Work: Temporal Factors in Work Scheduling. New York, John Wiley, 1985, pp 147–164.
90. Tepas DI: Do eating and drinking habits interact with work schedule variables? Paper presented at the 32nd Annual Meeting of the Human Factors Society, Anaheim, California, October, 1988.
91. Tepas DI, Walsh JK, Armstrong D: Comprehensive study of the sleep of shiftworkers. In Johnson LC, Tepas DI, Colquhoun WP, Colligan MJ (eds): The Twenty-four Hour Workday: Proceedings of a Symposium on the Variations of Work-Sleep Schedules. DHHS (NIOSH) publication no. 81-127, 1981, pp 419–434.
92. Tierney J: Personal communication from Personnel Specialist, Southern California Gas Company, 1987.
93. Turek FW: Circadian principles and design of rotating shift work schedules. Am J Physiol 251:R636–638, 1986.
94. Walker J: Social problems of shiftwork. In Folkard S, Monk TH (eds): Hours of Work: Temporal Factors in Work Scheduling. New York, John Wiley, 1985, pp 211–226.
95. Walsh JK: Using pharmacological aids to improve waking function and sleep while working nights. Paper presented at the 32nd Annual Meeting of the Human Factors Society, Anaheim, California, October, 1988.
96. Walsh JK, Muehlbach MJ, Schweitzer PK: Acute administration of triazolam for the daytime sleep of rotating shift workers. Sleep 7:223–229, 1984.
97. Walsh JK, Sugerman JL, Muehlbach MJ, Schweitzer PK: Physiological sleep tendency on a simulated night shift: Adaptation and effects of triazolam. Sleep 11:251–264, 1988.
98. Walsh JK, Tepas DI, Moss PD: The EEG sleep of night and rotating shift workers. In Johnson LC, Tepas DI, Colquhoun WP, Colligan MJ (eds): Biological Rhythms, Sleep and Shift Work. New York, Spectrum, 1981, pp 371–381.
99. Weiss B, Laties VG: Enhancement of human performance by caffeine and the amphetamines. Pharmacol Rev 14:1–36, 1962.
100. Wever RA: The Circadian System of Man. New York, Springer Verlag, 1979.
101. Wever RA: Light effects on human circadian rhythms: A review of recent Andechs experiments. J Biol Rhythms 4:161–185, 1989.
102. Williamson AM, Sanderson JW: Changing the speed of shift rotation: A field study. Ergonomics 9:1085–1096, 1986.
103. Wojtczak-Jaroszowa J: Physiological and psychological aspects of night and shift work. DHEW (NIOSH) publication no. 78-113, 1977.

AUTHORS' AFFILIATIONS

Roger R. Rosa, PhD
National Institute for Occupational Safety and Health
Division of Biomedical and Behavioral Science
Cincinnati, OH 45226

Richard R. Bootzin, PhD
Department of Psychology
University of Arizona
Tucson, AZ 85721

Timothy H. Monk, PhD
Western Psychiatric Institute and Clinic
3811 O'Hara Street
Pittsburgh, PA 15213

Donald I. Tepas, PhD
Department of Psychology
University of Connecticut
Storrs, CT 06268

Michael H. Bonnet, PhD
Sleep Laboratory (111P)
VA Hospital
5901 E. 7th Street
Long Beach, CA 90822

Charmane I. Eastman, PhD
Rush-Presbyterian-St. Lukes Medical Center
Psychology Department
1653 West Congress Parkway
Chicago, IL 60612

Patricia E. Penn, PhD
Department of Psychology
University of Arizona
Tucson, AZ 85721

James K. Walsh, PhD
Sleep Laboratory
Deaconess Hospital
6150 Oakland Avenue
St. Louis, MO 63139

Much of the information included in this report is based on presentations by participants in a symposium entitled "Designing Shift Work Systems to Improve Performance and Alertness: What Do We Know and What Do We Need to Know?" This symposium, sponsored by the National Institute for Occupational Safety and Health (NIOSH), took place at the 32nd Annual Meeting of the Human Factors Society, Anaheim, California, in October 1988. Symposium participants were: Michael Bonnet, University of California, Irvine; Richard Bootzin, University of Arizona; James Duchon, U.S. Bureau of Mines; Charmane Eastman, Rush-Presbyterian-St. Luke's Medical Center; Timothy Monk, Western Psychiatric Institute; Patricia Penn, University of Arizona; Roger Rosa, NIOSH; Donald Tepas, University of Connecticut; and James Walsh, Deaconess Hospital, St. Louis. Their specific contributions are noted throughout this report.

ONG C.N., PhD
KOGI K., MD

SHIFTWORK IN DEVELOPING COUNTRIES: CURRENT ISSUES AND TRENDS

Ong C.N, PhD
Department of Community Medicine
National University of Singapore

Kogi K., MD
International Labour Office
Geneva, Switzerland

Portions of this article are borrowed from Kogi K, Ong CN, Cabantog C: Some social aspects of shiftwork in Asian developing countries. Int J Ind Ergon 4:151–159, 1989.

Reprint requests to:
Dr. Choon-Nam Ong
Department of Community Medicine
National University of Singapore
Kent Ridge
Singapore 0511

Shiftwork is now commonly practiced in many developing countries. It is being increasingly used, not only because of technical and public needs, but also for economic reasons. Shiftwork can mean better return by continuous use of costly machinery, acceleration of production outputs, and the use of more manpower with relatively small additional investment. In developing countries, shiftwork is often regarded as a means of better using resources and of increasing employment.[1]

Shiftwork in the less developed, developing, and industrialized nations is similar in many respects. Shift schedules, however, are very much influenced by the socioeconomic background of the individual country[10,16,32] and by the traditions and customs of the local community.[5] Thus, the practical problems encountered by shiftworkers in developing countries can be quite different from those of their counterparts in industrialized countries.[19]

The impact of shiftwork on the health and social life of workers is of concern.[6] The effects of shiftwork in developing countries are aggravated by generally poor conditions of work and life, exhausting climate, transportation problems, inadequate housing, the lack of supporting community services, and other factors. Psychosocial factors also seem to affect the health and productivity of shiftworkers in these countries. A common problem, for example, is associated with the transfer of workers from traditional work methods in the rural areas to mechanized work on assembly lines in the urban settings. Such transfers give rise to difficulties in conforming to night and shiftwork patterns and often result in high turnover and absenteeism.[21]

Information on shiftwork in developing countries is limited, especially information about shift-scheduling patterns and their interaction with local working conditions. This chapter will review briefly a few shiftwork studies recently conducted in several countries in Asia and South America. Common problems and suggested ways to improve the lot of shiftworkers in these locations will be discussed.

Data available at the national level indicate that shiftworkers account for at least 10% of the industrial workforce, and their numbers are gradually increasing. It is estimated that about 6% of the total work force in Thailand, 10% in the Philippines, and 14% in Peru are involved with shiftwork; the percentage is higher in Malaysia and Singapore.[11]

On the basis of a survey of shiftwork practices among manufacturing industries in Singapore, about 37% of the workers in 419 firms surveyed were shiftworkers.[17] Close to two-thirds of the shiftworkers were in the machinery or electronics industry, apparently for economic reasons. As Figure 1 shows, the electronics industry employs about 50% of the total 16,107 shiftworkers surveyed. Comparison of the proportions of shift- and nonshiftworkers among the major industrial groups reveals, however, that the petroleum and petrochemical industry has the highest workforce participation—nearly 100%—in shiftwork.

Another noteworthy finding from this survey is the high degree of female participation in shiftwork, particularly in the permanent nightshift. Nearly three times as many female as male workers were found to have permanent night duties. The situation is reversed in industrialized nations, where the nightshift is traditionally worked by men.[9] It is also noteworthy that the majority of permanent nightshift workers were engaged in the microelectronics industry. They were usually women of reproductive age, about 18–45 years old. These findings suggest that female operators are generally in high demand in this kind of manufacturing industry and that female operators prefer permanent nightwork. The night schedule apparently makes it easier to keep up with home activities. Many married women find that night jobs give them more time for family commitments. They have more time for their children and can perform household duties, such as preparing meals, before and after reporting for work. Although the social and health effects on women of working nightshifts have not been studied in detail, both management and workers in the manufacturing sector believe that labor turnover and absenteeism for sickness are adversely affected.[19]

Quite often in Asian developing countries workers are given monetary benefits for shiftwork rather than better transportation or housing facilities.

SHIFTWORK AND SICKNESS ABSENCE: A STUDY IN TWO DEVELOPING COUNTRIES

Most of the studies in sickness absence in shiftwork have been conducted in industrialized countries. Sickness absence, or absence from work attributed to incapacity such as illness or injury, is known[26] to be an extraordinarily complex matter. Absence for sickness may have many causes, including especially spurious elements and social and personal factors. Medical reasons are often not the major factor in sickness absence.[28] Sickness absence of shiftworkers might be

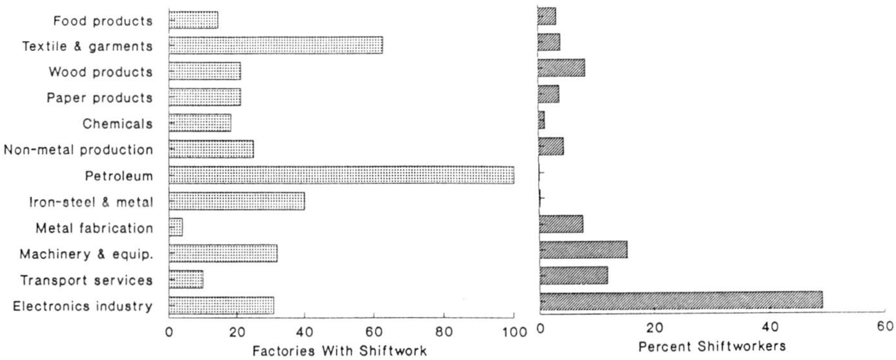

FIGURE 1. The percentage of industries adopting shift systems *(left)* and the proportion of shiftworkers in each industrial group *(right)* in Singapore. Source: Ong and Hoong[17] (unpublished data).

more related to social factors, which are probably of a different nature and magnitude than social factors in developed countries.

Studies conducted recently in industrial settings in Singapore and the Philippines analyzed personnel and medical records of 865 employees in a large metal industry and 324 workers in a refinery according to the variables of age, occupational activity, and workshift. In both plants studied, sickness absence was documented by medical certificates. A spell of absence meant an uninterrupted period of absence irrespective of duration, which was recorded in calendar days.

The following comparative rates were used: (1) mean spells per person, the ratio of total spells of absence during the study period to the population at risk; (2) mean days per person, the ratio of total days of absence during the study period to the population at risk; and (3) average duration per spell, the ratio of total days lost to total spells. The population at risk here was the number of persons employed throughout the study period of 12 months. Employees arriving or leaving during the study period were excluded.

The results are summarized in Tables 1–3. Table 1 shows that shiftworkers in the metal works in every age group (except for those 45 or more) had more spells and days of absence than nonshift dayworkers. Shiftworkers in this plant had an average of 4.6 spells and 8.7 days per person compared to 3.9 spells and 6.3 days per nonshift dayworker for the study period. For both shiftworkers and dayworkers, an increase in days taken was associated with increasing age.

TABLE 1. Sickness Absence of Dayworkers and Shiftworkers in a Metal Works, Singapore

	Dayworkers			Shiftworkers		
Age Group	%	Spell	Days	%	Spell	Days
24 or less	11	3.0	4.6	9	5.5	7.1
25–34	32	3.8	5.6	35	4.9	8.7
35–44	37	4.0	6.4	44	4.4	8.5
45 or more	20	4.4	8.2	12	4.1	10.4
All ages	100	3.9	6.3	100	4.6	8.7

Source: Kogi, Ong, and Cabantog[13]

TABLE 2. Sickness Absence of Dayworkers and Shiftworkers in an Oil Refinery, the Philippines

Age Group	Dayworkers			Shiftworkers		
	%	Spell	Days	%	Spell	Days
24 or less	10	0.9	1.9	5	2.1	6.3
25–34	52	2.2	4.1	62	3.6	7.3
35–44	22	2.4	5.4	13	2.3	4.1
45 or more	16	0.8	5.6	18	1.3	3.2
All ages	100	1.9	4.4	100	3.1	6.0

Source: Kogi, Ong, and Cabantog[13]

Table 2 shows that regular dayworkers in a refinery in the Philippines contributed a total of 881 (53.5%) days of sickness absence and 392 (51%) spells, giving mean spells of 1.9 and average days of 4.4 per employee. The shiftworkers had a total of 763 (46.5%) days of sickness absence and 374 spells, giving mean spells of 3.0 and mean days of 6.0.

The frequency of workers who reported sick in a metal works and oil refinery is summarized in Table 3. A significantly higher proportion of shiftworkers incurred more spells of sickness absence than nonshiftworkers. Shiftworkers were also more apt to be "repeaters," having more than one spell of absence during the one-year study period.

These findings in absence rates among shiftworkers and dayworkers are of considerable interest. The differences cannot be explained by age, as there are equal proportions of employees in the different age groups of both shiftworkers and dayworkers (Tables 1 and 2).

It should be noted that both plants in the Philippines and Singapore used three-shift rotational schedules with shifts changed every week. The slow rotation and the fairly long periods of nightshifts may be considered unsatisfactory[24] and potentially dangerous to health.[15,30] These factors could have led to the increased absenteeism among shiftworkers with certain health problems or occupational stressors.[13] Also of interest are the findings in the Philippines by Reverente and Ariosa,[23] who showed that shiftworkers in a detergent and an edible oil factory, on the average, visited medical clinics more often than dayworkers. Analyzing the sickness incidence records with respect to the nature of illness, they found

TABLE 3. Frequency by Workshift of Persons Ill in a Metal Works and an Oil Refinery*

Spells	Metal Works (%)		Oil Refinery (%)	
	Daywork	Shiftwork	Daywork	Shiftwork
0	17.0	13.5	53.5	40.4†
At least 1 spell	83.0	86.5†	46.4	59.5‡
At least 5 spells	24.0	32.0	24.6	44.1

* Sickness absence rate can be seriously distorted by the odd employee with an exceptionally high absence. The usual tests of statistical significance for comparison of means cannot be rigorously applied to mean rates of frequency (spells and days). It is more appropriate to base statistical comparison on percentage of employees exceeding certain levels of absence—for instance, the percentage of persons with one or more spells.

† The significance (χ^2) of the difference between daywork and shiftwork was $p < 0.05$.

‡ The significance (χ^2) of the difference was $p < 0.01$.

that the difference between the groups was mainly due to a greater incidence of respiratory and gastrointestinal diseases among shiftworkers.

In several studies related to sickness absence, Ferguson[3] found that very few of the "frequently sick" actually had chronic illness, and Taylor and Pocock[29] observed that many of the "never sick" rarely consulted doctors despite much ill health. These studies together with other findings suggest that sickness absence is multifactorial and can be influenced by both economic and human factors. Local social factors may have also been shown to influence sickness absence.[13] Fischer's analysis[5] of absences among shiftworkers in automotive plants in Brazil found that family burdens and the attitude of the workers were related to an increase in sickness and unjustified absences. In the case of the two plants in Singapore and the Philippines, the remote locations of the metal works and the refinery (the metal work is located about 5 miles from the nearest residential area and the refinery is in a rural location in the Philippines) would need to be taken into account. For both, the available means of public transportation was usually infrequent, especially during the "odd" hours when shiftworkers had to travel to work. All these factors may have contributed to the high absence rates among shiftworkers. The fact that absence rates can be higher among shiftworkers for a variety of organizational and social reasons deserves our attention.

SHIFTWORK AND WORK INJURIES

A fair number of studies of shiftwork in developing countries have focused on the relationship between health and shift system. In contrast, there are relatively few studies of injuries on different shifts. Although it has not been confirmed that more accidents happen during nightwork than during daywork, a few early studies on accidents and shiftwork indicate a trend in this direction. On the other hand, several recent studies suggest that accidents may be less frequent at night.

In view of a relatively unchanged production pattern throughout the 24-hour day, the same-size work force in each shift, and the similarity in job activities for shiftworkers in a steel production plant, a study was conducted in Singapore to analyze 921 accidents reported for the 5-year period from 1978 to 1982.[20] The results showed that more than 40% (383 cases) of the accidents happened during the morning shift, 210 occurred in the afternoon shift, and only 150 were reported during the nightshift (Table 4). Two injury peaks were noted throughout the study, one at midmorning (0900–1000) and the other toward midafternoon (1400–1500).

TABLE 4. Injury Frequency Rate and Man-Day-Loss at Different Shifts in a Steel Mill, 1978–82

Shift System	No. Workers	No. Accidents	Injury Frequency Rate	Average Man-Day-Loss per Accident
Shift I (0700–1500)	141	383	266.04	3.26
Shift II (1500–2300)	141	210	142.00	3.55
Shift III (2300–0700)	141	150	107.84	3.80
Nonshift (0830–1700)	241	178	71.85	0.74
Total	664	921	146.93	2.84

Although the work force is the same size on all shifts, there is a statistically significant difference (χ^2) in the injury frequency rate, $p < 0.01$

It was also observed that although the work activities and task functions of those in shiftwork were the same as those of the dayworkers, the work injuries were quite different; hand injuries were more common during the morning and afternoon shifts, and foot injuries normally occurred at night.

Another interesting aspect of this study was that although more accidents happened during the morning and afternoon shifts, work injuries that occurred at night generally required longer sick leave. The man-day-loss for the morning shift was 1,249 days. On the second shift, 210 accidents gave a 747 man-day-loss. The 152 accidents on the nightshift give a total man-day-loss of 570, suggesting that accidents that happened at night were more serious (Table 4). It is believed that, during the nightshift, alertness and speed of response may be decreased in comparison to the dayshift. Thus nightworkers would tend to make more errors. Poor visibility may also contribute to the seriousness of night accidents in the steel mill.

On the other hand, at night, the mill's medical and emergency facilities were less accessible. Thus nightworkers may tend to report only accidents that are serious and require urgent medical attention.

In many small- and medium-sized industrial settings in developing countries, working conditions are still far from satisfactory. The above study is just an example illustrating that the shift system and work environment can have a substantial influence on work injuries.

SHIFT SCHEDULING

In most developing countries, rotating shifts are the predominant work schedule. Rotation usually is weekly but both shorter, more rapid, and slower, longer, rotation cycles are also common.[6] In the above-mentioned 1982 survey conducted in Singapore, 63% of shiftworkers were on two-shift rotation, 18% on three-shift rotation, 6% on permanent second shift, and 12% on permanent nightwork.[17] In Brazil, a popular rotation schedule is three shifts with either weekly or 2-day (2 × 2 × 2) rotation, followed by two shifts of 12 hours each.[4] In the case of continuous systems with weekend work, as in many iron, steel, or chemical plants, rapid rotation seems to be increasing. In several Asian countries, the dayshift begins early in the morning. In Bangladesh, Indonesia, and Sri Lanka the first shift begins at 0600.

Although a shift usually lasts 8 hours, many industries also have extended shifts or overtime work to cope with production demand. A recent experience in Singapore involving 12-hour shifts has revealed an adverse impact of long shifts on the health and social life of workers. The results confirm earlier reports of significant fatigue and performance deficits on 12-hour shifts.[7,14] Although the 12-hour shift system was first considered to have some favorable effects, such as lower absence rates, compared with 8-hour shift systems,[33] serious deleterious effects have necessitated a reconsideration.

Some of the shift systems in the developing countries of Asia and South America have been studied with regard to health and social problems. Table 5 describes health-related problems of a weekly rotated three-shift system in textile mills in Thailand,[32] biweekly or monthly rotated and fixed systems in Bangladesh,[8] biweekly or monthly rotated and fixed systems in automobile plants in Brazil,[4] and a continuous three-shift system in a power plant in Thailand.[22] Disturbed sleep, fatigue due to nightwork, health complaints, and frequent absence among shiftworkers were noted by these reports. A more recent study conducted in

TABLE 5. Reports Indicating Health and Social Problems of Shiftworkers in Some Developing Countries

			Health-Related Information					Social Aspects*
Country	Industry	Shift system	Sleep loss	Fatigue	Subjective health	Gastric trouble	Absenteeism	
Singapore	Manufacturing	12-hour/4 days	•	•	•	•	•	1, 2, 3
Bangladesh	Jute, tobacco	Fixed 3-shift/ weekly 3-shift	•	•	•		•	2, 3
Thailand	Textile	Weekly 3-shift	•	•	•			1, 2, 4
Brazil	Automobile	Fixed 2- or 3-shift/biweekly or monthly 3-shift	•	•			•	2, 3, 4
Thailand	Power plant	Continuous 4-crew 3-shift	•	•	•	•		2, 3, 4
Singapore	Electronics industry	Weekly and permanent night	•		•	•	•	Not studied

* 1, Conditions interrupting daytime sleep (heat, insects, conversation); 2, clashes with family routine; 3, fewer family get-togethers; 4, reduced social contacts and training opportunities.

Singapore of 594 female electronic production operators also indicated that workers on weekly rotated shifts have significantly more complaints related to sleep, indigestion, and tiredness.[2] Work-related social problems were also common among workers studied. Such problems can be separated into four categories: (1) conditions interrupting daytime sleep, such as heat, insects, and conversation; (2) clashes with family routines; (3) insufficient family contacts; and (4) reduced social contact. Categories 2 and 3 are noted in all the reports listed (see Table 5), indicating that family relations are particularly affected by shiftwork.

Summarizing these findings, it is obvious that shiftworkers in developing countries are not better able than those in developed countries to tolerate the operational conditions of some of the shift systems. Effects on their health and general well-being relate to phase-shifting and sleep hours, as well as to other job-related, environmental, and social factors.

An International Labour Organization (ILO) seminar[6] held in Bangkok recently pointed out that the major problems of shiftwork in developing countries are (1) organization of shift schedules, including shift patterns, holidays, and working hours, shift-related absenteeism, and supervision at night; (2) effects on health among nightworkers, in particular sleep disturbances and fatigue; (3) disruption of social and family life, particularly the lack of basic services and facilities for shiftworkers. "Long working hours" was also one of the issues discussed.

Singapore's Experience with 12-Hour Shifts

Twelve-hour shifts have been introduced in several developing countries in Asia. The effects of the 12-hour system are not well understood. Nevertheless, the experience of Singapore workers revealed that long shifts require cautious consideration.

Around 1983, the 12-hour shift system was introduced to many industries in Singapore.[31] It was believed that 12-hour shifts worked consecutively for 3 or 4 days followed by time off would give workers more free time, reduce commuting time, contribute to energy conservation, and also reduce traffic congestion. "Work 12 hours a day for 4 consecutive days and get the next 3 or 4 days off. On top of it, earn 35% more in salary" was the common arrangement factories offered employees. Usually there were two working shifts: 0700–1900 and 1900–0700.

The system was short-lived. Most factories abandoned it after less than a year. The main reasons for giving up long shifts were (1) the physical health of shiftworkers and (2) social factors.

Effects on Health

Although there has been no conclusive evidence that working 12 hours a day is unfavorable to health, the results from factories that applied the 12-hour schedule suggest higher labor turnover rates and maladjustment problems.

A large, multinational electronics factory abandoned the 12-hour scheme after 2 months and reverted to the 8-hour shift system owing to worker complaints of tiredness and difficulty in concentrating.

A survey conducted in 1984 showed that more than 45% of workers engaged in the 12-hour system said their health deteriorated after starting the 12-hour shifts. The main complaints were insufficient sleep, loss of weight, and gastric troubles.[25] The hot, tropical climate and noisy dwelling units of Singapore were not conducive to sound sleep for shiftworkers, who need to sleep in the daytime. Sleep was often disturbed by children, radio or television, and noises from neighbors and traffic. Such circumstances adversely affected productivity for a long work schedule on the following day.

A number of employers were reported to have been severely inconvenienced by problems arising from 12-hour shifts. A significant fall in productivity, high labor turnover, and moonlighting on days off were more prevalent among the 12-hour shiftworkers than among 8-hour shiftworkers.

Social Implications

The social implications of 12-hour shifts were also significant. According to the survey, about 64% of the 12-hour shiftworkers said they spent less time with their families because their working hours clashed with normal family routines. Some workers felt that when spouses were working on different shifts, they saw less of each other. Working mothers found it even harder to organize or juggle marketing, housework, and looking after their children. Consequently, children saw less of their parents.[27] Therefore, the concern was raised that long-hour shifts would adversely affect family cohesiveness, which the government of Singapore had been trying hard to preserve. Thus, many enterprises mentioned the effects on family life as a major reason for abandoning the 12-hour shifts.

This experience in Singapore is summarized in Figure 2. The experience showed that not even increased benefits attracted or motivated workers to endure long working hours. While it is clear that shiftwork can offer more employment opportunities, the experience in Singapore demonstrates that the social life and physical health of the work force cannot be ignored. Consideration should be given to the inherent cultural and social practices that may affect working hours and shift systems.

Long Shift Cycle

Industrial groups in developing countries not uncommonly use a long shift cycle (slow shift rotation). It is often adopted by enterprises in remote areas

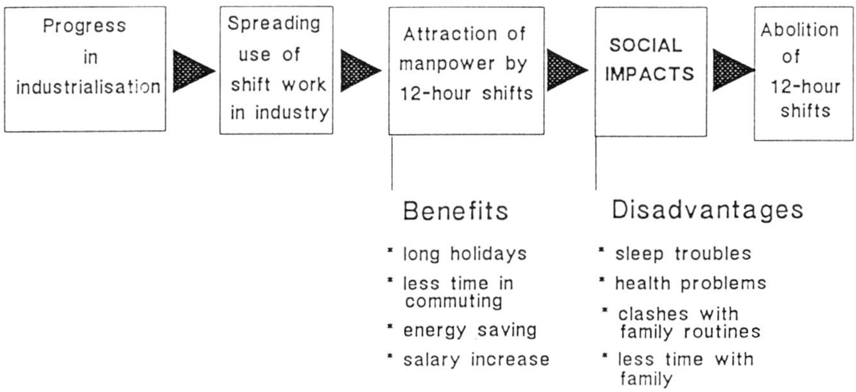

FIGURE 2. The Singapore experience with 12-hour shifts in the 1980s. Source: Kogi K, Ong CN, and Cabantog C: Some social aspects of shiftwork in Asian developing countries. Int J Ind Ergon 4:151–159, 1989.

isolated from residential districts: power plants, mines, offshore oil explorations, and factories, for example. Workers in these enterprises are forced to live for many years isolated from their families and relatives. They tend to prefer longer holidays rather than scattered ones, creating problems in the organization of shift schedules.

An example of such "combination holidays" was reported for a power plant[22] and for an open-cast coal mine[1] in Thailand. The three-shift system with four crews was applied in both cases, with a cycle period of 12 days in the former and 20 days in the latter. To accommodate workers' preference, holidays were gathered together within the cycle period. In the power plant, each crew worked three afternoon shifts (1600–2400), three night shifts (2400–0800), and three morning shifts (0800–1600) with 24 hours of rest at each shift change, followed by a holiday period of 72 hours. In the coal mine, the 20-day shift cycle consisted of 5 days of the afternoon shift (1600–2400 hours), five days of morning shift (0800–1600 hours), five days of the nightshift (2400–0800 hours), and five days off.

Fatigue was notable during the continued workshifts in both cases, and the managements undertook a field study on the effects of the shift schedules with the cooperation of an occupational health service. The results showed an accumulation of fatigue particularly for the nightshift. The results from the power plant indicated that both body temperature and the critical flicker fusion (CFF) frequency measurement of fatigue reached the minimal level around 0400–0600 during the nightshift; these tendencies remained similar throughout the three days of the nightshift. In addition, fatigue feelings were common during the nightshift, and their mean frequency increased from the first night to the third night. The rate of workers' fatigue feelings decreased during the following morning shifts, but increased again considerably in the third morning, which was the last day before the 72-hour holiday. Similarly, the results from the coal mine revealed that the circadian minimal level of CFF frequency around 0400 was retained throughout the nightshifts and that "fatigue feelings" were the most common complaint for the nightshift. The percentage of workers having fatigue feelings was greatest at around 0400 during night duty.

In a questionnaire study done at the power plant, 49% of the shiftworkers said that working nightshifts consecutively had caused increasing sleepiness and fatigue. About half of the married workers (accounting for 51% of the shiftworkers) indicated that they had little time with their families. Forty-four percent of the shiftworkers also reported that nightwork interfered with social activities.

SOME SOCIAL ASPECTS OF SHIFTWORK IN DEVELOPING COUNTRIES

Several earlier studies have indicated that poor hygiene at workplaces, overcrowded workplace housing, and diet deficiencies are common problems among shiftworkers in Asia.[13,16] The psychosocial implications of nightwork and changing schedules, including those involving family and social life, are often regarded by the workers themselves as most troublesome. The negative effects of nightwork, permanent or on rotation, are especially significant with respect to (1) inadequate facilities and services for daily activities and transportation and (2) interferences with local customs, particularly those related to family life and social values.[12] Particularly important factors are discussed below.

Supply of Meals. Workers who must take meals at irregular hours cannot get nutritious food provided in a family setting. Canteen facilities at the workplace are usually limited. Meals, if provided, are not necessarily of sufficient quality. Often workers have to buy food from outside vendors.[27] Many workers eat at or near workplaces because eating places are not provided or are unhygienic. The work schedule also makes it difficult to arrange nutritious meals.

Transportation Facilities. Transportation for irregular working hours is usually insufficient. This was also shown in the sickness absence study mentioned earlier. Public transportation facilities rarely take into account shiftworkers who return home at odd hours. Furthermore, travel to and from work is less secure during night hours, particularly for female shiftworkers. Shiftworkers often need a long commuting time to visit families and friends during holiday periods.

Overcrowded Workplace Housing. Heat, noise, and insects often disturb the resting period at home. The dormitories provided in some countries are often overcrowded and lack appropriate sanitary and bathing facilities.

Health Care/Child Care Services. Lack of adequate health care or child care services should be mentioned. Health services provided by employers, if any, are quite often limited to certain daytime treatments. The care of young children presents a serious problem for female workers.[5]

Interference with Local Customs. Interference with family life and with local values and customs has important implications for shiftworkers in developing countries.[12] Shiftworkers are apparently in an unfavorable situation for taking family responsibilities and having opportunities for family get-togethers. At times, special arrangements become necessary in the farming seasons for some workers' participation in family farmwork.

CONCLUSIONS

Both occupations and countries differ significantly in shift schedules used and problems related to shiftwork. The basic problems appear to be related to the reasons for adopting shiftwork. As important as the basic shift patterns, however, are the social aspects of shiftwork in the local context.

More and more developing countries are turning to continuous industrial production. Shiftwork is therefore no longer a minor problem, but one of increasing importance. Because of its economic consequences and its adverse effects on worker health and social and family life, the developing countries need a different approach to managing shiftwork. Particular attention needs to be given to the lack of adequate facilities and support services and to interferences with local customs. It is also necessary to pay particular attention to the health and the social and psychological consequences of shiftwork for the large proportion of female workers involved in permanent nightwork.[18]

Flexible guidelines for adopting and operating shiftwork need to take into account specific aspects of shiftwork in developing countries.[20] Possibilities for improving shiftwork, particularly its social consequences, are significant in developing countries.

REFERENCES

1. Chaiyakul K, Pongkad S, Petchart P, et al: Fatigue testing as a means to improve working conditions of shift workers in lignite mine. In Symposium on Conditions of Work and Environment in Developing Countries, 6–8 November 1985, Proceedings, Bangkok National Institute for the Improvement of Working Conditions and Environment, 1985, pp 40–53.
2. Chan OY, Gan SL, Phoon WH: Health of night workers in the electronics industry. Singapore Med J 28:390–399, 1987.
3. Ferguson D: Some characteristics of repeated sickness absence. Br J Ind Med 14:266–274, 1972.
4. Fischer FM: Working conditions of the shift workers of the metropolitan area, Sao Paulo, Brazil. J Hum Ergol 11(suppl):177–194, 1982.
5. Fischer FM: Absenteeism among shift workers of the automotive plants. In Haider M, Koller M, Cervink R (eds): Night and Shiftwork: Long-term Effects and Their Prevention. Frankfurt, Verlag, 1986, pp 189–196.
6. International Labour Office: Shift Work and Related Issues in Asian Countries. Geneva, ILO, 1985.
7. Kelley RJ, Schneider MF: The twelve-hour shift revisited: Recent trends in the electric power industry. J Hum Ergol 11(suppl):369–384, 1982.
8. Khalefue A, Rahman A: Sleep disturbances and health complaints of shift workers. J Hum Ergol 11(suppl):155–160, 1982.
9. Knauth P, Rohmert W, Rutenfranz J: Systematic selection of shift plants for continuous production with the aid of work-physiology criteria. Appl Ergon 10:9–15, 1979.
10. Kogi K: Shift work in developing countries. Phillipines Labor Rev 2:29–40, 1977.
11. Kogi K: Shift work in different occupations and different countries with reference to its social aspects in developing countries. In Haider M, Koller M, Cervinka R (eds): Night and Shift Work: Long-term Effects and Their Prevention. Frankfurt, Verlag, 1986, pp 141–148.
12. Kogi K: The organisation of work and shift work in developing countries. Proceedings of the XX International Conference on Occupational Health, 1987, pp 210–223.
13. Kogi K, Ong CN, Cabantog C: Some social aspects of shift work in Asian developing countries. Int J Ind Ergon 4:151–159, 1989.
14. Kogi K, Takahashi M, Onishi N: Experimental evaluation of frequent eight-hour versus less frequent longer nights. In Colquoun P, et al (eds): Experimental Studies of Shift Work. Frankfurt, Verlag, 1975, pp 103–112.
15. LaDou J: Health effects of shift work. Western J Med 137:525–530, 1982.
16. Mahathevan R: Overview of shift work in developing countries. J Hum Ergol 11(suppl):139–145, 1982.
17. Ong CN, Hoong BT: Shift work in manufacturing industries in Singapore. J Hum Ergol 11(suppl):209–216, 1982.
18. Ong CN, Kogi K: Some social aspects of rotating shift systems in developing countries. Proceedings, 8th International Symposium on Night and Shift Work, Krakow, 1987.
19. Ong CN, Kogi K: Ergonomics for developing countries. In Jeyaratnam J (ed): Occupational Health for Developing Countries. New York, Oxford University Press, in press.
20. Ong CN, Phoon WO, Iskandar, Chia KS: Shift work and work injuries in an iron and steel mill. Appl Ergol 18:51–56, 1987.
21. Perera SEG: Industrial shift and night work practices in Asian developing countries. J Hum Ergol 11(suppl):201–208, 1982.

22. Poliwattana P, Rojanajin P, Retcharat P, et al: A study on health, living, sleeping and fatigue problems of shift workers of Bank Pakong Gas Turbine Plant. In Symposium on Conditions of Work and Environment in Developing Countries, 6–8 November 1985, Proceedings. Bangkok, National Institute for the Improvement of Working Conditions and Environment, 1985, pp 19–30.
23. Reverente BR, Ariosa L: Sickness absence among shift workers in an industrially developing country. J Hum Ergol 11(suppl):195–200, 1982.
24. Rutenfranz J: Occupational health measures for night and shift workers. J Hum Ergol 11(suppl):67–86, 1982.
25. Seet K: Support to call to ban 12-hour shift. Straits Times, Singapore, 25 January, 1985.
26. Shepherd RD: Absenteeism and presenteeism in industry. Arch Environ Health 21:670–677, 1970.
27. Tan TC: The Health of Working Mothers in Hong Kong. Department of Community Medicine, Chinese University of Hong Kong, 1985.
28. Taylor PJ: Absenteeism: Causes and control. In Encyclopeida of Occupational Health and Safety. Geneva, International Labour Office, 1985, pp 5–8.
29. Taylor PJ, Pocock SJ: Sickness absence: Its measurement and control. In Schilling RSF (ed): Occupational Health Practice. London, Butterworth, 1981, pp 339–358.
30. Winget CM, Hughes L, LaDou J: Phsyiological effects of rotational work shifting: A review. J Occup Med 20:204–210, 1978.
31. Wong AK: The new work day. Straits Times, Singapore, 23 August, 1983.
32. Wongphanich M, Saito H, Kogi K, et al: Conditions of working life of women textile workers in Thailand on day and shift work systems. J Hum Ergol 11(suppl):165–175, 1982.
33. Zee KO: Twelve hour shift work and health. In Lai CS, Lee HP, Low WF, Ong CN (eds): Proceedings of the 10th Asian Conference on Occupational Health. Singapore, 1983, pp 241–245.

INDEX

Entries in **boldface type** indicate complete chapters.